THE METAPHYSICAL PHYSICIAN

THE METAPHYSICAL PHYSICIAN
The Symbolic and Hermetic Basis of the Western Herbal Tradition

Dylan Warren-Davis

AEON

First published in 2026 by
Aeon Books

British Library Cataloguing in Publication Data

A C.I.P. for this book is available from the British Library

ISBN-13: 978-1-91280-797-0

Typeset by Medlar Publishing Solutions Pvt Ltd, India

www.aeonbooks.co.uk

DEDICATION

To my wife Stella, who has been a constant companion on our herbal journeys.

Without her love and support this book would not have come into being.

CONTENTS

LIST OF ILLUSTRATIONS

Introduction

Chapter 1

Chapter 2

Chapter 3

Chapter 4

Chapter 5

Chapter 6

Chapter 7

Chapter 8

Chapter 9

Chapter 10

Chapter 11

Chapter 12

Chapter 13

Chapter 14

Chapter 15

Chapter 16

Chapter 17

Chapter 18

Chapter 19

Chapter 14

Chapter 15

Chapter 16

Chapter 17

Chapter 18

Chapter 19

Chapter 20

Chapter 21

Epilogue

ACKNOWLEDGEMENTS

I would like to thank my astrologer friends and herbal colleagues who have encouraged and inspired me over the years in my herbal research: Maggie Hyde, Geoffrey Cornelius, Derek Appleby, Olivia Barclay, Deb Houlding, Graeme Tobyn, Nick Campion, Steve Taylor, Beata Bishop, Sharon Knight, Thomas Bartram and Christopher Hedley.

An especial thanks must go to Oliver Rathbone, who after hearing me speak at a seminar commissioned me to write this book, and for being so understanding, while keeping the faith in me when I spectacularly missed its original deadline, about five years ago! Thanks too to all the staff at Aeon Books for their involvement in the production of this book. In particular, to Matthew Seal for his discerning editorial tightening of the text. A belated thank you goes to herbalist and garden writer Ann Freeman, who presciently gave me copies of the original plans to the L'Orto Botanico di Padova over 30 years ago. As she handed them to me, she said, "these plans contain symbolism that I cannot understand, perhaps with your expertise, you will be able to make sense of them."

A particularly warm thanks to Izzy Seaton and Ellie Kirkby at Aeon Education, for their help and support in getting the "Living History of Western Herbal Medicine" webinar series together. The "Living History" lectures were instrumental in structuring the ideas included in *The Metaphysical Physician* and also provided the opportunity to expand on themes beyond the framework of the book. It is recommended to watch these webinars in conjunction with reading this book.

A special shout-out to all the artists who have given me permission use their artwork and photographs, including Liz Downey, Stephen Middleton, Jasmin Grant, Leo Delavega and Kaye Miller-Dewing (https://www.redbubble.com/people/kamide/shop).

Finally, I would like to acknowledge the support of English Heritage, who were very helpful in providing access to a 19th-century detailed study by a young architectural student, named Buckler. His drawing clarified the lost elements of the masonry from Winchester Palace Rose Window and provided the template for the geometric graphics used in Chapter 1.

FOREWORD

The term "Medieval" is often used pejoratively, to describe practices or standards which are outdated, rudimentary, barbaric, unscientific, or harmful. As Dylan Warren-Davis magnificently demonstrates in this book, this is a grossly inaccurate libel. No doubt many things deserve to remain in the past, but others urgently need re-appraisal. This baby-bathwater issue is frequently encountered today, when all but the most objective historians and researchers are biased by contemporary revisionism, and suffer from presentism, hubris, and—in the words of Michael Foley, author of *The Age of Absurdity*—"chronic general ingratitude". Post-enlightenment science has revealed much to us and elevated the average standard of living (for those living in more privileged countries, at least) to that of Medieval kings and queens; but the accompanying global fall-out in terms of environmental and social harms is often grossly understated. These harms may not be unrelated to the dismissal of past practices that cannot presently be scientifically ratified, or which seemed to the colonial-era authors of post-enlightenment science to be anachronistic and superfluous.

Those of us with an interest in improving the odds of humanity's survival today have powerful incentives to study the lessons of the past, before the age of technology amplified the possibility of human auto-extinction. It is our responsibility to closely investigate the means by which our ancestors navigated through and made sense of their (and, by extension, our) brief human lives: how they addressed and sought to foresee, forestall or remedy the "slings and arrows of outrageous fortune" that everybody must endure, the vagaries of illness and misfortune. As Henry Longfellow wrote and Ella Fitzgerald famously sang, "into each life a little rain must fall". Long before the invention of the umbrella, our predecessors had methods of literally and figuratively predicting the weather and protecting themselves from it. Chief among these was astrology, arguably the most sophisticated form of prediction and analysis of phenomena affecting human existence in the pre-modern era.

Few other disciplines associated with the most educated strata of society have been more highly regarded, or more thoroughly vilified. No other ancient technology with such a venerable pedigree and central position in the evolution of city-dwelling civilisations worldwide has been so airbrushed from history in the present day—whether that be in archaeology, religion, or medicine. Wikipedia articles and history books frequently describe ancient sites, placed so as to align with specific asterisms or planetary bodies at particular times of year, in terms of their 'astronomical', rather than astrological, importance. Religious characters, stories, and calendars are described only in terms of their 'allegorical' or 'cultural' significance. Ancient medicine may be derided for its 'superstition' or 'irrationality' or praised for its 'pre-scientific' empiricism. The common central axis in many of these descriptions, blinding in its invisibility and deafening in its silence, at least minimized to the point of absurdity, is astrology—a single word describing a diverse set of highly variable context-dependent divinatory systems based on the observation of celestial phenomena, enormous in scope and incalculable in their effect on ancient and pre-modern civilisations from Asia to Europe to the Americas. Astrology was an inescapably pre-eminent force in all pre-modern philosophies, religion, education, science, culture, and medicine.

This book expertly salvages what is hidden in plain sight in pre-modern edifices and historical documents, revealing how central astrology was in philosophy and medicine. *The Metaphysical Physician* goes way beyond archaeoastronomy (study of the astronomical knowledge of historical and pre-historical cultures) or even archeoastrology, delving into the fine detail of the symbolism woven into ancient art and sacred sites, revealing their underlying metaphysics. This book explores the principles of prescribing herbal medicine alongside astrology; a sophisticated art reduced to parody by some armchair historians who have little or no practical experience with either medicinal plants or the practice of astrology. Contemporary studies frequently reveal the effectiveness of ancient and medieval remedies, such as the recent demonstration of the MRSA-killing effect of an Anglo-Saxon eye salve against styes made with a mixture of garlic, wine and ox gall infused and fermented for nine days in a brass vessel.[i] This formula was discovered to be a much more effective bactericidal agent on animal tissue than Vancomycin, the reference antibiotic; moreover, the formula was only effective when the original recipe and preparation was followed carefully.

This sort of thing is, of course, no surprise to herbalists from any tradition, who frequently have empirical (clinical) experiences to validate our ancestors' herbal formulations, but may be shocking to contemporary pharmacists who presume that microscopy and molecular biology could only ensure the superiority of modern medicines over messy traditional compositions. To an astrologer, this eye salve formula contains a good dose of Mars (garlic, gall and brass) with some Sun (wine made from grapes)—and Mars is the planet primarily correlated with inflammation and infection. According to Cornelius Agrippa, the 15th century doctor and metaphysician, the nine-day infusion may also be significant, as the number nine relates to the symbolism of both Mars

[i]Harrison, F., Roberts, A., Gabrilska, R., Rumbaugh, K., Lee, C., & Diggle, S. (2015) *A 1,000-Year-Old Antimicrobial Remedy with Antistaphylococcal Activity*. mBio 6, (4):e01129–15.

and the Moon[ii]—the Moon, along with the Sun, symbolises the eyes. As always, the astrological symbolism does not obviate the necessary medicinal action of the salve's ingredients—what would once have been described as their 'occult virtues', which we would nowadays largely ascribe, reductively, to their pharmacology—but adds another layer of significance to their selection and manufacture, resulting a in a product which objectively outperforms contemporary antibiotics.

Anyone who has done a sufficiently deep dive into traditional medicine or metaphysics anywhere in the world will accrue plenty of first-hand evidence to show that there is a great deal of truth and utility in such systems, proving that our forebears weren't all idiots. While astrology has failed many scientific tests of replicability, there is some favourable scientific evidence—the work of the Gauquelins[iii] provides tangential support, or the studies collated by Robert Currey (editor of *Correlation* magazine) on his website astrologer.com offer more direct testimony.[iv] The apparent statistical failings of astrology are, as Dylan amply illustrates, largely due to a paradigm clash between the ancient model of a living universe imbued with meaning and purpose (teleology), versus the post-enlightenment mechanistic one. Contemporary investigators are looking for replicable results from astrology, rather than treating it as a context-dependent divinatory art; no matter how many 'trials of prediction' astrology fails in artificial scenarios that treat it like a numbers game, it frequently performs very well in real life, as our ancestors well knew. In this book, Dylan has produced an invaluable primer for contemporary students of herbal medicine, astrology, the history of medicine, and even the general medical practitioner—because in order to see where we need to go, we first need to accurately perceive where we have been. This work is an excellent and much-needed step towards rediscovering and reclaiming a medical heritage which has been sadly neglected, as well as resuscitating the best aspects of ancient 'Western' medicine which served humanity well for thousands of years.

Marcos Patchett,
13th February 2026

[ii] Agrippa, H. (1651). *Three Books of Occult Philosophy*. Edited & annotated by Tyson, D., (2012), for Llewellyn, Woodbury, NM.

[iii] Gauquelin, M. (1994). *Cosmic Influences on Human Behaviour: The Planetary Factors in Personality*. Aurora Press, Santa Fe, NM.

[iv] Currey, R. (2022). *Astrology & Science*. https://www.astrologer.com/about Equinox Astrology, UK.

INTRODUCTION

When the human race learns to read the language of symbolism, a great veil will fall from the eyes of men [and women].

Manly P. Hall

A lot of the ideas in this book have been going around in my head for more than four decades, having evolved from various studies, writings, travels and meditations. Part of the delay in getting it written sooner was not having a clear sense of where to start.

One weekend I was walking through London's South Bank, on the way to visit the Globe Theatre to obtain tickets to see Shakespeare's "As You Like It". I was looking at all the new developments in the area when I spotted the rather forlorn Winchester Palace Rose Window. I had absolutely no idea that such a Palace had existed. In stark contrast to the recent construction of high-tech, glass and steel buildings, this Gothic window, suspended midair in a crumbling medieval stone wall, seemed well out of place. I photographed it and went on my way.

Looking at my weekend snaps on the laptop, I became more and more intrigued by the broken geometry of the Rose Window. A breakthrough happened when I realised that with my graphics program, I could digitally "repair" the missing components of its stonework and bring it alive by adding some coloured glass, from a previous photographic study.

As soon as I saw the dynamism of Elemental symbolism incorporated into its geometry, I realised the cultural importance of this window. It had a catalytic effect on my research and became the nidus around which this work started to take shape and fall into place. It was like a single crystal being dropped into a supersaturated salt solution, suddenly precipitating myriad other crystals.

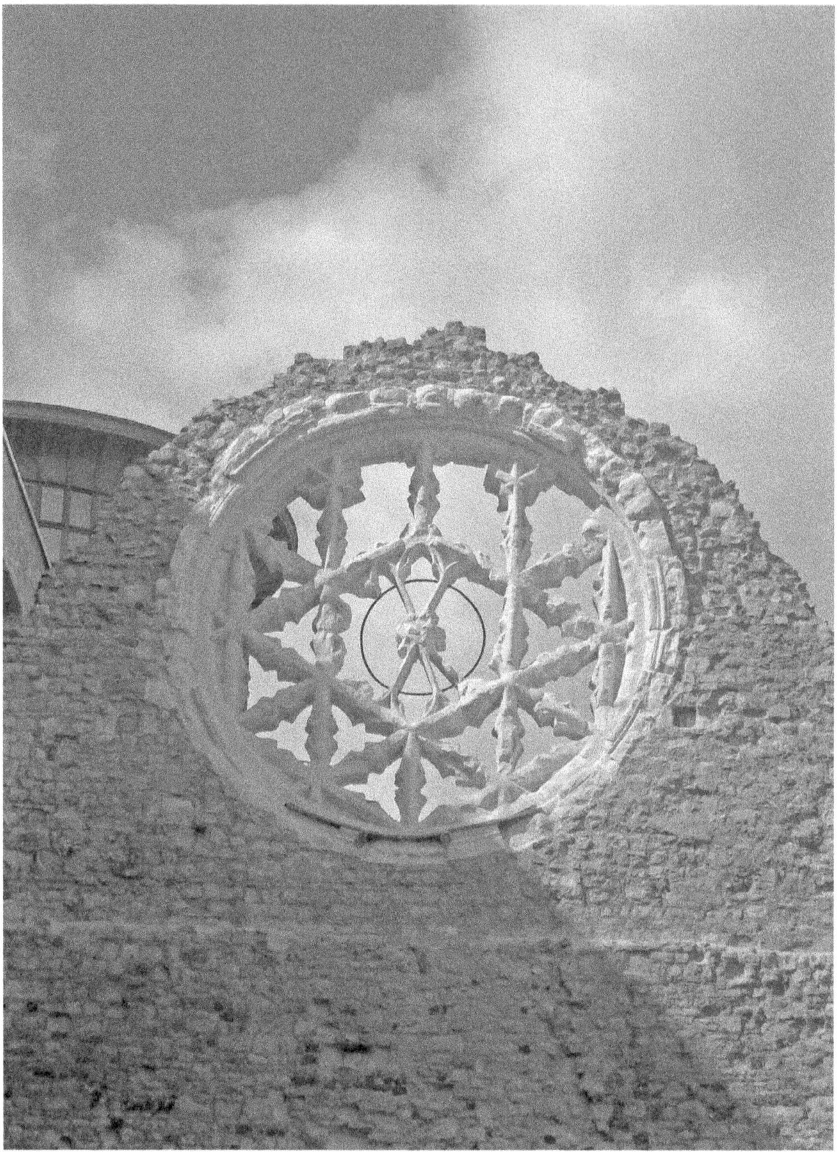

Winchester Palace Rose Window, Lambeth, London

I could also see that the current forlorn condition of the window is also symbolic of how much of this knowledge has fallen into decline and subsequently been lost, in the approximately 900 years since the window was first commissioned.

The reader will soon notice a lack of references to many of the ideas in this work. This is deliberate. For though there is historical detail to the material, it is important to see this knowledge solely in the present. Symbolism is timeless, since symbols evoke ideas that lie beyond the rational mind and its logical ordering of ideas in time and space. Water, for example, is just as wet today as was in the time of Plato and Hippocrates, and will be for generations to come.

To quote Manly P. Hall again:

> *Symbolism is the language of the Mysteries; in fact, it is the language not only of mysticism and philosophy but of all Nature, for every law and power active in universal procedure is manifested to the limited sense perceptions of man* [kind] *through the medium of the symbol. Every form existing* [in] *the diversified sphere of being is symbolic of the divine activity by which it is produced. By symbols men* [and women] *have ever sought to communicate to each other those thoughts which transcend the limitations of language.*

Symbols have multiple meanings, which can be seen at different times in different situations, therefore their study requires repetition—an essential part of cultivating awareness of their meanings. However, each time they are contemplated, your understanding should be perceived as continually expanding. In fact, every time you reread sections of this book you will discover "new insights" that you will have not noticed before.

As a literary device, I have capitalised every symbol in the text, for that is when I intend you to "refer" to your own evolving understanding of the symbols. For it is in your own mind's eye that the knowledge contained in this book will come "alive". It is a work that seeks to speak to and nourish your higher intuitive mind, so that you can connect with the source to the wealth of knowledge of the Western herbal tradition.

The true definition of a physician is a practitioner of physic. Physic is the largely forgotten traditional name for the art and skill of making medicines from plants and herbs. Though herbal medicine has survived into the 21st century, much of the traditional knowledge of physic has become lost. So while Western herbalists today continue using herbs, often in ways that have been identified centuries ago, the principles on which this knowledge was based are largely forgotten, even eschewed by a scientific, pharmacological perspective that has been superimposed onto the herbal kingdom. Much of the knowledge of physic was worked out using metaphysical ideas that evolved over millennia within different cultural contexts, and coalesced into a highly sophisticated organisation of knowledge.

For this reason, the title of this book is "The Metaphysical Physician". It will explore the symbolic and metaphysical ideas central to the practice of physic. It will explain these principles within a European historical perspective and then show how different major events in history have conspired against its survival, including the Black Death, the witch hunts, the dissolution of the monasteries, the Reformation, the age of Enlightenment, the birth of chemistry and the development of the pharmaceutical industry.

The book starts in the Gothic era, for resulting from the proliferation of monasticism was a whole cultural explosion of knowledge in the 11th and 12th centuries, and the foundations of institutionalised learning were established. This was an era when many of the metaphysical ideas central to understanding the philosophy of physic were plaited together. Once the full complexity of all the symbolic and metaphysical ideas is expounded, then the impact of the major historical events on herbal medicine can be more fully appreciated.

For readers wanting to see all the illustrations in full colour and more.... then please subscribe to my webinar The Living History of Western Herbal Medicine Discount 50% for readers who have purchased a copy of The Metaphysical Physician.

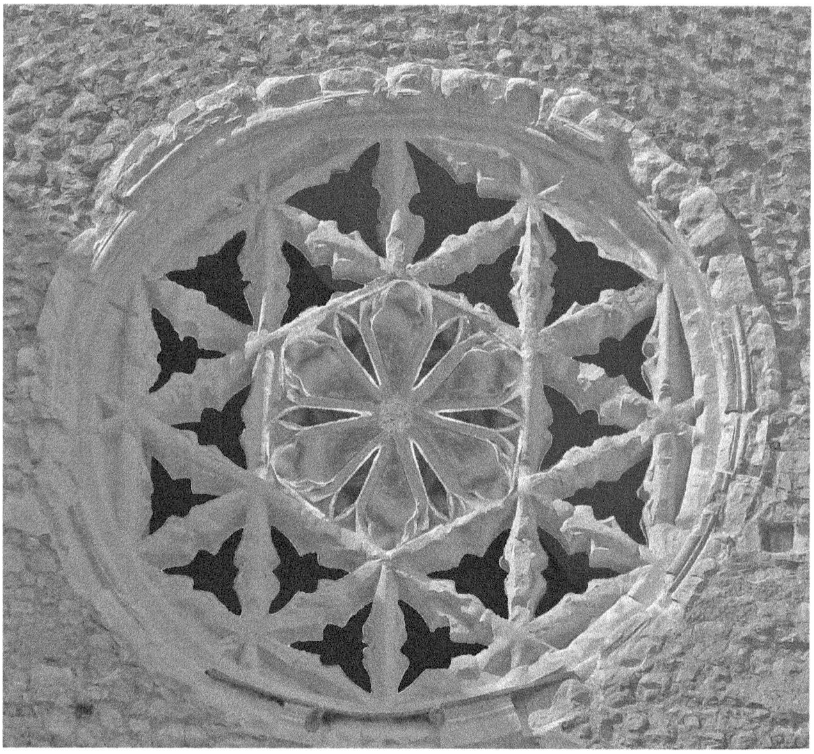

Figure 1.1: Winchester Palace Rose Window, digitally reconstructed by D. Warren-Davis

CHAPTER ONE

Westminster Palace Rose Window—a window into the medieval mind

Geometry was used in medieval era to elevate the mind to spiritual ideals, as described in Plato's words: "*Geometry will draw the soul toward truth and create the spirit of philosophy.*" Accordingly, geometry was included as a key topic of the Seven Liberal Arts. When the geometric shapes are used symbolically, they can articulate the metaphysical ideas that emerged in the Gothic era. It is in the carving of the Rose Windows that arguably the masons achieved some of their most sublime forms. Consequently, these windows encapsulate the genius of the medieval mind.

The ruin of Winchester Palace is located on what is now Clink Street, in the parish of Southwark, on the south bank of the River Thames. It was built in the 12th century and functioned as the London townhouse of the Bishop of Winchester. Henry of Blois, who was the first Bishop of Winchester, built the palace as his luxury and high-status London residence.

Henri de Blois (c. 1096–1171), was the youngest of four sons of Stephen Henry, Count of Blois by Adela of Normandy, daughter of William the Conqueror and Matilda of Flanders. Hence, he was a younger brother of King Stephen. Henry was born at Blois c. 1096, before his father left on the First Crusade. Henry's father died while on crusade in 1102, leaving a considerable estate with many castles and large properties in France. Most importantly it included property at Chartres. Henry was educated at Cluny and upheld the principles of the Cluniac reform, which encouraged intellectual freedom of the Seven Liberal Arts in conjunction with the high standards of devotion within monastic discipline.

The Cluniac reforms came about through the desperate need to reform monasticism in Europe, which had descended into disarray. On the one hand the reforms reemphasised the importance of the strict adherence to the rules of St Benedict, while on the other hand they encouraged the education of monks and nuns through the study of the Seven Liberal

Arts, the use of stained glass as medium of communication to those who were illiterate, as well as promoting work in service to the community, rather than retreating from it.

With his education and family connections, Henry was invited to England by King Henry I to become Abbot of Glastonbury in 1126. On 4 October 1129, he was also given the bishopric of Winchester, while allowed to remain as Abbot at Glastonbury.

When his brother Stephen of Blois was crowned King Stephen in 1135, essentially Henry was second in command so that when his brother was unavailable, he took over. Henry became the most powerful, and quite possibly even the wealthiest, man in England.

With Henry's education and family connections to Chartres, doubtless he would have been a witness to the building of the magnificent cathedral. There was an important cathedral school at Chartres, which trained the masons in physical skills needed for the construction of the building, along with the principles of geometry, mathematics and engineering. Additionally, they were educated in metaphysical and theological ideas. A translation of Plato's *Timaeus* was a key text studied there.

Such was the magnitude of cathedrals, they often took several centuries to complete, so the sheer scale of the task involved several generations of stone masons. The knowledge and masonry skills were thus passed on from father to sons and their apprentices. Though the liberal arts were to be found in Egyptian and Roman times, it was at Chartres that the Seven Liberal Arts were arranged into the metaphysical order that ultimately became the basis of monastic and university education in the early Gothic era.

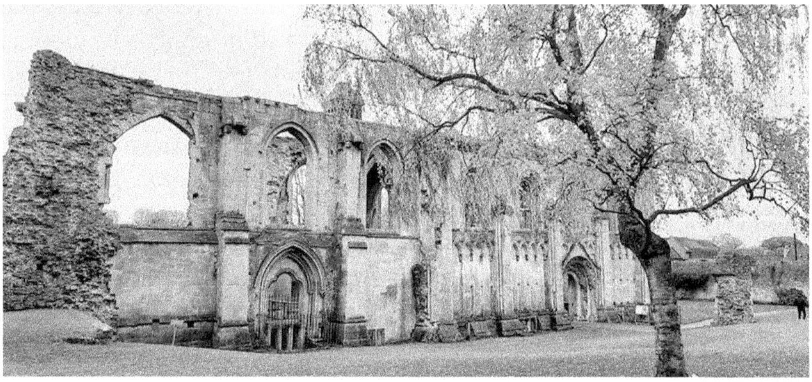

Figure 1.2: The ruins of Glastonbury Abbey. Photo credit Yasmin Grant

When Henry of Blois started work on building Winchester Palace, it was natural that he should commission masons at Chartres to construct the rose window. Not unsurprisingly its design is replete with Platonic ideas. An examination of the geometric construction and symbolism incorporated in the design of this window provides powerful insights into the spirit of the Gothic era. Indeed the very name "Gothic" is derived from the Greek word *goete*, which means "hidden meaning".

Accordingly, the Gothic style was encouraged in Britain by Henry of Blois. At his London residence, Henry would have entertained bishops, abbots and other prominent members of the clergy. The rose, through its association with Venus, the goddess of love, was used in Christian teachings as a symbol of the flowering of knowledge within the heart through love. The rose window would have been designed to encourage much philosophical discussion, which in turn would have then inspired the construction of abbeys and cathedrals to incorporate these neo-platonic principles.

This window is not only quite literally a window into the philosophical ideas of the medieval mind but also records the defining moment that started the infusion of the new ideas of the Gothic era into Britain.

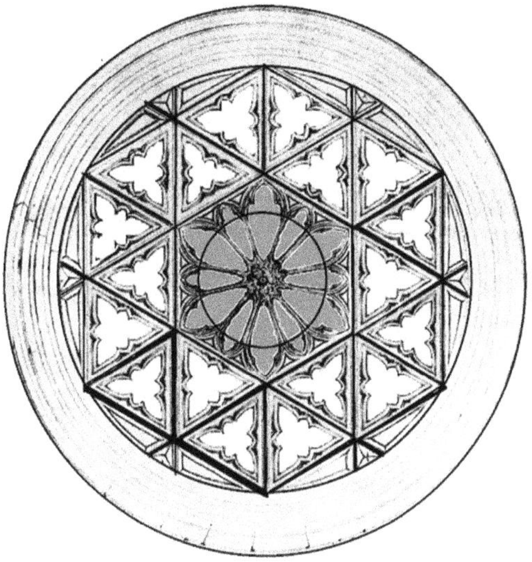

Figure 1.3: Winchester Palace Rose Window. Graphic, after Bucker

In the exploration of the hidden meaning, the construction of the window is primarily based on the Solar glyph (⊙), comprised of the Circle of the Soul enclosing a central Dot. From this central point the Light of Creation is visualised as manifesting the physical material world. This primary symbolism becomes animated by the Sun outside, shining through the window.

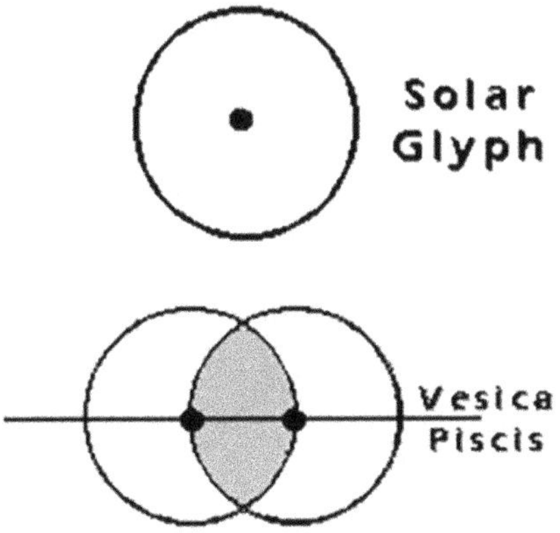

Figure 1.4: The relationship of the Solar glyph to the Vesica Piscis

Closely related to the Solar symbol is the ovoid shape of the Vesica Piscis (fish bladder), which is generated by two overlapping Solar glyphs, so that their respective circumferences touch the central point of each glyph. The Vesica, resembling a vulva, symbolically gives birth to the material (L. *mater*, meaning "mother") world.

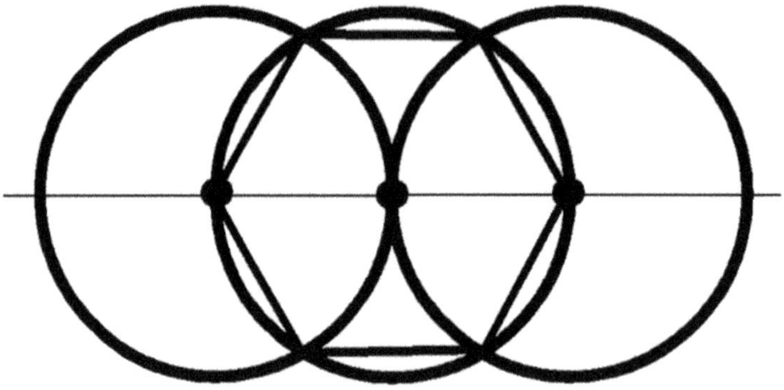

Figure 1.5: The relationship of the Solar glyph to the hexagon

When three Solar glyphs are aligned horizontally, a hexagon is generated from the interconnecting points. Six is the number associated with the Sun, so it is highly symbolic that the hexagon should be born in this way.

Flower of Life—interconnectedness of all life

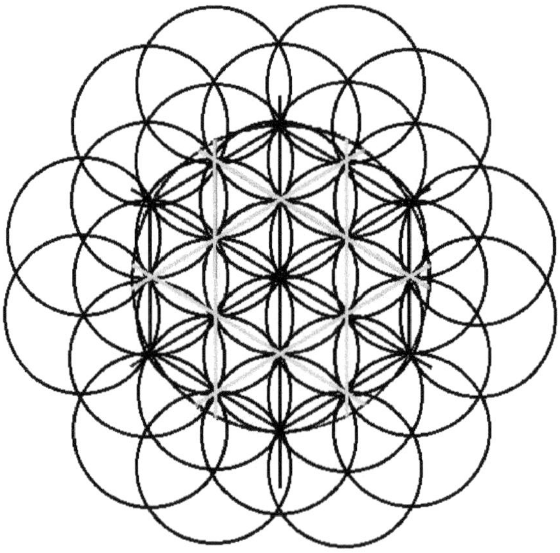

Figure 1.6: The relationship of the Solar glyph to the Flower of Life

From the corners of the hexagon, using a compass with the same radius as the original Solar glyph, six more circles are created. In turn from their intersections, more circles can be created. The sequence can be repeated ad infinitum, whereby a whole web of intersections is generated. The shapes of the Vesica Piscis thus formed are much more slender than the original one formed by the intersection of two Solar glyphs, and consequently have been thought to resemble the petals of flowers. The resultant pattern, common to many cultures, is called the Flower of Life.

Since the Sun symbolises the Soul and the generation of the Vital Force within, then the composite symbol of the Flower of Life essentially shows the interconnectedness of all life. The Flower of Life constitutes the template from which the geometries of the Winchester Palace Rose Window are generated.

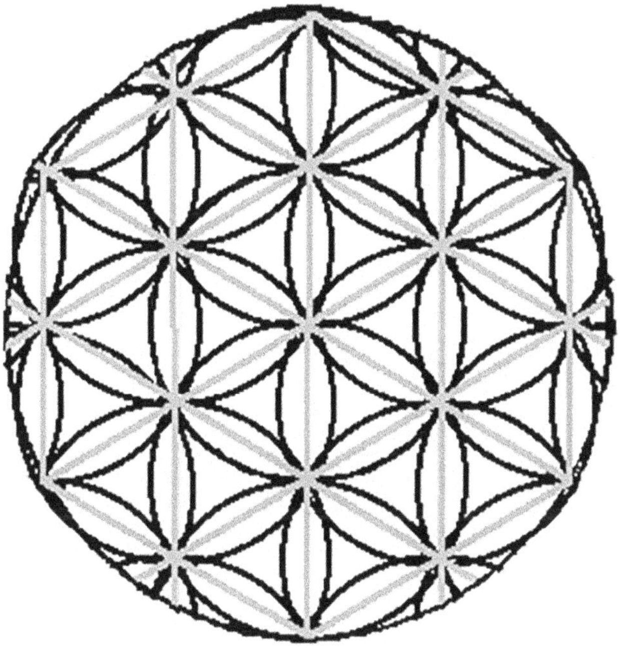

Figure 1.7: The Flower of Life Template of Winchester Palace Rose Window

The symbolism of the elements

With the knowledge that the masons at Chartres were trained in neo-platonic ideas, the first set of symbols to consider in the window are the Five Elements. For Plato the four material Elements—Earth, Water, Air and Fire—represented the universal forces upon which life depends:

- Earth stands for the *terra firma* beneath our feet, which nourishes, supports and sustains our bodies.
- Water irrigates the soil, allowing vegetation to grow, and provides the medium of all biochemical processes.
- Air is the atmosphere we breathe and derive life-sustaining oxygen from.
- Finally, Fire is the Sun in the sky, which provides heat, warmth and light, and energises living systems through the transformative process of photosynthesis.

Ether is the non-material Element representing Life and the Vital Force. In his *Timaeus*, Plato divides the Elements into two worlds: the inner subjective world of Ether he calls the *"World of Being"* and the outer objective world of the four material Elements he calls the *"World of Becoming"*. Ether represents the pure light of consciousness. It has a quintessential relationship with four material Elements, which can be perceived when they are in balance and harmony.

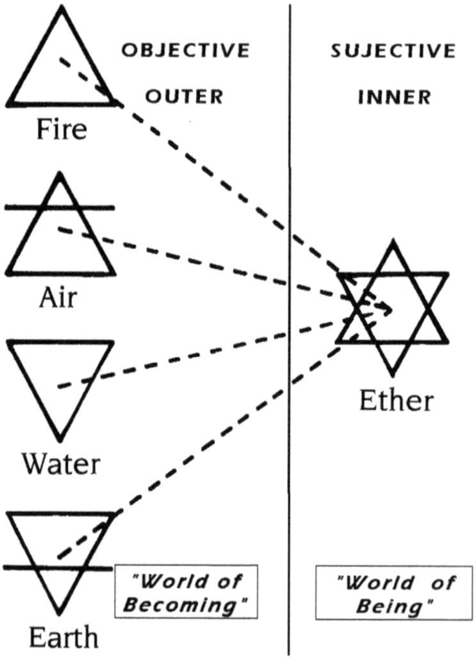

Figure 1.8: The generation of the four Elements and their corresponding Plato's Solids from the geometry of Winchester Palace Rose Window

This relationship is symbolically encapsulated in the triangular glyphs used to represent the Elements. If they are imagined as being made of wire hoops, then the glyphs for Earth, Water, Air and Fire can be stacked on top of each other, forming the composite star shape for Ether. This quintessential relationship can be imagined as analogous to beam of white light shining through a prism, causing the light to be split into the seven colours of the spectrum. These seven colours can be shone through another prism and then reunited as a beam of white light.

In essence the symbolism of the five Elements described the interrelationship of consciousness and matter, whereby the material Elements are continually being born out of the Ether—into the "World of Becoming"—and dissolving back again into Ether—the "World of Being".

The geometry of the Winchester Palace Rose Window generates two orders of Elemental symbolism. The first order is shown in the geometry of the inner hexagon—the World of Being. The second order is shown within the outer circumference—the

World of Becoming. The second order is indicated by the three-dimensional geometric figures known as Plato's Solids, which can be found within the window and symbolically represent the manifestation of the Elements in the Material World.

Thus, by understanding the Elements within, you can simultaneously understand the Elements manifested in the Material World outside us. The Sun shining through this window would visually bring all this symbolism alive in the interior of the Palace.

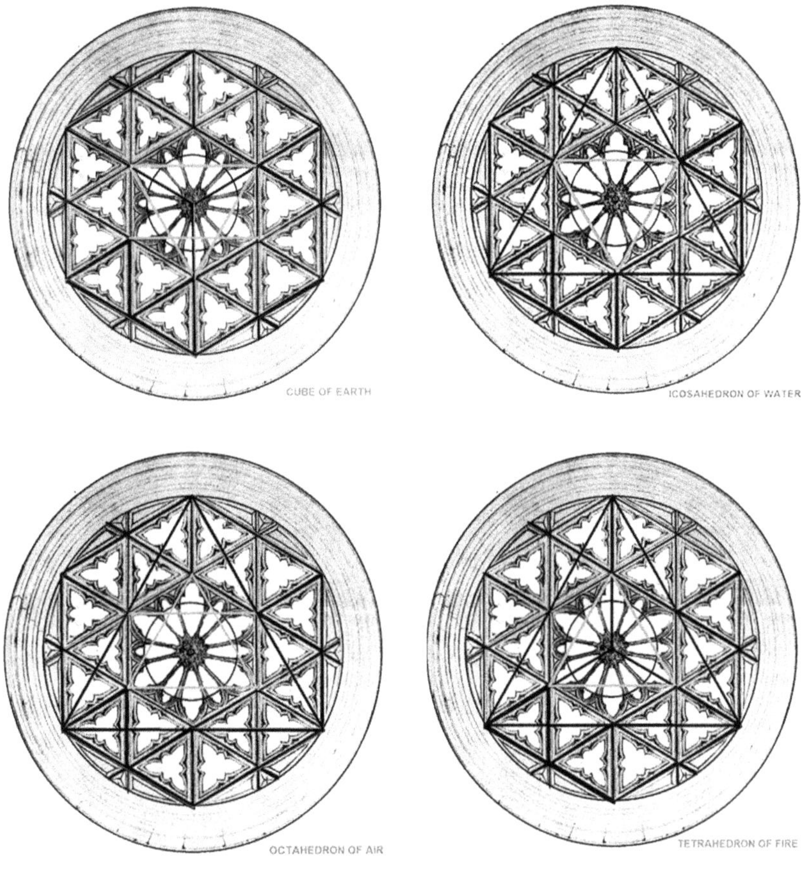

Figure 1.9: The quintessential relationship of the Elements as described by Plato

In the Winchester Palace Rose Window, the Earth Element is symbolised by the grey inverted triangle with a horizontal line dissecting it. The corresponding Platonic solid for Earth is the Cube, delineated by the black line. The Water Element is symbolised by the grey inverted triangle. The corresponding Platonic solid for Water is the black Icosahedron. The Air Element is symbolised by the grey triangle with a horizontal line dissecting it. The corresponding Platonic solid for Air is the black Octahedron. The Fire Element is symbolised by the grey triangle. The corresponding Platonic solid for Fire is the black Tetrahedron or pyramid. Finally, the Ether Element is symbolised by the grey hexangular star. The corresponding Platonic solid for Ether is the black Dodecahedron.

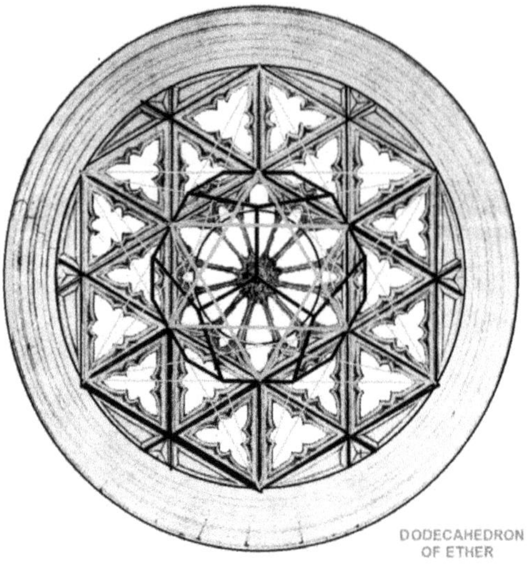

Figure 1.10: The generation of the Fifth Element Ether and its corresponding Plato's Solid from the geometry of Winchester Palace Rose Window

The Hermetic Three Worlds

The Rose Window also reflects the Hermetic Three World view, which underpinned the theology of the medieval era. The Elements were used to visualise the Hermetic Three Worlds. This will be more fully explained later in Chapter 4.

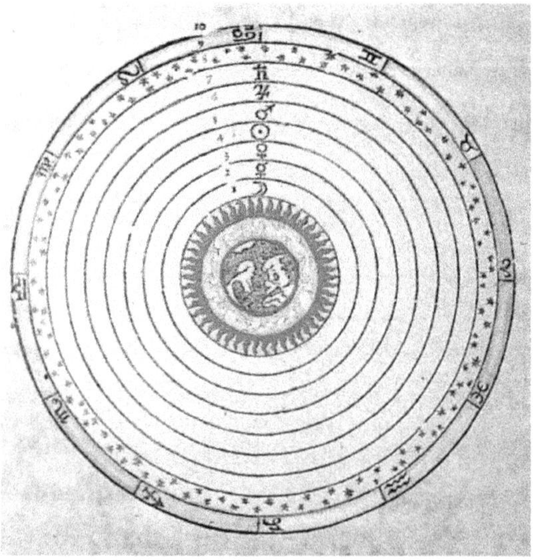

Figure 1.11: The cosmology of Spheres from the *Divine Pymander of the Corpus Hermeticum of Hermes Trismegistus*, 2nd century, published by John Everard, 1650

Outside the circles is the realm of Divine Fire, the Light of Creation, willing the Universe into being. The outer two circles show the signs of the Zodiac and the constellations of the Intellectual World. This is the realm of Divine Air.

The next concentric rings show the glyphs of the Planetary Spheres of the seven Planets of the Celestial World: Saturn (♄), Jupiter (♃), Mars (♂), Sun (☉), Venus (♀), Mercury (☿) and the Moon (☽). This is the realm of Divine Water.

The final four concentric rings show representations of the four Elements of the Elemental World: Fire, Air, Water and Earth. This is the realm of Divine Earth.

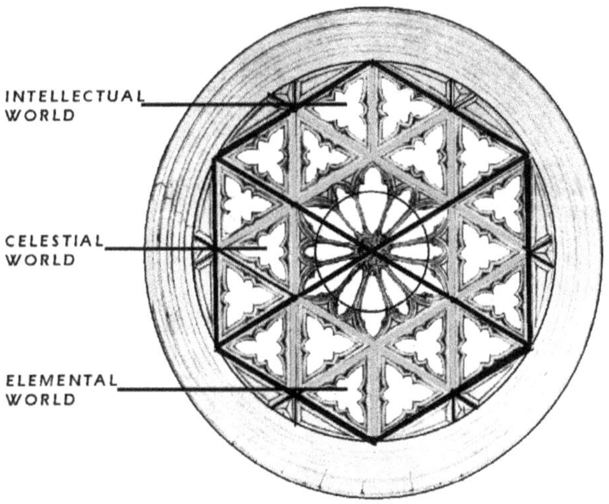

Figure 1.12: The Hermetic Three Worlds reflected in the geometry of Winchester Palace Rose Window

Twelve signs of the Zodiac

The third order of symbolism that the Flower of Life generates is the 12 points around the periphery of the Rose Window. The number 12 immediate corresponds to the 12 signs of the Zodiac. This is highly appropriate since the predominant geometric motif of the window is the creation and manifestation of the Elements from the Flower of Life.

Since the signs of the Zodiac are in turn composite symbols of the Elements, their superimposition into the window is most revealing. In the traditional sequence:

Aries (♈) – Cardinal Fire
Taurus (♉) – Fixed Earth
Gemini (♊) – Mutable Air
Cancer (♋) – Cardinal Water
Leo (♌) – Fixed Fire
Virgo (♍) – Mutable Earth
Libra (♎) – Cardinal Air

Scorpio (♏) – Fixed Water
Sagittarius (♐) – Mutable Fire
Capricorn (♑) – Cardinal Earth
Aquarius (♒) – Fixed Air
Pisces (♓) – Mutable Water

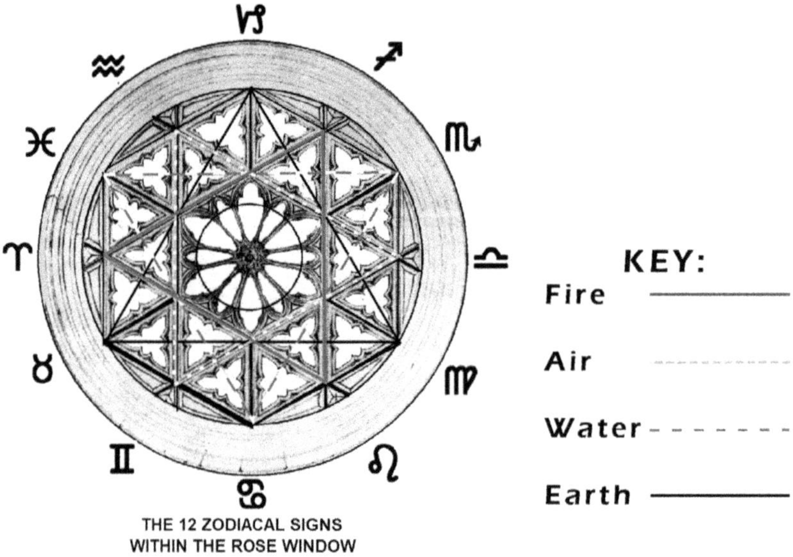

Figure 1.13: The Zodiacal signs reflected in the geometry of Winchester Palace Rose Window

Their Elemental triplicities highlight the Star motifs. When the triangles are drawn showing the triplicities, the lines exactly bisect 12 of the 18 star-shapes located in the window.

Thus, there is a symbolic concordance between the Elements of the Zodiacal signs at the periphery of the window and those Elements generated at the centre of the window, along with the generation of Plato's Solids:

- The triplicity of Fire signs in the Zodiac—Aries (♈), Leo (♌) and Sagittarius (♐)—delineated by the dark gray triangle, concord with the Fire Element within the inner Circle and the Tetrahedron.
- The Earth signs—Taurus (♉), Virgo (♍) and Capricorn (♑)—delineated by the black triangle, concord with the Earth Element within the inner Circle and the Cube.
- The Air signs—Gemini (♊), Libra (♎) and Aquarius (♒)—delineated by the light gray dashed triangle, concord with the Air Element within the inner Circle and the Octahedron.
- The Water signs—Cancer (♋), Scorpio (♏) and Pisces (♓)—delineated by the dark gray dashed triangle, concord with the Water Element within the inner Circle and the Icosahedron.

Collectively, all 12 Zodiacal signs and the 12 star-shapes concord with the 12 sides of the Dodecahedron, generated from the Ether Element within the inner Circle.

The whole Rose Window was framed by seven stone rings. The combined effects of the Palace being burned down and acid rain on the limestone through the centuries has largely destroyed this feature of the window. Fortunately, however, Bucker's 19th-century architectural sketch clearly depicts the presence of these rings. The seven rings obviously correspond to the seven traditional Planets, alluding to their orbits through the Zodiacal signs. In the Hermetic vision, as they move through the Elemental signs in the heavens, the Planets mediate their influence down to the Elements on Earth, in accordance with the Hermetic maxim, "As above, So below."

The three Alchemical Principles

The geometry of the Rose Window also encapsulates the polarity of the three Alchemical Principles—Salt, Sulphur and Mercury—by means of three diamond shapes, as can be seen in the diagram. These will be explained more fully later in Chapter 17.

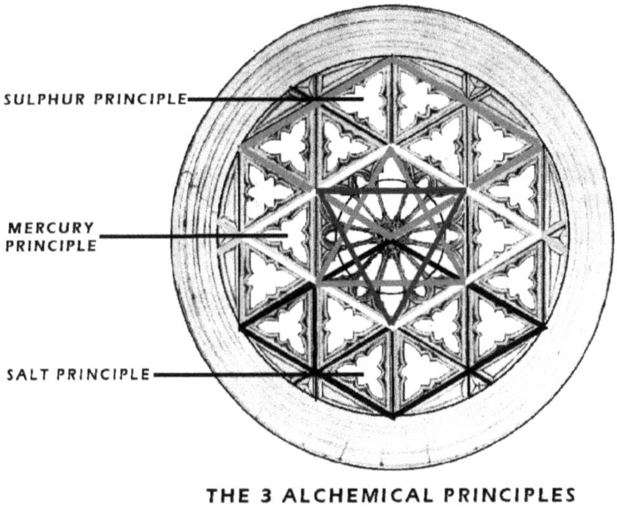

Figure 1.14: The Alchemical Principles reflected in the geometry of Winchester Palace Rose Window

The Mercury Principle is synonymous with the Fifth Element of Ether and symbolises the Vital Force. Fittingly, the central white diamond shape for the Mercury Principle encapsulates the central hexagonal shape of the window, which, as been shown above, is linked to the six-pointed star of Ether (defined by the black and dark grey triangles).

The "Philosophical Mercury", as the Alchemists referred to it, was symbolised by the fluid, shiny nature of quicksilver—the liquid metal. It was also called Hydragyrium, derived from the Greek term meaning "the Water that joins things together".

This explains why Hg is the chemical symbol for mercury, one of the irregular symbols for metals in the periodic table.

The Sulphur Principle is shown by the upper dark gray diamond shape. The golden yellow colour of Sulphur symbolically links it to the Sun and to the masculine Elements of Fire and Air. Fittingly, the apex of the dark gray triangle of the Fire Element focuses its energy into the centre of the gold diamond shape for the Sulphur Principle. The Sulphur Principle represents burning, volatile, sublime and expansive energy. Hence the diamond of the Sulphur Principle is located in the upper half of the window.

The Salt Principle is shown by the lower black diamond shape. The silvery colour of Salt symbolically links it to the Moon and to the feminine Elements of Water and Earth. Fittingly, the apex of the black triangle of the Water Element focuses its energy into the centre of the black diamond shape for the Salt Principle. The Salt Principle represents cooling, precipitating, contractive and crystallising energy. Hence the diamond of the Salt Principle is located in the lower half of the window.

The Mercury Principle represents the balance and synthesis of both the Sulphur and Salt Principles. Fittingly, the lower point of the dark gray diamond shape of the Sulphur Principle and the upper point of the black diamond shape of the Salt Principle both converge at the centre of the Rose Window, at the heart of the white diamond shape of the Mercury Principle.

The Tree of Life

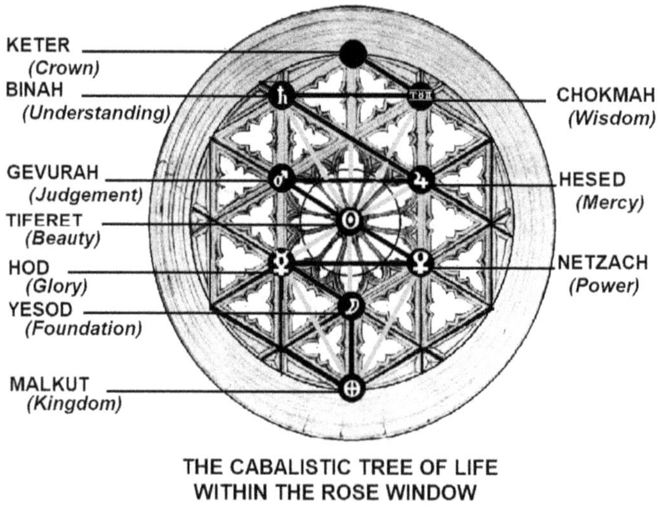

Figure 1.15: The Tree of Life reflected in the geometry of Winchester Palace Rose Window

The geometry of the Rose Window also reflects the Cabalistic Tree of Life. The name "Cabala" is a Hebrew word meaning "to receive". It is a system of knowledge and spiritual illumination that is traditionally said to have started in Egypt and later taken by the prophet Moses when he led the Israelites out of Egypt. Since then, the Cabala has taken on many different forms as it has spread through different cultures, though today it is generally represented as the Tree of Knowledge, as in the diagram.

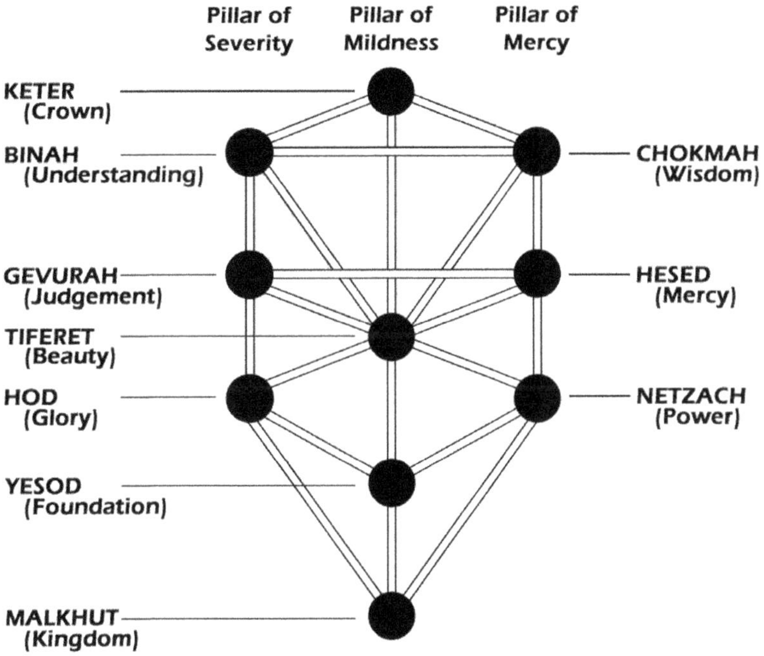

Figure 1.16: The Sephirot of the Cabalistic Tree

As in the Hermetic vision, the Tree describes the process of God willing creation into being from a realm of Divine Light, in a lightning flash. In this emanation, ten sepirot or stages are manifest. Starting at the top with Keter, the manifestation progresses down through Chokmah, Binah, Hesed, Gevurah, Tiferet, Netzach, Hod, Yesod and ends with Malkut. Each sephira is visualised as one of the ten fruits upon the tree. The English translations of the sephirot are shown in Figure 1.16, from which the last line of the Lord's Prayer can be recognised, *"for thine is the kingdom, the power and the glory"*.

In the Bible, the Tree of Knowledge is alluded to in the second chapter of Genesis in the myth of Adam and Eve in the Garden of Eden:

> *And the Lord God planted a garden eastward in Eden: and there he put the man he had formed.* Ch2 v8

The next verse states:

> *And out of the ground* [Malkut] *made the Lord God to grow every tree that is pleasant to the sight, and good for food; the tree of life also in the midst of the garden, and the tree of knowledge of good and evil.* Ch2 v9

Of this tree Adam is instructed:

> *But of this tree of knowledge of good and evil, thou shalt not eat of it: for in the day thou eatest thereof though shalt surely die.* Ch2 v17

In the Jewish tradition, Adam Kadmon is a name for the Cabala. Adam in the Bible should be seen as a symbolic "blueprint" for mankind, rather than the naïve idea of being the original person on the Earth. When the structure of the Tree is visualised as a sort of skeleton or scaffolding, then the idea of Eve being formed from one of Adam's ribs does not sound so ridiculous and should now be seen as alluding to the structure of the Cabala, rather than an erroneous statement of biological fact.

> *And the Lord God caused a deep sleep to fall upon Adam and he slept; and he took one of the ribs and closed up the flesh instead thereof:* Ch2 v21
>
> *And the rib, which the Lord God had taken from man, made he a woman, and brought her unto the man.* Ch2 v22
>
> *And Adam said, This is now bone of my bones, and flesh of my flesh: she shall be called Woman because she was taken out of Man.* Ch2 v23

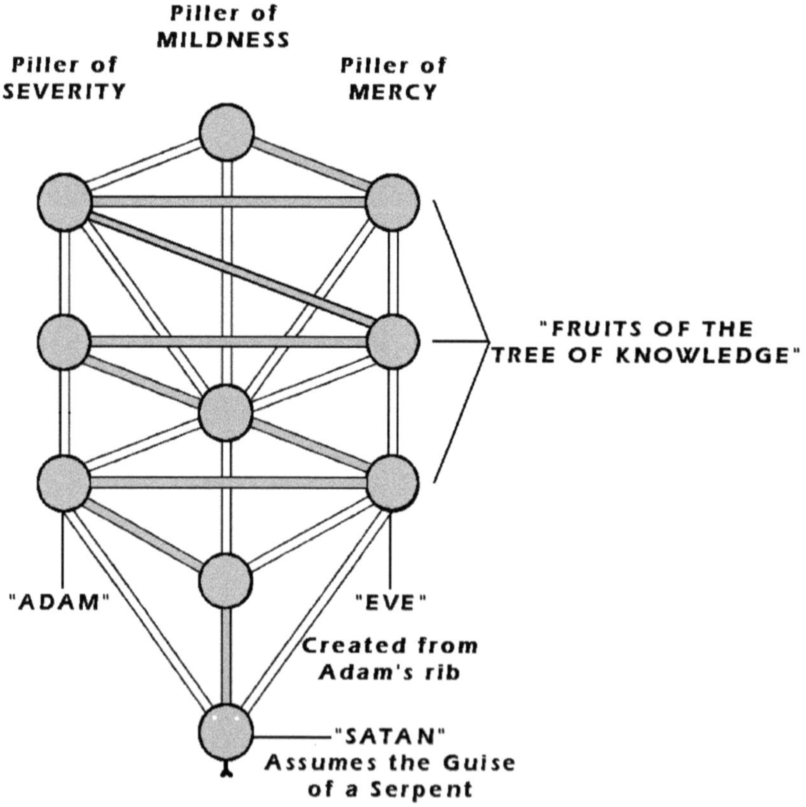

Figure 1.17: The myth of "Original Sin" reflected in the Cabalistic Tree

From the above description, key components of the myth can be recognised as joining together: Adam and Eve, as a couple, form the left and right pillars of the Tree.

> *Now the serpent was more subtle than any beast of the field which the Lord God had made. And he said unto the woman, Yea hath God said, Ye shall not eat of every tree in the garden?* Ch3 v1
>
> *And the woman said unto the serpent, We may eat of the fruit of the trees in the garden:* Ch3 v2
>
> *But of the fruits of the tree which is in the midst of the garden, God hath said, Ye shall not eat of it, neither shall ye touch it, lest ye die.* Ch3 v3
>
> *And the serpent said unto the woman, Ye shall not surely die:* Ch3 v4
>
> *For God doth know that in your day ye eat thereof, then your eyes shall be opened, and ye shall be as gods, knowing good and evil.* Ch3 v5
>
> *And when the woman saw that the tree was good for food, and that it was pleasant to the eyes, and a tree to be desired to make one wise, she took of the fruit thereof and did eat, and gave also unto her husband with her; and he did eat.* Ch3 v6
>
> *And the eyes of them both were opened, and they knew they were naked; and they sewed fig leaves together, and made themselves aprons.* Ch3 v7

In the Cabalistic Tree, the body of the serpent is depicted as following the path of the lightning flash of creation down through the sephirot. When it is seen that the Garden of Eden symbolically refers to the Empyrean—the realm of Divine Light beyond manifestation—the eating of the fruit of the Tree of knowledge thus precipitates the soul's fall from grace, whereby the soul is dragged back down to Earth. This loss of grace is referred to as the "Original Sin". The original sin is simply nothing more than describing a soul that has descended from the spiritual world through the sephirot into human form. The study of Cabala involves retracing the soul's journey back to the Empyrean.

Metaphysical Fusion

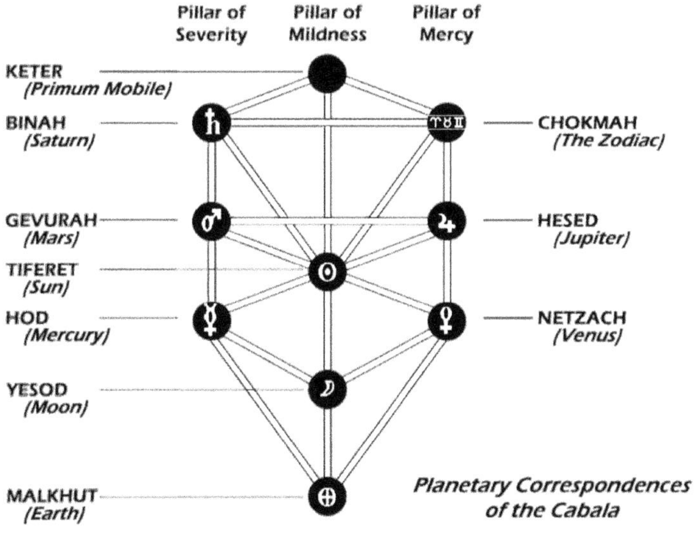

Figure 1.18: The planetary correspondences reflected in the Cabalistic Tree

When the *Corpus Hermeticum* was translated by scholars in the 12th century, they noted the remarkable similarities between the descriptions of creation in Genesis and the Poimandres—the first section of the *Corpus Hermeticum*—with the result the planetary spheres found in both Hermetic and Plato's teachings were fused with the sephirot of Judaic Cabala.

As can be seen in the diagram, Chokmah was linked to the 12 signs of the Zodiac, Binah was linked to the Planet Saturn (♄), Hesed to Jupiter (♃), Gevurah to Mars (♂), Tiferet to the Sun (☉), Netzach to Venus (♀), Hod to Mercury (♀), Yesod to the Moon (☽) and Malkut to Planet Earth (⊕).

Seen in terms of spiritual evolution, each sephirah represented a stage in the journey back to the divine. At each stage the soul was visualised as having to learn particular lessons before it is able to move onto the next sephira. Each sephira was seen to be linked to particular angels, who were considered to impart the knowledge to the receptive aspirant, necessary for them to complete their understanding. To this end the angelic orders of Pseudo-Dionysius were thereby linked to the sephirot.

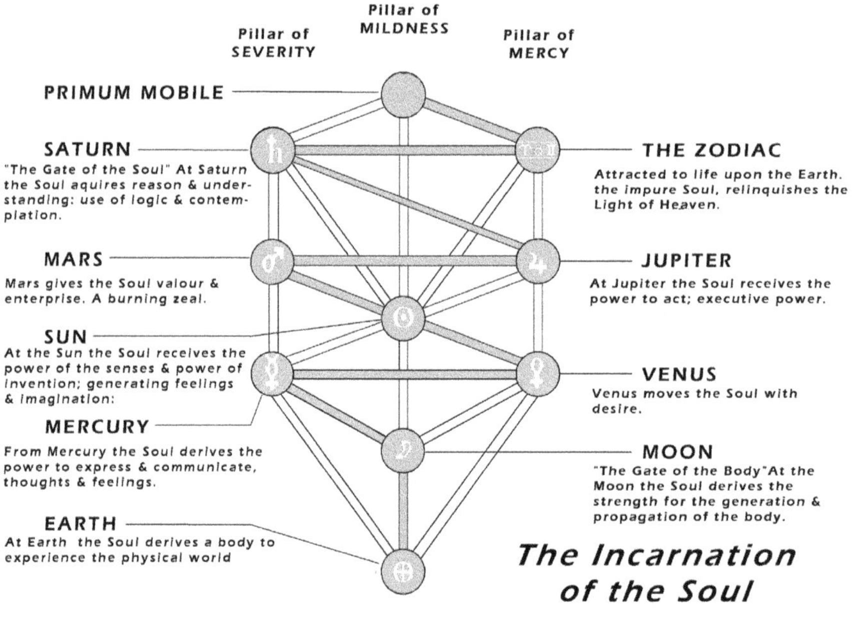

Figure 1.19: The Ascension of the Soul reflected in the Cabalistic Tree

This synthesis of several strands of metaphysical knowledge being plaited together would have provided a huge inspirational impetus to the Gothic era. As the sunlight shone through the Winchester Palace Rose Window it would have become a stunning visual mandala of the metaphysical knowledge that was at the heart of the medieval world. It shows how the Sun was considered the source of all creation, and how within the Solar glyph all the interacting geometries can be found, along with their correspondences to the different metaphysical teachings that were woven together by the scholars and theologians of the early Gothic era.

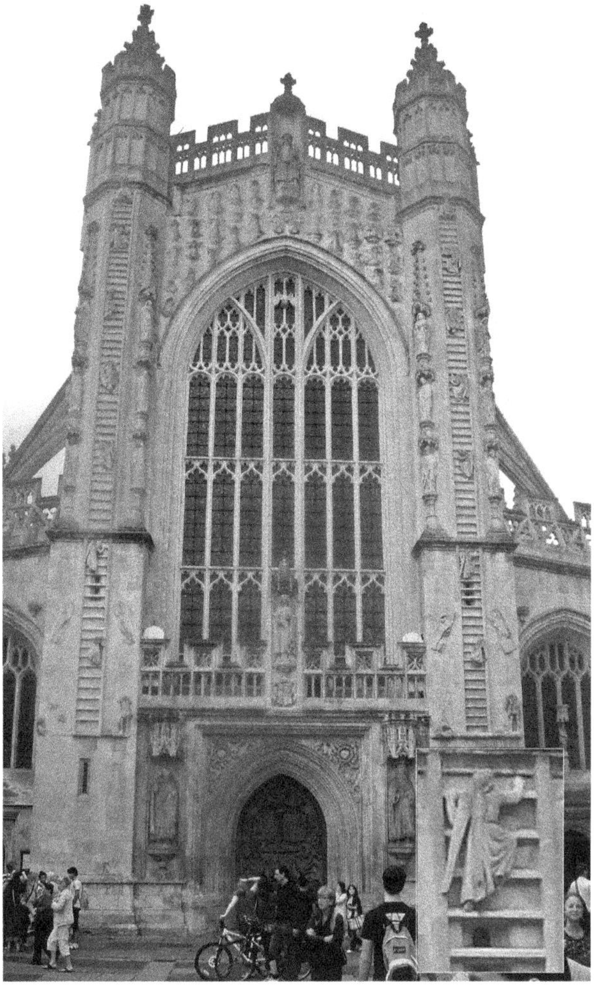

Figure 1.20: The West Door of Bath Abbey, showing Angels climbing up and down the ladders of the Angelic Orders

Such was the precision of the masons that the orientation of the window was deliberately constructed so that the orb of the Sun would perfectly align with the aperture of the window—probably exactly fitting into the central rose. In accordance with the Cluniac reforms, this alignment would be due West, coinciding with position of the Sun at sunset on the Autumnal Equinox.

In an era long before large, flat plasma screen televisions, this spectacular window must have been the source of enormous inspiration and philosophical discussion for Henry of Blois, in his role of Bishop of Winchester, while entertaining his clerical guests. In turn it would inspire them to return to their abbeys and priories to execute and explore these ideas within their own monasteries and nunneries. As Plato put it, *"It is through geometry that one purifies the eye of the soul."*

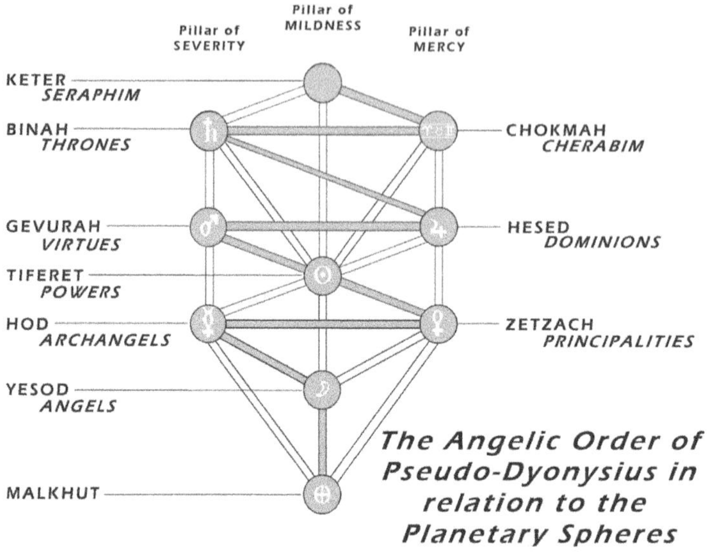

Figure 1.21: The angelic orders reflected in the Cabalistic Tree

As has been demonstrated, these metaphysical ideas underpinned medieval knowledge and learning. Later chapters will explore how these ideas were transposed into education, medicine and, more specifically, the art of physic. But first it is necessary to explore the ideas of Hippocrates and Galen, whose writings lay the foundation of the of the principles of physic.

CHAPTER TWO

Hippocrates and the birth of humoral medicine

Hippocrates (c. 460–380 BC) was a Greek physician, born on the tiny island of Kos. He is often referred to as the "Father of Medicine" in recognition of his lasting contributions to medicine. He was the founder of the Hippocratic School of Medicine, which revolutionised Ancient Greek medicine, thus establishing it as a profession. A body of medical texts, known as the Hippocratic Corpus, survives and though bearing his name is written in several different styles, which suggests that most of the texts were written and compiled by his students.

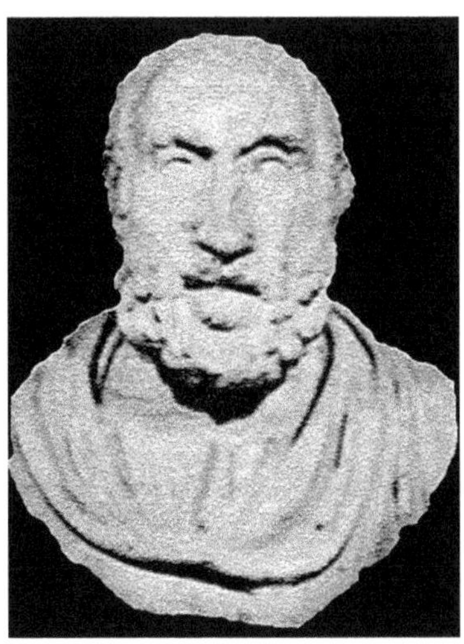

Figure 2.1: A bust of Hippocrates—a replica of one found at Ostia in the tomb of Marcus Demetrius, a 2nd-century AD physician. Its base was inscribed with the famous Hippocratean phrase: "Ars Longa, vita brevis"

Hippocrates was the son of the physician Herakleis and Phainarete. While he must have learned about medicine from his father, he studied physic principally with Herodikos from Selymbria, along with the philosophers Gorgias, Prodikos and Demokritos. Of these men Prodikos is likely to have exposed him to the teachings of Plato.

While a young man Hippocrates left Kos and worked for a time as a doctor in Thessaly. During the Peloponnesian War he is known to have helped the Athenians in the great plague. He also worked in the court of the Persian king Artaxerxes, and died in Thessaly in 380 BC.

His name is often held up as a shining example of the ideal physician, who is credited with composing the Hippocratic Oath, an ethical code still sworn by medical herbalists today. He is also credited with formulating the principles of humoral physiology, thereby greatly advancing the systematic study of clinical medicine. The texts of the Hippocratic Corpus importantly influenced the medical practices of physicians for millennia.

The Hippocratic Oath

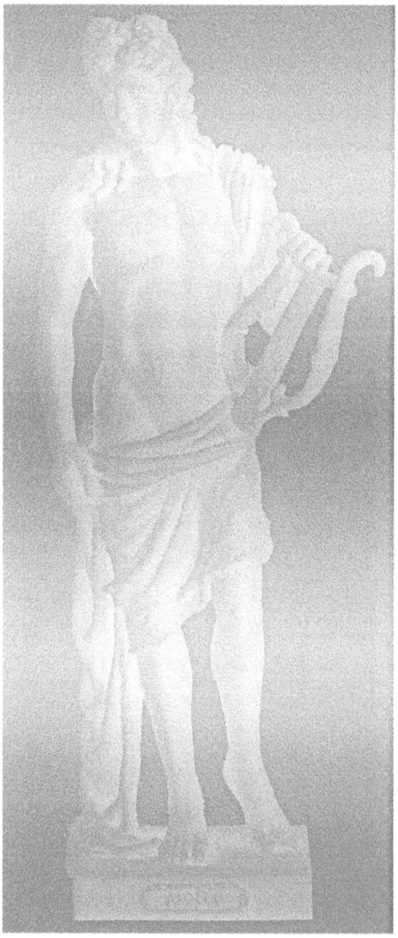

Figure 2.2: Statue of Apollo bearing his harp

The Hippocratic Oath, though still taken by doctors today as an ethical ideal, has radically changed from the original oath as attributed to Hippocrates. Formerly the Oath opened with the invocation,

> *I swear by almighty Apollo, by Asclepius, by Hygeia and Panacea, and call all the gods and goddesses to witness, that I will observe and keep this underwritten oath, to the utmost of my power and judgment.*
>
> *I will reverence my master who taught me the art. Equally with my parents, will I allow him things necessary for his support, and will consider his sons as brothers. I will teach them my art without reward or agreement; and I will impart all my acquirement, instructions, and whatever I know, to my master's children, as to my own; and likewise to all my pupils, who shall bind and tie themselves by a professional oath, but to none else.*
>
> *With regard to healing the sick, I will devise and order for them the best diet, according to my judgment and means; and I will take care that they suffer no hurt or damage.*
>
> *Nor shall any man's entreaty prevail upon me to administer poison to anyone; neither will I counsel any man to do so. Moreover, I will give no sort of medicine to any pregnant woman, with a view to destroy the child.*
>
> *Further, I will comport myself and use my knowledge in a godly manner. I will not cut for the stone, but will commit that affair entirely to the surgeons.*
>
> *Whatsoever house I may enter, my visit shall be for the convenience and advantage of the patient; and I will willingly refrain from doing any injury or wrong from falsehood, and (in an especial manner) from acts of an amorous nature, whatever may be the rank of those who it may be my duty to cure, whether mistress or servant, bond or free.*
>
> *Whatever, in the course of my practice, I may see or hear (even when not invited), whatever I may happen to obtain knowledge of, if it be not proper to repeat it, I will keep sacred and secret within my own breast.*
>
> *If I faithfully observe this oath, may I thrive and prosper in my fortune and profession, and live in the estimation of posterity; or on breach thereof, may the reverse be my fate!*

Apollo is the Sun god in the Greek pantheon, and consequently is far removed from most people's beliefs and understanding today. But taking the god Apollo symbolically as a representation of the Sun, then the Sun represents the Soul, the source of light within. In deep meditation or silent prayer when the mind becomes still and concentrated, the light of the Soul spontaneously becomes visible. As the inner stillness grows, so the light becomes brighter, to the point where the mind becomes absorbed into the light.

Once an individual has experienced this inner connection to the light of their Soul, a profound change of perception takes place. Throughout your daily life, you can then see this light permeating everything. It creates an aesthetic awareness of the beauty in life. In short, it enables you to see the spiritual within the material. You can see the interconnections between all life, whether it is between people or within nature.

This is this perception that is behind the Hippocratic Oath, from respect to his teachers, students, patients and colleagues. Medicine literally means "the art of healing", relieving the pain and suffering of patients. As Hippocrates stated: "*Wherever the art of medicine is loved, there is also a love of humanity.*" Furthermore, he said: "*Whenever a doctor cannot do good, he must be kept from doing harm.*"

Apollo's son was Asclepius, the god of medicine. His mother was Koronis, daughter of the Thessalian king, Phlegyas. Koronis was killed by the goddess Artemis when Apollo learnt of her love affair with the mortal Ischys. Asclepius was then entrusted to the care of the Centaur Chiron, who taught him the art of medicine.

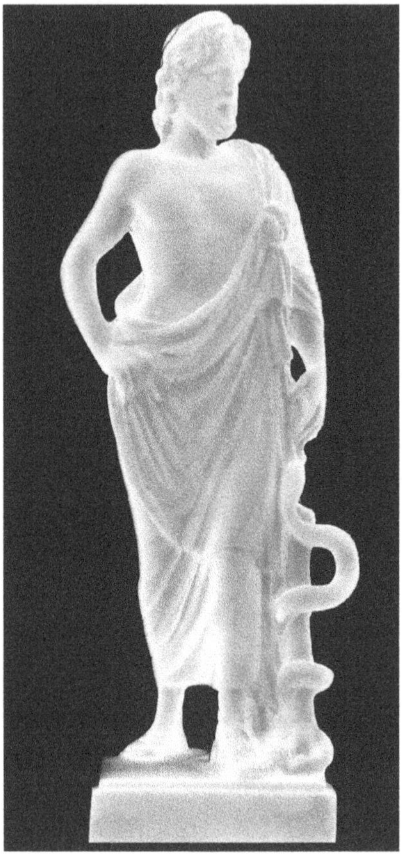

Figure 2.3: Statue of Asclepius with his signature python and stave

Asclepius married his wife Epione (the mild one), and they had four daughters: Hygeia, Iaso, Aceso (those who heal) and Panacea (she who cures all). In the initial invocation of the Hippocratic Oath, the names of two of Asclepius' daughters are found. Such is the warped genealogy of Greek myths, however, that Hygeia was also becomes Asclepius' consort. She was associated with the balance of nature and a representation of health.

Hygeia's name gave rise to the term "hygiene", which in a post-microbial world refers to conditions and practices conducive to maintaining health and preventing the spread of infectious disease. However, in Hippocrates' day hygiene would have referred to the ritual cleansing of the body in preparation for healing within the temple.

The term "panacea" has come down to us a mythical remedy for all disease or a cure-all, but in the Asclepiad tradition it related to the power of the Sun. The light of the Sun sustains all life on Earth; therefore, the Sun symbolically represented the generation of

Vital Force—the healing mechanism of the body—hence the concept of panacea as the universal medicine that heals all mankind.

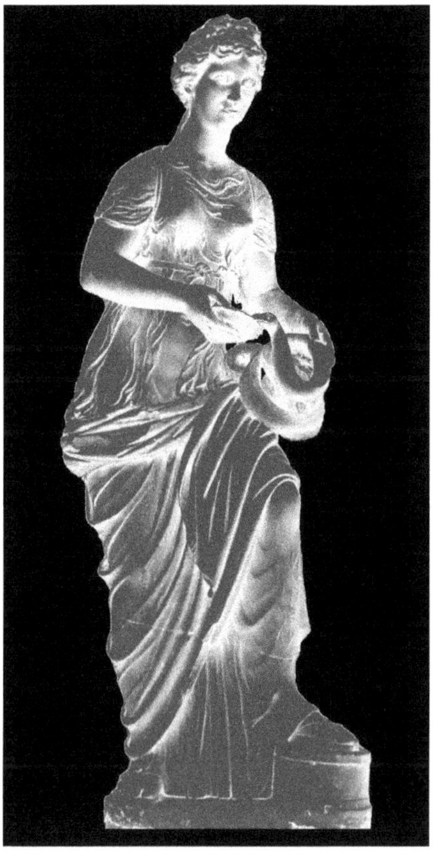

Figure 2.4: Statue of Hygeia feeding a python

Chiron the Centaur is a mythological beast who is half man and half horse. Chiron, being an archer, is associated with the Zodiacal sign of Sagittarius, which is ruled by Jupiter.

At the request of Pluto, lord of the underworld, Jupiter had Asclepius die because he cured the sick and hell stayed deserted. However, Apollo requested that Asclepius be immortalised, remaining among the stars as the constellation of Ophiuchus, the snake.

The Sun, as the source of all life on the planet, symbolically represents the generation of the Vital Force in the body. Hence the Asclepiad tradition was primarily a vitalistic perspective of medicine. As Hippocrates stated, *"The natural healing force within each one of us is the greatest force in getting well."*

The fact that this opening section of Hippocratic Oath is now missing reflects how doctors today lack the humility to respect the Vital Force in the healing process. Worse still, they even eschew the idea of its existing. Hippocrates made the apposite comment: *"Foolish the doctor who despises the knowledge acquired by the Ancients."* The story of how this has happened will become clear later, in Chapter 19.

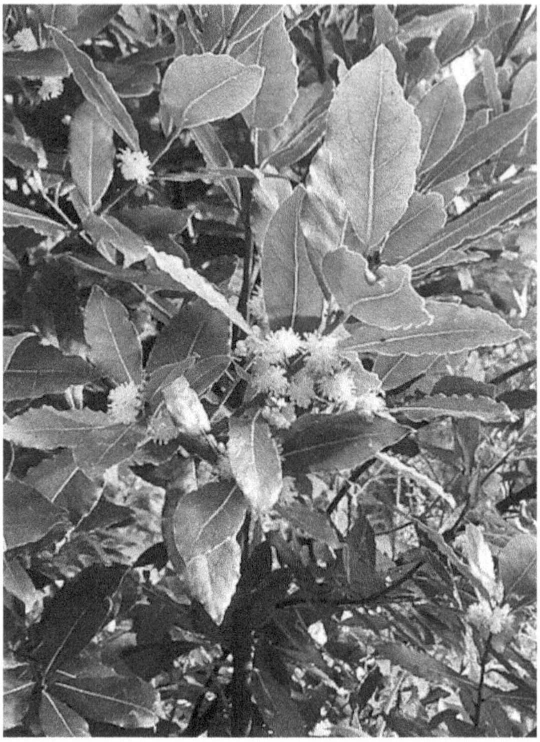

Figure 2.5: The golden complexion of the bay tree in flower

These ideas are demonstrated in the bay tree (*Laurus nobilis*), which is sacred to the Greek god Apollo. Despite the tree having a dark complexion from the deep, evergreen leaves, it does have a golden aura about it. The shiny leaves have golden margins and central veins. The flowers too are golden in colour, and when the sun shines on the tree in full blossom, it really displays its regal magnificence. It is totally appropriate that the tree should be connected to Apollo, the Solar deity of the Greek pantheon.

The Pythia, the priestesses who officiated at the Apollonian temple in Delphi, before going into a trance burnt bay leaves as incense and even chewed them. This was an important part of the ritual for invoking the presence of Lord Apollo, before imparting wisdom and instruction to whoever came to enquire of the Oracle.

Apollo is the God of beauty, music and harmony, for his emblem is a harp. As a Sun god, Apollo represents the Soul, the source of inner light, which can be perceived in deep meditation. Once consciousness is absorbed into your inner light then a profound peace and harmony pervades your whole being, within and without. In the afterglow of the meditation, everything around you seem to shine, creating an aesthetic sense of the beauty in the world. The bay tree captures this amphoteric quality, with its dark green complexion, yet it shines with a golden aura in the sunshine.

Artists, musicians, poets and orators who have connected with their inner light become inspired. Their creations and performances are infused with this light, displaying a mastery or magnificence. In turn they are celebrated by being feted with a wreath of bay leaves being placed on their head, symbolising their inner illumination.

In medieval Europe when the first universities were founded, students were rewarded, on the completion of the Seven Liberal Arts, by being named a Bachelor of Arts. The word "bachelor" is derived from the Latin *bacca* and *Laurus*, meaning "berries of the laurel". In other words, the graduates had achieved the fruits of their labours and were ready to set seed by imparting their knowledge to others.

Humoral physiology

It was Hippocrates' application of Plato's metaphysical ideas to the body that transformed the medical thinking of his day. Essentially the symbolism of the Five Elements was applied to analyse the blood, the components of which were visualised as the Four Humours. Physicians in Hippocrates' day did not have microscopes and biochemical tests to evaluate the blood, but by using Elemental symbolism they were able to have profound insights into the physiology of the body and formulate the therapeutic principles on which the Western herbal tradition was based.

Since the flow of blood in the body was synonymous with life, the Elements were easily transposed to evaluate the nature of the blood. The Four Humours are all contained in the blood. They were symbolically perceived and differentiated using the Four Elements:

- the Sanguine humour (L. *sanguineus* = bloody) corresponds to Air
- the Choleric humour (Gk *chole* = bile) corresponds to Fire
- the Melancholic humour (Gk *melanchole* = black bile) corresponds to Earth
- and the Phlegmatic humour (Gk *phlegma* = phlegm) corresponds to Water.

ELEMENT	HUMOUR	DESCRIPTION	PHYSIOLOGY
EARTH	*MELANCHOLIC (Black Bile)*	*"The Sediment of the Blood"*	Plasma proteins: Blood viscosity, clotting & thrombus formation.
WATER	*PHLEGMATIC (Phlegm)*	The Fluid Portion of the Blood	Blood plasma: formation of mucus, lymph, sweat, synovial fluid, CSF, urine, humours of the eye.
ETHER	*VITAL FORCE*	The Flow of Vital Force through the Blood	Electrical properties of the Blood.
FIRE	*CHOLERIC (Yellow Bile)*	*"The Spume & Froth of the Blood"*	Blood cells: Erythrocytes Role in tissue respiration heat & energy production.
AIR	*SANGUINE (Blood)*	The Totality of the Melancholic, Choleric & Phlegmatic Humours	Total composition of the Blood: Transportation of respiratory gases, nutrients, hormones. Immune function.

Figure 2.6: A table of the four elements and corresponding humours within the blood

Of all the Elements, Earth is the most solid and material. Thus, symbolically the Earth portion of the blood is that which precipitates from the bodily fluid. In Culpeper's writings he defines the Melancholic humour as the *"sediment of the blood"*. In contemporary physiology, this symbolic description would concord with the plasma proteins that contribute to the blood's viscosity. When the blood vessels are cut, these proteins form clots, helping to seal and repair the damage to the vessel, conserving the loss of blood, thereby preserving the life of the body.

However, in the physiology of several diseases, the precipitation of the clotting proteins within the blood vessels leads to the formation of clots, known as thrombi. These travel in the circulating blood to points where the lumen of the blood vessel becomes smaller than the diameter of the thrombi, where they then become lodged. Blood is prevented from flowing past this blockage, leading to a lack of blood, or ischaemia, reaching critical tissues in the organs. The brain, lungs and heart are notably vulnerable in this respect, leading to strokes, pulmonary embolism and heart attacks respectively.

Water is a fluid Element, flowing and connecting things together. If you imagine two drops of water touching, then they immediately coalesce into a larger drop. When Water is symbolically transposed into the blood, it concords with the blood plasma, the fluid medium in which all the different blood cells are carried and into which various nutrients, electrolytes, hormones and waste products are dissolved. Through the medium of the blood plasma all the cells throughout the body are essentially connected together.

When the blood supplies all the different tissues of the body, the plasma perfuses out of the capillaries, leaving the blood cells behind, thereby forming the interstitial fluid that bathes the cells constituting the various tissues. As the plasma continually perfuses into the tissues, so the lymphatic system, through a series of vessels, drains the surplus interstitial fluid and returns it once more to the circulating blood.

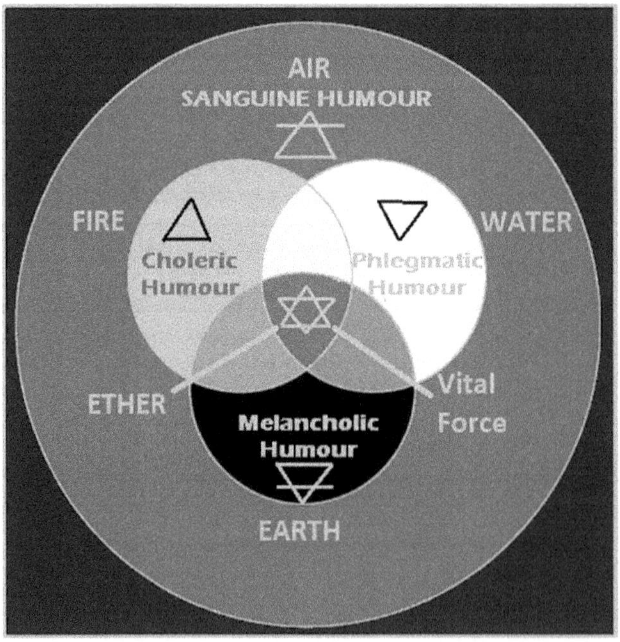

Figure 2.7: The relationship of the four humours within the blood

So too, the plasma draining through the sweat glands in the skin forms sweat. Similarly, the plasma is linked to the secretion of cerebro-spinal fluid in the brain and spinal column, the formation of mucus by the mucous membranes, the secretion of synovial fluid in the joints as well as the vitreous and aqueous humours within the eye. Thus, the concept of Phlegmatic humour embraces what in contemporary physiology is described as the blood plasma, lymph, sweat, phlegm, synovial fluid and the formation of urine.

Fire is the most dynamic Element—captured by Culpeper's phrase, the "*spume and froth of the blood*". Today most physicians would perhaps more easily recognise the dynamism as the "lub dub, lub dub" sound heard when listening to the heart.

This sound is in part created by the blood cells brushing against the walls of the blood vessels as they circulate around the body, punctuated by the opening and closing of the heart valves, as the heart beats. Erythrocytes are the predominant blood cells contributing to the sound.

Since the Choleric humour is linked to the generation of heat and energy, then an excess of choler is linked to the generation of a fever. Since most pathogenic organisms that cause disease in the body flourish at normal body temperature, raising the body temperature provides the first line of defence, for it inhibits their proliferation. The extra heat speeds up the physiological response of the immune system in attacking the offending organism. Once the fever has subsided it often leaves a rejuvenated sense of clarity and vitality.

The expansive nature of the Air Element makes it unique among the Four Elements in that it is able to embrace the other Elements—Earth, Water and Fire—within it. Air sits upon the Earth and pervades its spaces, Water evaporates and condenses within it, while Fire is sustained by it while its heat moves it. Similarly, Air symbolically connects to the totality of the blood—described as the Sanguine humour.

The Sanguine humour thus represents the balance or temper of the three constituent humours: Melancholic, Choleric and Phlegmatic. Arguably, the most important function of the blood is the transportation of oxygen, inhaled from the air in the lungs and distributing it to all the cells throughout the body, supporting cellular respiration, enabling the cells to generate energy. In the reverse process carbon dioxide, formed by cellular respiration, is removed in the blood and expelled out of the body via the lungs back into the air. The expansiveness of the Air Element is also reflected in how the blood distributes cellular nutrients, immune cells, hormones and other key chemicals throughout the body.

The balance of the four humours within the blood is important to enable the Vital Force (Ether) to flow through it. The more balanced the humours are, the stronger a person's vitality becomes. The evenness of flow to the Vital Force through the blood was seen as being important for healing and maintaining balance of mind, emotions and body. Thus, the adjective "sanguine" is synonymous with a state of health—a balance of mind, emotions and body.

In health the harmonious combination of humours is held in balance, or temper, which allows the Vital Force or Ether to flow freely through the body, whereas in disease the temper of the humours is lost. A particular humour predominating over the others causes a characteristic distemper. The humour can be identified by the symptoms it produces, whether they are hot or cold, dry or moist. The "common cold", for example, is classically a Phlegmatic condition, which should more accurately be diagnosed as a cold and moist!

Hippocrates said, *"We must turn to nature itself, to the observations of the body in health and in disease to learn the truth."* Just as the balance of the Four Elements is important for life (Ether) to flourish in nature, so too the therapeutic objective of humoral physiology is to counteract the dominant humour and so restore the temper to the blood. For example, a fever is a hot and dry condition, which is helped by medicines that are cooling and moistening. One of the herbs identified in the Hippocratic writings for dealing with fevers is the willow. It is easy to see how a tree with such an affinity for the Water Element should have been chosen to extinguish the Fire of a fever. As Hippocrates described the healing role, *"The physician treats, but nature heals."*

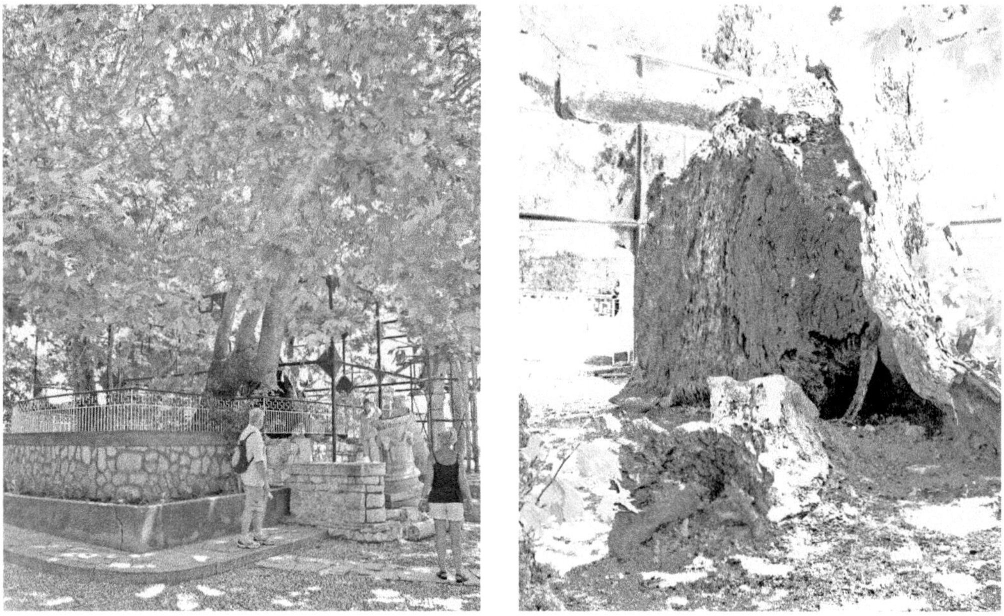

Figure 2.8: The Hippocratic tree in Kos, where in its shade Hippocrates taught his students the principles of humoral physiology

There is an old plane tree, located just a stone's throw away from the harbour in the town of Kos, known as the Hippocratic tree. Underneath the shade of this tree Hippocrates taught students his principles of medicine, including his humoral physiology. Today there is a line of four mature trees at the site, their trunks clearly little more than 150 years old.

However, just behind a public platform, enclosed in a protective cage, the remaining one third of the outer circumference of a trunk can be seen. This decayed, hollowed-out trunk was formerly about 6 feet in diameter and would easily have been a tree that would have survived for more than 2,500 years. A single surviving branch emerging from what remains of the old trunk has collapsed onto the ground, from which suckers have taken and evolved to form the line of the four mature trees seen today.

Amazingly, the survival of the Hippocratic tree can be seen as a living botanical homage to the four humours of the blood, formulated by the physician. Whether by accident or design, they have even grown in such a way that one of the two suckers has formed three trunks in contrast to the other one, which has remained as a single trunk—a symbolic echo of the three humours within the blood. It is a fitting living symbol of the renewed interest in Hippocratic teachings.

The plane tree or *Plátanos* has long been associated with the god Apollo, as shown in the words of Pausanias from the 2nd century AD: *"As you go along a mountain road by way of this rock, you reach a temple of Apollo surnamed Platanistius,"* which means "god of the plane tree grove". Plane trees are commonly located in meeting places throughout Greece, for they offer shade and cool from the heat of the midday sun, and it is fitting that Hippocrates taught his students, within the Asclepiad tradition, the principles of the humours from its protective shade. Plato too had previously taught his students under the shade of a plane tree.

The Asclepion temple on Kos

The island of Kos is famous for its Asclepion temple, situated on the mountain above the town of Kos. The site is huge, as big as any metropolitan hospital today, with a commanding view across the Aegean Sea to Bodrum on the present-day Turkish coast. When it was built, in the late 4th century to early 3rd century BC, Kos and much of Turkey were all part of the kingdom of Phrygia.

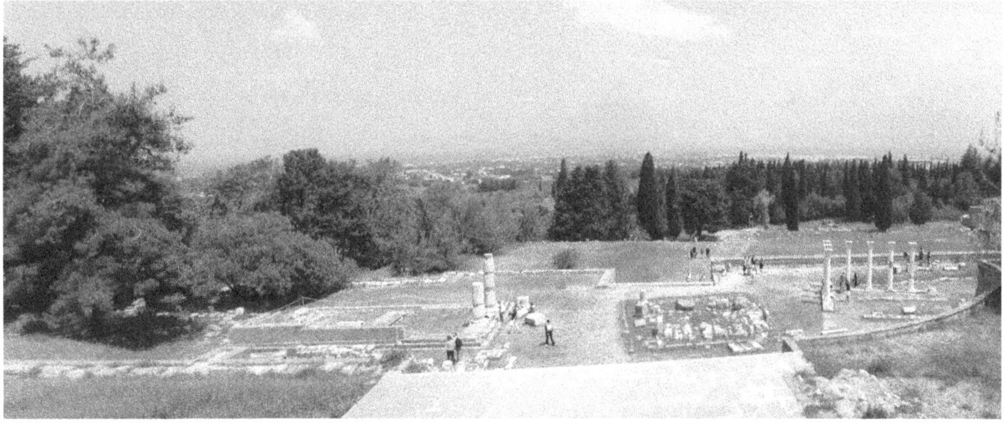

Figure 2.9: The view from the top terrace of the Asclepion at Kos

This site in Classical Greece was famous for its healing and medical expertise. It was here that Hippocrates worked as a physician and would have given clinical instruction to his students.

The site takes advantage of the gradient of the mountain, and intentionally incorporated in three distinct levels of the facility interconnected by stone steps. These three levels reflected the Hermetic order of Body, Soul and Spirit.

The site has been ravaged by earthquakes since its heyday. Kos is located just 20 miles away from the neighbouring island of Nisyros, which is an active volcano. Minor tremors are felt weekly on Kos and are accepted as part of daily life there. Much of what is visible today has been reconstructed by archaeologists from the rubble.

However, what survives of the site is still very impressive. The lower terrace has a stone wall below the second level, with a series of arches. In one of these arches (3rd left from the stairs) is a vulval-shaped stone, with a statue of the god Pan in its upper arch. A small cascade of water emerges from the lower arch, then falls and collects in a small pool. The vulval symbol would be connected to Hygeia, the goddess representing the balance of nature.

The middle terrace has the ruins of a dormitory block on the left-hand side, while on the right a few columns are found standing from a temple dedicated to the god Apollo. The upper terrace contains the ruins of a temple dedicated to Asclepius, the god of medicine.

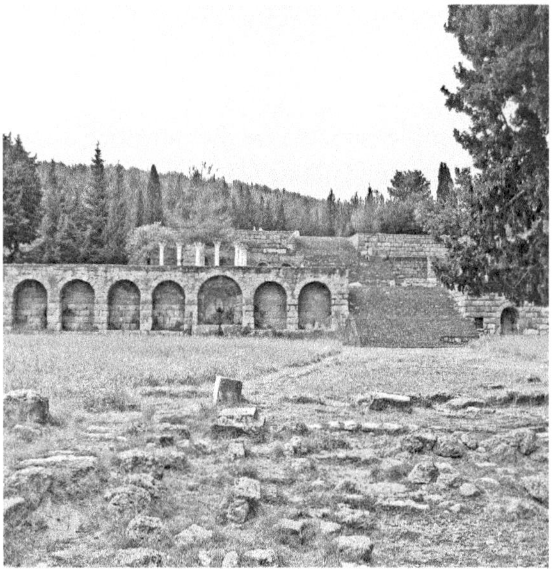

Figure 2.10: The view from the bottom terrace of the Asclepion at Kos

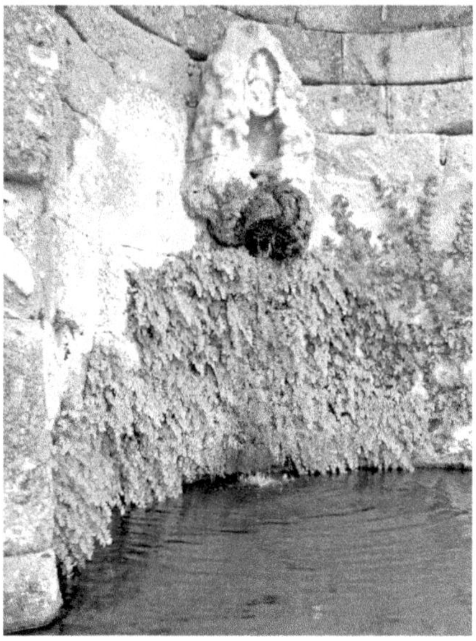

Figure 2.11: The ablutional pool at the Asclepion

When people arrived for healing, they fasted and abluted in the temple's spring water. The ritual cleansing was a precursor to balancing the humours in the body. Having been physically cleansed, the aspirant was then permitted to ascend the steps to the temple of Asclepius, where after making an offer of flowers, they then prayed to the god for healing and guidance.

Next came the incumbent stage of the healing when aspirants were instructed to go to the dormitory area and await the arrival of the god in their sleep. If the patient was successful in their prayers, Asclepius would appear to them in their dream and instruct them according to their illness.

Asclepius was identified in the dream by his signature emblem of a single python curling around his staff. Being touched or licked by the snake in their dream describes their direct healing by Asclepius. The patient was then expected to remember any instruction and inform the priest on waking. The name clinic, as a place of medical practice, is derived from the Greek word *kline*, meaning "to dream".

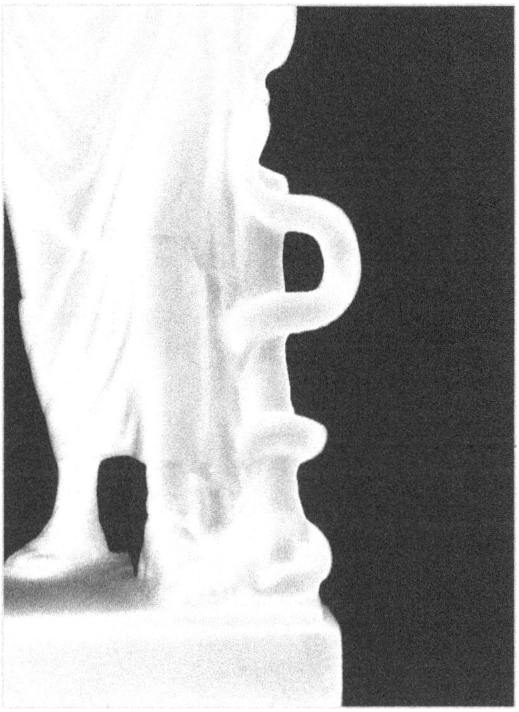

Figure 2.12: The python, symbolic of the healing power of Asclepius

Where no clear instructions were obtained, then the priests derived insights into the balance of the patient's humours, from the key Elements in their dream. Thus, if a dream was about crossing water, that would indicate that the Phlegmatic humour was predominating. By contrast, if the dream showed a house in flames, that would indicate the Choleric humour was predominating.

According to the dreams, so different combinations of diet, herbs and exercise were prescribed by the priests.

The two different temples of Apollo and Asclepius, located on the middle and upper terraces respectively, must have also been significant. The Apollonian temple, on the middle level of the soul, suggests this is where patients prayed, seeking to balance their humours and strengthen their vitality. The Asclepiad temple, on the upper terrace of spirit, suggests this was where patients prayed, seeking more specific instruction on the spiritual factors contributing to their illness.

Patients stayed in the vicinity of the Asclepion, eating fresh food (Earth), drinking the spring waters (Water), inhaling the fresh sea air (Air) and taking gentle exercise, especially walking, in the sunshine (Fire), till they were cured—in other words, getting the balance of the Elements right to enhance the flow of the Vital Force and enable healing.

According to Greek myth, Asclepius was taught medicine by Chiron the Centaur. Chiron suffered a severe, mortal wound from an accident while out hunting with Hercules. Being an immortal, this wound caused him to experience the pain and suffering of mankind. There are different myths concerning the healing of Chiron's wound, but the one most interesting from a herbal perspective is the use of the herb centaury

(*Centaurium erythaea*) to heal it. Both the common and Latin names clearly allude to the importance of this myth.

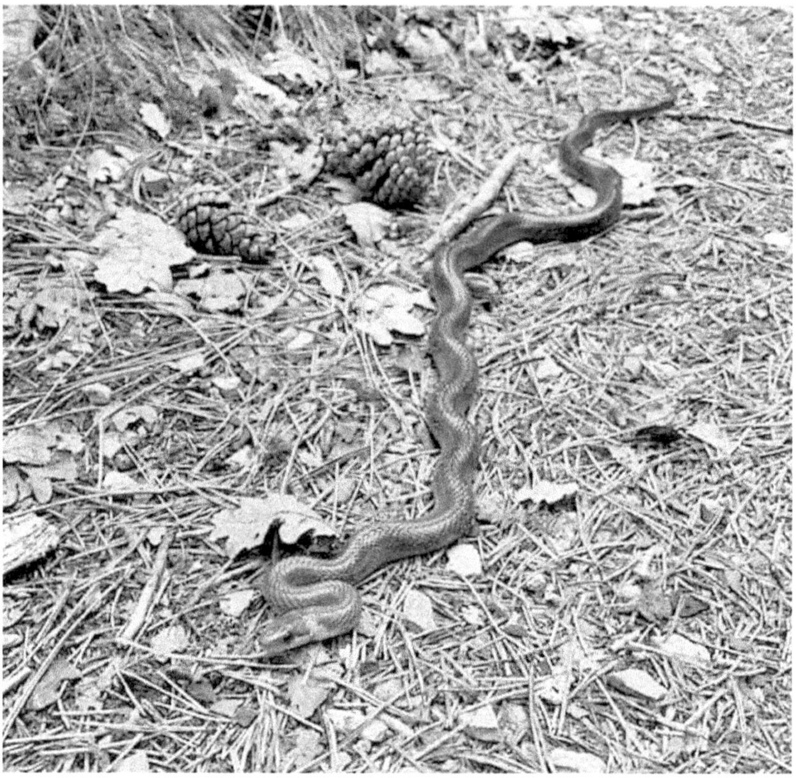

Figure 2.13: The harmless Asclepian snake.
The snakes were encouraged to freely roam the temple grounds.
Photo credit Valerie Hobson

Today the temple of Asclepius largely lies in ruins, but the altar stones survived and have been reassembled. Such is the power of the Asclepius myth that people still visit the temple site for healing from the Greek god of medicine. Behind the altar a small patch of centaury can be found growing—the remains of a votive offering to Asclepius, which ties the god to his teacher Chiron. The small herb is traditionally linked to the Sun.

The name "Hippocrates" literally means the "power of the horse", which clearly alludes to the myth of Chiron, who taught medicine to Asclepius. It is a powerful epithet, implying the physician was seen to embody the knowledge of the Asclepiad tradition.

With the Asclepion complex at Kos having such a commanding view over the Aegean Sea, it is hardly surprising that Hippocrates was inspired there to incorporate the Elements into his therapeutics. He encouraged his patients to take plenty of exercise (Fire), eat good food (Earth), drink plenty of water (Water), and enjoy regular sunlight (Fire) and fresh air (Air), all balanced with sound sleep to enhance healing of the body (Ether). As he put it, *"If we could give every individual the right amount of nourishment and exercise, not too little and not too much, we would have found the safest way to health."*

He stated, *"Health is the greatest of human blessings."* Accordingly, he strongly encouraged his patients to take responsibility for their own health: *"If you are not your own doctor, you are a fool."* In essence, he taught them to become their own doctor, especially through sound nutrition: *"Let food be thy medicine, thy medicine food."* Furthermore, he said, *"The greatest medicine of all is teaching people how not to need it."*

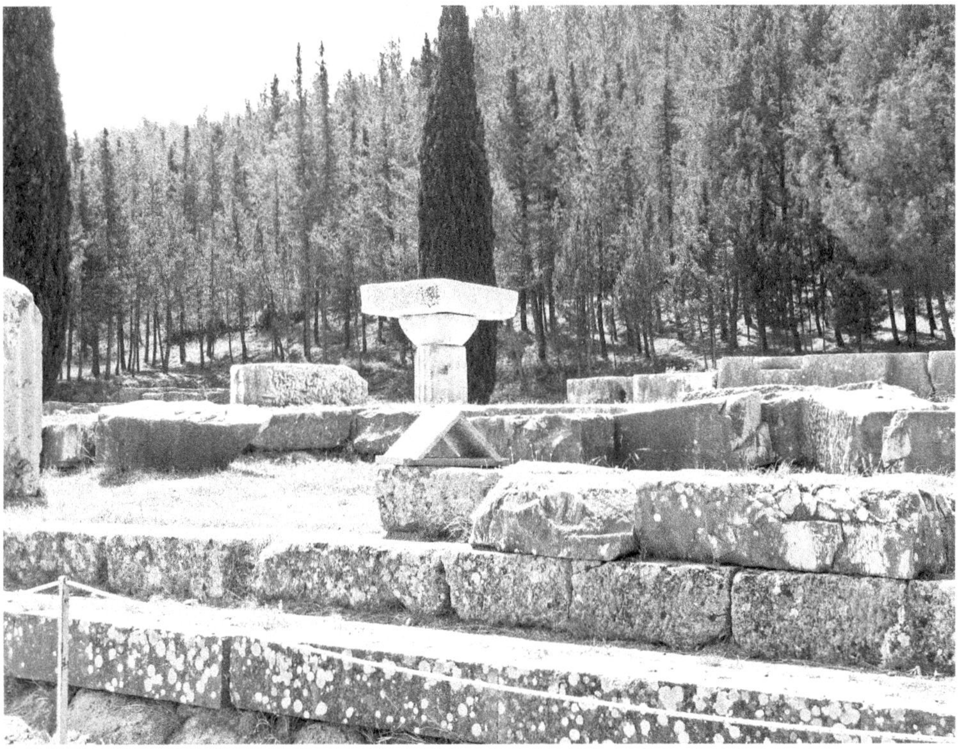

Figure 2.14: The altar stone of the temple dedicated to Asclepius

Hippocrates clearly had a holistic vision of his patients, for he emphasised, *"It is more important to know what sort of person has a disease, than know what sort of disease a person has."* To this end, he utilised particular herbs to enhance the balance of their humours. These herbs collectively have come down to us as the docks, which are the subject of the next chapter.

Reflecting on his long life as a physician, Hippocrates summed up his work in the phrase *Ars Longa Vita Brevis*, meaning "Art is long, life is short." It implies that it takes a long time to master the principles of medicine, by which time your own may be ending. In Hippocrates' day, medicine meant the art of healing.

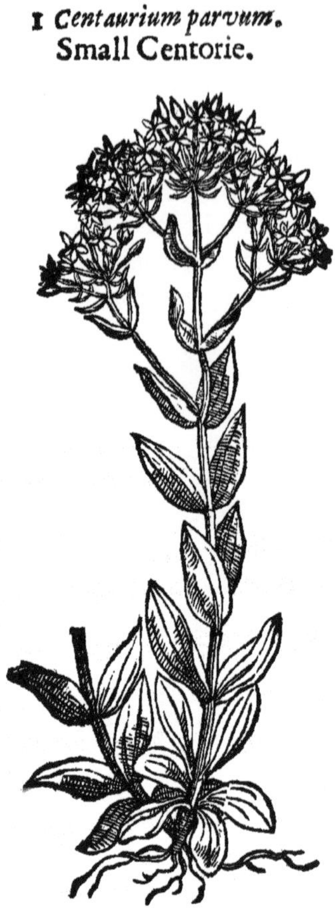

Figure 2.15: Woodcut of centaury from *The Herball* by John Gerard, 1633 Edition

CHAPTER THREE

The docks

The therapeutic objective of humoral medicine was all about identifying the predominating humour and then weakening it or identifying the weakest humour and then strengthening it, in order to restore temper to the Sanguine humour, thereby enhancing the flow of the Vital Force.

To this end, patients were taught how to take responsibility for their health, through diet, exercise and particular herbs. These herbs were known collectively as the docks, their name being derived from the Latin verb *doceo*, meaning "to teach". It can now be seen that docks originally provided a mnemonic that has been used to teach the herbal principles of humoral physiology to people who were largely uneducated within the community. This association of docks to a particular humour was done largely by colour, linking the herb to a corresponding humour in the blood.

First of these is the red or bloody dock (*Rumex sanguineus*), so called because it has a prominent red venation to its leaves, thereby linking it to the red or Sanguine humour of the blood. Since the Sanguine humour represents the totality of the blood and the harmonious balance of the other three humours within it, the red dock was used as blood tonic, strengthening the blood and enhancing the flow of Vital Force though it.

Bloody dock has largely fallen from current herbal use, though it is going through a resurgence of interest again, being promoted as a salad vegetable, under the name "red sorrel".

Next, the yellow or curly leaved dock (*Rumex crispus*) derives its name yellow dock from the cortex of the root, which in the winter months, when the aerial herb dies down, becomes a striking yellow. The yellow colour links the herb to the yellow bile or Choleric humour within the blood. The Choleric humour was seen to have its seat in the gall bladder. Jaundice, when the skin and whites of the eyes turn markedly yellow, was a clear example of the yellow bile predominating.

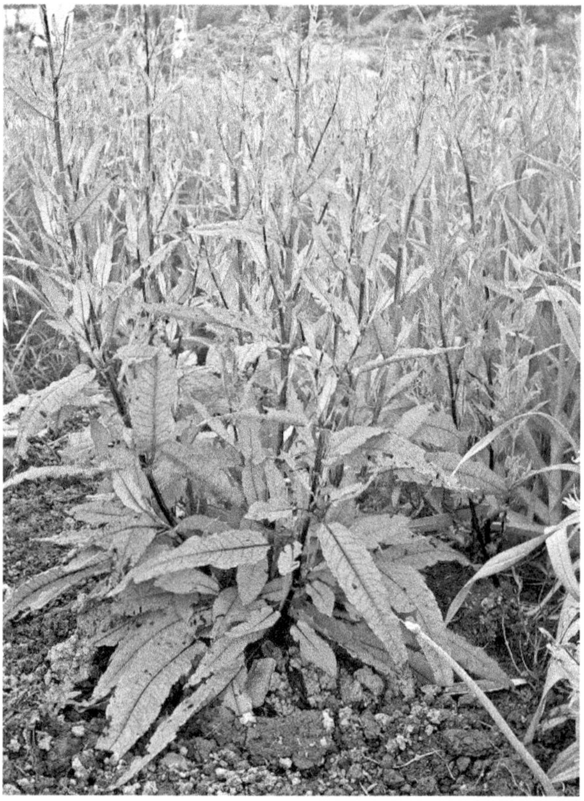

Figure 3.1: Red dock (*Rumex sanguineus*)

Today herbalists still use yellow dock for stimulating the gall bladder and releasing bile, thereby helping the digestion of fatty foods, aiding the elimination of toxins by the liver and promoting regular bowel function where there is mild constipation. Few are aware this plant was one of Hippocrates' key herbs.

Next, the blue dock or common mallow (*Malva sylvestris*) derives its name from the bluish hue in the pink/mauve colour of its petals. In the Mediterranean sunshine, the mallow has a distinct blue coloration, in contrast to those plants that grow in more northerly latitudes. It was linked to the cooling Phlegmatic humour in the blood. The Phlegmatic humour was seen to have its seat in the lungs. Hence the blue dock was used to soothe a cough and help clear phlegm from the chest.

Today herbalists seldom use the blue dock, and its use as a demulcent remedy for the chest has largely been replaced by its relative, the marshmallow (*Althaea officinalis*), to soothe inflammation in the lungs, bowels, urinary tract and bladder.

The leaves of the blue dock are an important, delicious vegetable commonly used in Middle Eastern cuisine, known as "molochia". This use of the vegetable probably had its origins in the Hippocratic teachings.

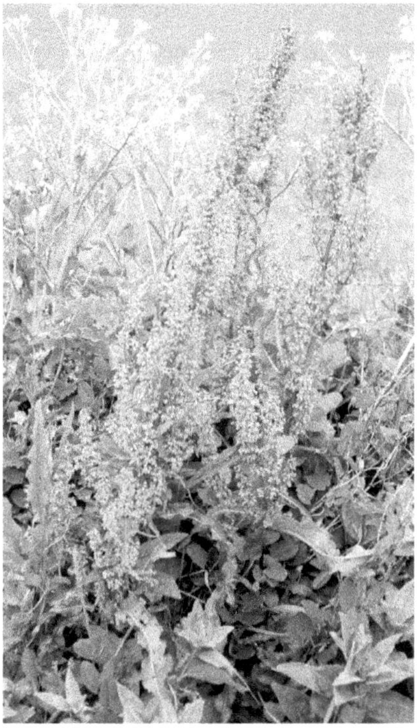

Figure 3.2: Yellow dock (*Rumex crispus*)

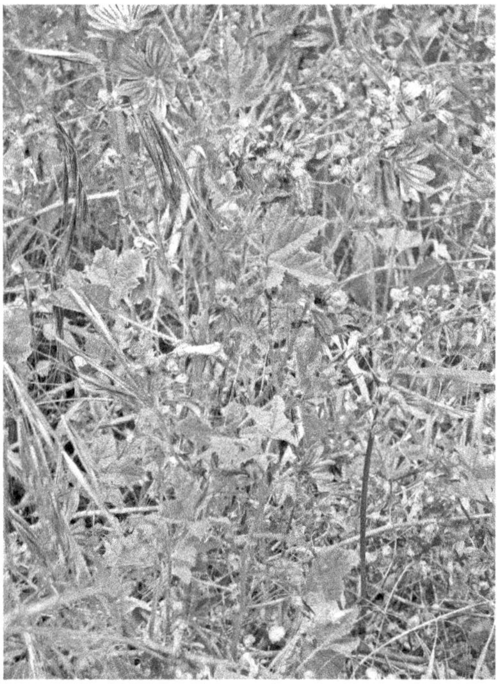

Figure 3.3: Blue dock or common mallow (*Malva sylvestris*)

The identification of a black dock by name, to complete the picture of the examples of docks being linked to the four humours, is notable by its absence. However, there are a few contenders for the role. These include black medick (*Medicago lupulina*), which does grow freely at the Asclepion on Kos. The adjective "black" comes from its black seeds. As the name also implies, "medicks" herbs were also used for doctoring various diseases. The black seeds would have linked the herb to the black bile or Melancholic humour.

When the Melancholic humour predominates people feel depressed, lacking motivation and vitality. It was associated with constipation. The virtue of the black medick, with its cheery golden flowers, was visualised as dispelling the gloom of the Melancholic humour and uplifting the spirits.

Another similar medick species is the spotted medick (*Medicago arabica*), which possesses a little heart-shaped black dot. Its black heart shape would represent the "blackness" of the Melancholic humour gripping the heart. The spotted medick too has golden-yellow flowers, so it was similarly used, perhaps more specifically, to dispel melancholia.

A third contender for the role of black dock is comfrey (*Symphytum officinale*). Though it was not found growing at the Asclepion complex, comfrey is such an important healing herb that it is hard to imagine Hippocrates did not use it. A lesser-known common name for the herb is blackwort, for when you harvest and process the herb, the blackness becomes increasingly apparent as the herb dries out.

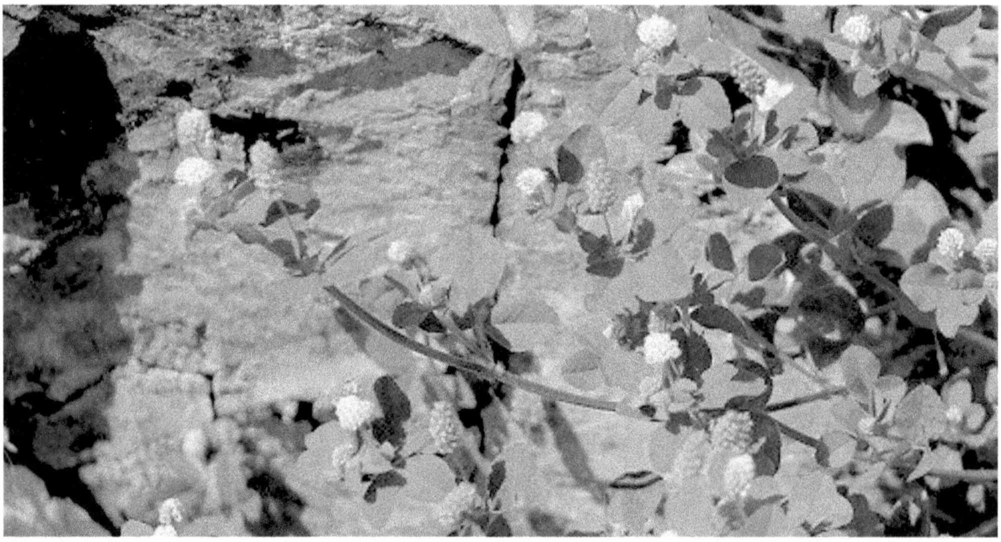

Figure 3.4: Black medick (*Medicago lupulina*)

Certainly, comfrey is used for treating the Melancholic humour, for when its predominates, one of the symptoms is melaena. These are the black tarry stools formed when there is bleeding from the upper digestive tract. As the blood leaks into the digestive system, it too gets broken down, forming the "black tar". Comfrey has a long history for treating gastric and duodenal ulcers.

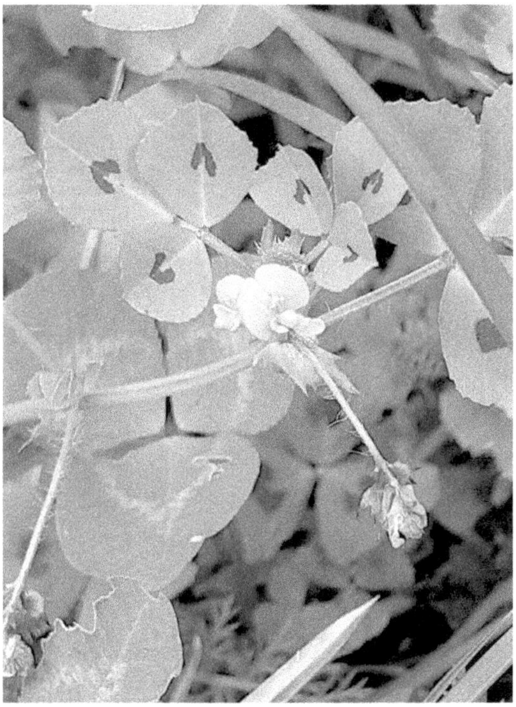

Figure 3.5: Spotted medick (*Medicago arabica*)

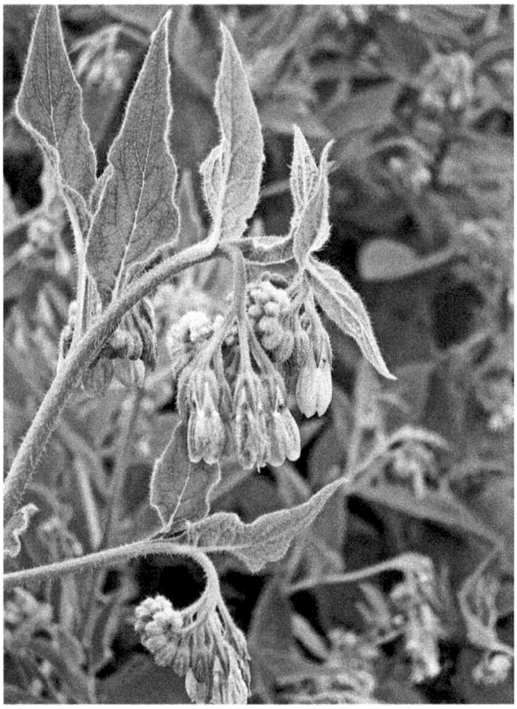

Figure 3.6: Comfrey or blackwort (*Symphytum officinale*)

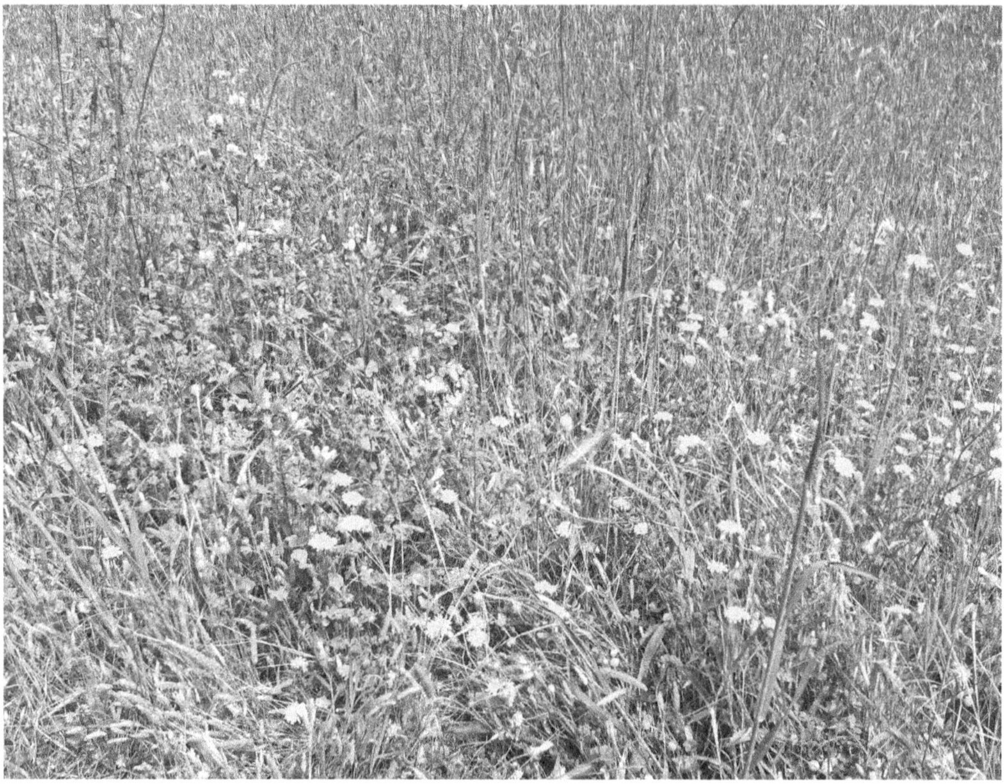

Figure 3.7: The rich floral carpet of the Asclepion at Kos

It is fitting to conclude this chapter with a photograph of the rich diversity of herbs growing wild that carpet the Asclepion at Kos. Most notably the pinkish flowers of the blue dock stand out. Doubtless, 2,500 years on these are descendants of the blue docks that would have been used by Hippocrates and his fellow physicians and students as they administered herbs to their patients.

CHAPTER FOUR

Claudius Galen

Claudius Galenus, Galen (AD 129–216), was born in the ancient city of Pergamon, in Asia Minor, now Bergama in Turkey. He was the son of Aelius Nicon, who was a successful, wealthy Greek architect.

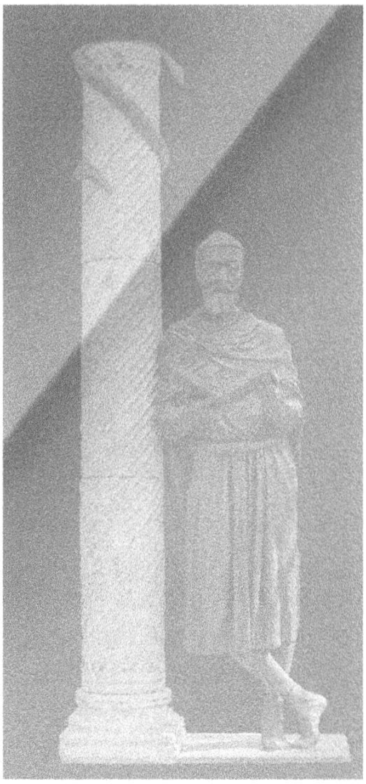

Figure 4.1: Statue of Galen at Pergamon (Bergama)

The young Claudius had the benefit of a privileged liberal education, in a city boasting the library of Eumenes II, which was then the second largest in the ancient world after the library at Alexandria.

A key part of his education was being exposed to the main schools of philosophy of the day, including Aristotelian, Platonic, Epicurean and Stoic schools.

In keeping with the Asclepiad tradition, Claudius' father had a dream in which the god Asclepius appeared and commanded Nicon to send his son to study medicine. In accordance with his father's dream, Claudius entered the Asclepion at Pergamon as an apprentice for four years.

At the Asclepion, he came under the tutelage of Aeschrion, from whom he learnt about Hippocrates' teachings, his humoral physiology and principles of healing. From this initial training at the Asclepion in Pergamon, he understood the importance that Hippocrates placed on diet, fitness, hygiene and preventive measures.

Tragedy struck when his father suddenly died while Claudius was only 19 years old. As a consequence, he got to inherit considerable wealth from his father's estate.

He used this wealth wisely, travelling widely, furthering his medical education in such destinations as Smyrna (Ismir), Corinth, Crete, Cilicia (Anatolia), Cyprus and Alexandria, studying at their respective medical schools. Such an astonishing range of education would have been denied to many of lesser means.

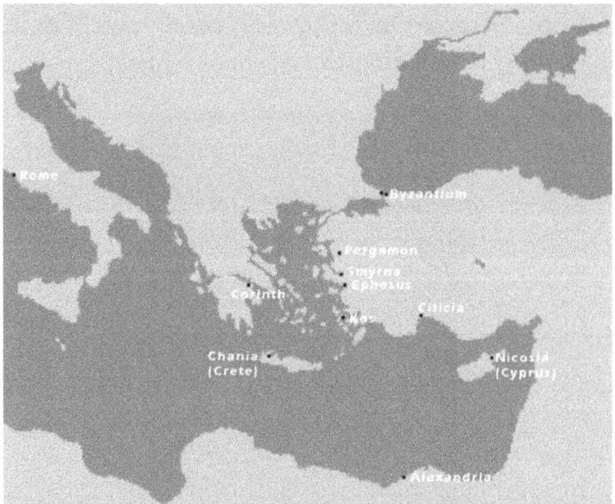

Figure 4.2: The principal locations of Galen's travel and centres of learning

However, it was the legendary school of medicine at Alexandria that was to have the most profound influence on him. For under the tutelage of Heraklianos, Stratonicus and Satyrus, he was exposed to the Hermetic metaphysical ideas that had evolved within Egyptian culture.

In AD 157, Galen returned to Pergamon to act as the physician to the gladiators for the High Priest of Asia. His treatment of the wounds and fractures sustained by the gladiators gained him a considerable reputation for being a healer.

In Roman times, there was a stricture on dissecting the human body. This experience revolutionised Galen's understanding of anatomy—he described the gladiators' wounds as "windows into the body".

Galen finally settled in Rome, where he formed a flourishing practice serving the wealthy and famous within Roman society. One patient was Flavius Boezius, a consul who in turn introduced him to the tribunal, where he became physician to the court of the Emperor Marcus Aurelius.

In turn, Galen became the physician to Lucius Verus, commadore of Emperor Septimus Severus. He spent the rest of his life living in and working for the court where he had a number of scribes at his disposal, writing down his teachings.

His imperial connections must have boosted his status as a physician and his authority as an author. Essentially, his position would have enabled him to become the physician to the Roman armies. His knowledge of healing the wounds of gladiators would have been especially valuable for the wounds sustained by soldiers in battle.

Galen's final resting place is uncertain. It has been suggested that his body was interred in Misilmeri, near Palermo in Sicily.

Six hundred years after Hippocrates, Galen took his humoral physiology and incorporated it into the Hermetic cosmology of Egypt. Hermeticism is based upon the teachings of Hermes Trismegistus, who was linked to Thoth, the scribe of the gods, in the Egyptian pantheon. Thoth is the deity depicted with the head of an ibis. The ibis is a shoreline bird, which uses its distinctive long-curved beak to probe for food in the alluvial silt on the banks of the River Nile. The patterns left after its beak has trawled through the mud were thought to be sacred writing being brought down from the heavens by the bird.

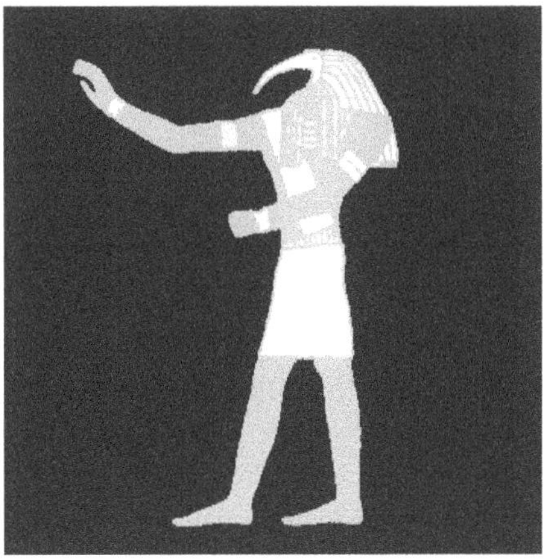

Figure 4.3: Thoth

The Greek deity equivalent to Thoth is Hermes, and in the Hellenistic period when Egypt was under Greek rule, Thoth was known as Hermes Trismegistus or "Thrice Great Hermes". The "thrice great" refers to the Hermetic Three World view.

Just as Hippocrates used the Five Elements to analyse the blood, so too the Hermetic teachings took the Elements to conceptualise the cosmology of the Three World view.

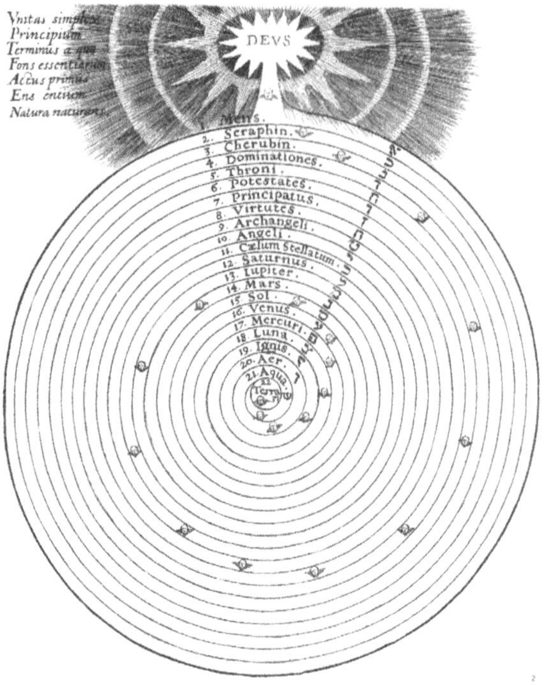

Figure 4.4: The Hermetic Three World view from Robert Fludd's *Utriusque cosmi maioris scilicet et minoris, metaphysica, physica atque technica historia on the Microcosmic Arts* (Oppenheim, 1619)

Robert Fludd, a Hermetic philosopher in the Elizabethan era, in an illustration from his history of the Microcosmic Arts, depicts God or Deus, as a Realm of Light. This is the Divine Fire of creation. The spiral shows God willing the creation of the Universe into being.

The outer ring of the spiral starts with *Mens*—the Universal Mind—and descends through the Angelic Orders to the *Caelum Stellatum*—the constellations. This describes the Intellectual World, which corresponds to the Divine Air.

Next the spiral descends through the seven traditional Planets: Saturn, Jupiter, Mars, Sun, Venus, Mercury and Moon. This describes the Celestial World that corresponds to the Divine Water.

Finally, the spiral descends through the four material Elements of Fire, Air, Water and Earth. This defines the Elemental World that corresponds to the Divine Earth.

In the Hermetic vision, the Planets, in passing through the Zodiacal signs, mediated God's will down to Earth. This is the astrological conception that underlies the line in the Christian Lord's Prayer, "Thy will be done on Earth as it is in heaven." Not unsurprisingly, the earliest version of the Lord's Prayer is found in the hieroglyphs of the Pyramidal texts. Since Jesus was educated in Egypt, a lot of Hermetic ideas are found in Christian teachings.

In the Roman pantheon, Hermes is linked to Mercury, the god of communication, healing and medicine.

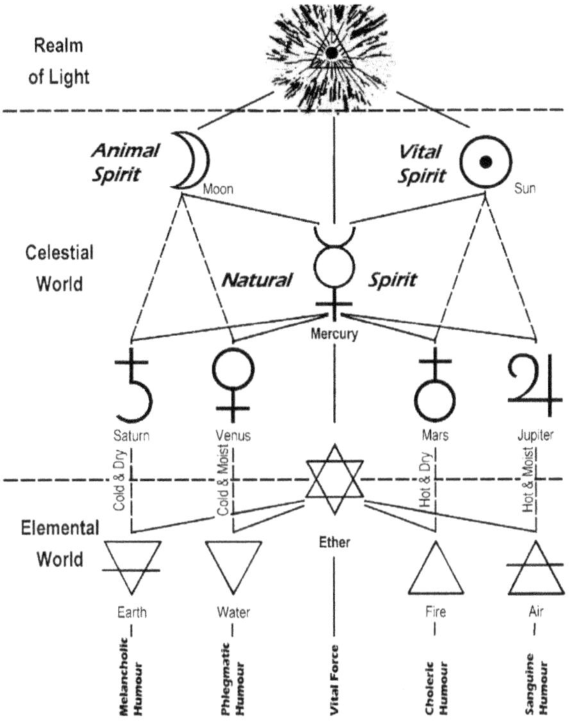

Figure 4.5: The hermetic vision: as above, so below

The uniting factor of the Hermetic Three World view is the fifth Element, Ether, in the Elemental World, which is symbolically linked to the Planet Mercury in the Celestial World.

Mercury and Ether can be considered as synonymous. For, just as Ether is the quintessence of the four material Elements, so too, Mercury encapsulates the other six Planets.

All the Planets in the Celestial World have their counterparts in the Elemental World. By means of a symbolic concordance, Galen visualised the Planets above, influencing the Elements and Humours below.

Aristotelian philosophy ascribed the primary qualities of the Elements as: hot, cold, moist and dry. Thus:

- Fire is hot and dry
- Air is hot and moist
- Water is cold and moist
- Earth is cold and dry.

Similarly, the Planets were also ascribed the primary qualities:

- Jupiter is hot and moist, and concords with the Air Element and the Sanguine Humour.
- Mars and the Sun are hot and dry, and concord with the Fire Element and the Choleric Humour.

- Saturn is cold and dry, and concords with the Earth Element and the Melancholic Humour.
- Venus and the Moon are cold and moist, and concord with the Water Element and the Phlegmatic Humour.

The viral infection causing fever and phlegm of the ear, nose and throat, which we now call influenza, derives from "la influenza", implying the influence of the Moon or Venus on the Phlegmatic humour.

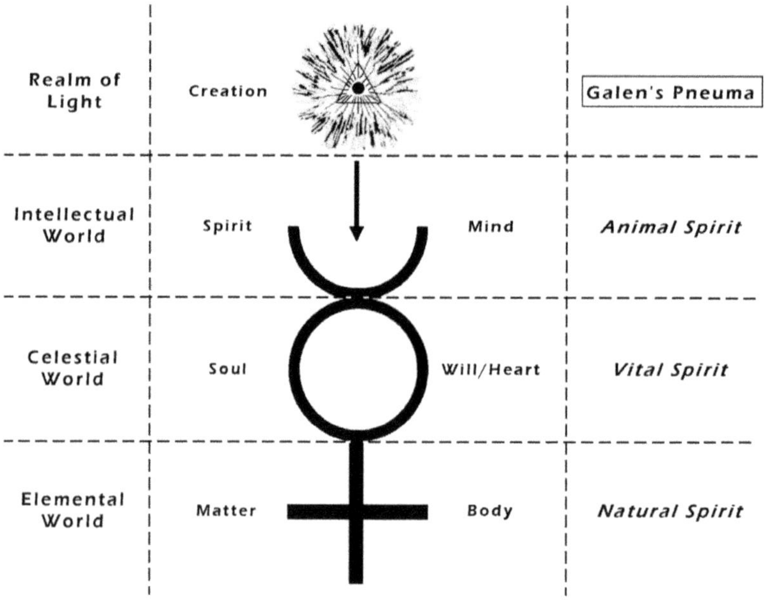

Figure 4.6: Correspondences within the Glyph of Mercury

The glyph for Mercury is composed of the three primary shapes: Crescent of Spirit, Circle of the Soul and Cross of Matter.

This triplicity of shapes correspond to the Hermetic Three World view and, furthermore, in Galen's writings, to his concepts of the Three Pneumas or breaths.

- The Cross of Matter connects Mercury to Ether, the Vital Force that sustains, heals and repairs the physical body.
- The Circle of the Soul connects Mercury to the generation of the Vital Force within the heart, along with its flow through the blood, which creates the medium of emotional experience.
- The Crescent of Spirit connects Mercury to the receptiveness of the mind to the Light of Creation, forming the substance out of which ideas are generated.

After Galen had incorporated Hermetic cosmology into Hippocrates' humoral physiology, the constituent humours can now be seen with their respective Planetary Rulers.

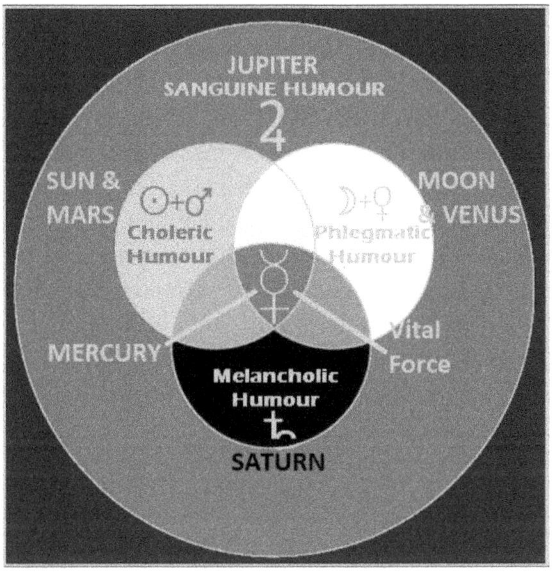

Figure 4.7: Galen's planetary rulerships of the four humours

Galen saw that health is associated with the temper or balance of the humours, which he called *eucrasia*. This temper, which enables the free flow of the Vital Force through the blood, facilitates mental, emotional and physical health, bringing them into a state of harmony.

The imbalance of the humours was associated with the Planets. Galen termed these imbalances *dyscrasias*. From this we have the word "crazy", when someone loses their mind and behaves irrationally.

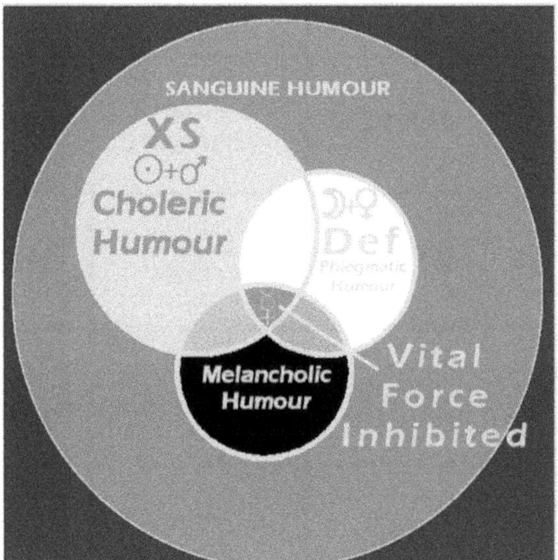

Figure 4.8: A Choleric *dyscrasia*

Thus, for example as in the diagram, an excess of the Choleric humour is connected with the Sun and Mars. The excess of choler causes the weakening of the Phlegmatic humour and inhibits the flow of Vital Force.

Imagine a time when you have had a childhood infection. The excess of Fire is shown in the accompanying fever and exhaustion that means you have to go to bed. The deficiency of Water is linked to the profuse sweating and need to keep drinking, in order to preserve body fluids. The weakening of the Vital Force in the febrile state is reflected in sleep becoming restless and uncomfortable, with intense dreams or nightmares.

Excess choler is thus linked to fevers, inflammation and acute disease, especially of the gall bladder—the seat of the Choleric humour. Galen drew up lists of diseases for each Planet, and these have come down through the ages. For example, the diseases for Mars include pestilence (plague), quotidian and tertian agues (malaria), migraines, yellow jaundice and shingles.

Seats

There was a Roman stricture on studying the anatomy of dead bodies, as we have seen. However, from his time as physician to the gladiators in Pergamon, Galen was able to gain anatomical insights denied to other physicians. Hence his description of these wounds as "windows into the body".

ELEMENT		HUMOUR	SEAT
🜃	EARTH	*MELANCHOLIC (Black Bile)*	SPLEEN
🜄	WATER	*PHLEGMATIC (Phlegm)*	LUNGS
✡	ETHER	*VITAL FORCE*	HEART
🜂	FIRE	*CHOLERIC (Yellow Bile)*	GALL BLADDER
🜁	AIR	*SANGUINE (Blood)*	LIVER

Figure 4.9: Galen's attribution of the seats for each humour

From his observations Galen attributed each humour a "seat" in the body:

- The Sanguine humour had its seat in the liver.
- The Choleric humour had its seat in the gall bladder.
- The Phlegmatic humour had its seat in the lungs.
- The Melancholic humour had its seat in the spleen.

The idea that the humours have seats sounds somewhat simplistic in a modern medical context, but given the anatomical limitations of the day, there is considerable physiological sense to these observations. Peering through the wounds into the abdomen, Galen would have easily noticed that the liver is the largest organ within the abdominal cavity, corresponding to Jupiter being the largest planet in our Solar system. Observing the two portal veins leading into it, alongside the hepatic artery and vein, Galen must have deduced its importance for maintaining the temper of the blood or Sanguine humour. Given we now know the myriad enzymic functions that the liver performs in relation to the blood, it is true to say that the total function of the liver is directly related to the composition of the blood.

Close to it, underneath the organ, is located the gall bladder. A wound here that punctured it would have released a notable quantity of yellowy-green bile. It is easy to see why Galen would have attributed the gall bladder to being the seat of the Choleric humour or yellow bile. We now know that the yellow colour in the bile is formed from the breakdown products of the haemoglobin inside destroyed red blood cells. The abundance of these contributes to the "lub-dub" sound heard with a stethoscope.

Galen's attribution of the spleen being the seat of the Melancholic humour or black bile is less straightforward to explain, since in the living body it is a large organ saturated with blood, giving it a reddish colour. We now know that one of its functions is being an emergency reserve of blood, so that when the body haemorrhages, the organ contracts, making up the blood loss, thereby preserving haematological functions. Given that Galen was inspecting wounded and dead bodies, the loss of blood from the wound will have triggered the collapse of the spleen, which now resembles a black pudding, hence linking it to the black bile.

The lungs being the seat of the Phlegmatic humour is readily seen in chest infections and long being recognised by physicians. The common cold should be more accurately diagnosed in Phlegmatic terms as a symptom of cold and moist humour predominating!

The Virtues of Herbs

Using the Hermetic cosmology, Galen classified the virtues of herbs into two different categories: Hidden and Manifest Virtues.

The virtue describes the Vital Force within a herb that embodies its medicinal properties. The Hidden Virtue, which corresponds to the Celestial World, is perceived with Planetary rulers. The Manifest Virtue, which corresponds to the Elemental World, involves the temperatures, hot, cold, moist and dry, perceived through taste and smell. These will be explained in Chapter 5.

Today Galen is perhaps most recognised for classifying the herbs of the Western *materia medica* according to different temperatures. The skill of a physician lies in being able to visualise both these aspects of a herb's virtue simultaneously.

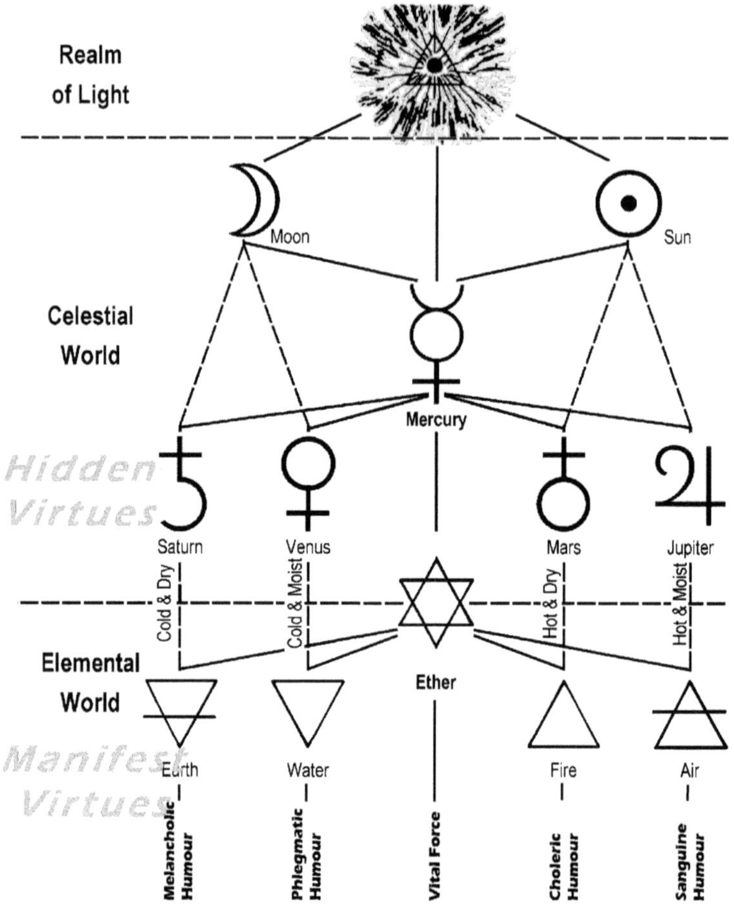

Figure 4.10: Galen's classification of the Hidden and Manifest Virtues of Each Herb

This statue of Galen at the Asclepion in Pergamon (Figure 4.1) commemorates his life and work. Galen is depicted standing against a pillar with the Python of Asclepius entwined around it. The pillar can be seen as alluding to the Stave of Asclepius; however, the sheer mass of its stones here implies that Galen built on the foundations of Hippocratic tradition.

The column consists of three vertical stones, representing the Hermetic Three World view that Galen incorporated into the Hippocratic teachings. The upper stone, which corresponds to the Intellectual World, has the Python entwined around it. This alludes to the myth of Asclepius who in the afterlife became the constellation of Ophiuchus—the serpent—in the sign of Scorpio.

Galen holds a book in both hands, while staring directly at you. The hands and arms are linked to the Zodiacal sign of Gemini, which is ruled by Mercury, the Roman god of medicine and communication. Furthermore, Galen leans against the middle stone, which corresponds to the Celestial World—the statue symbolically communicating to the beholder that his writing and teachings can lead you to the heart of the Art of Physic.

CHAPTER FIVE

Galen's temperatures of Herbs

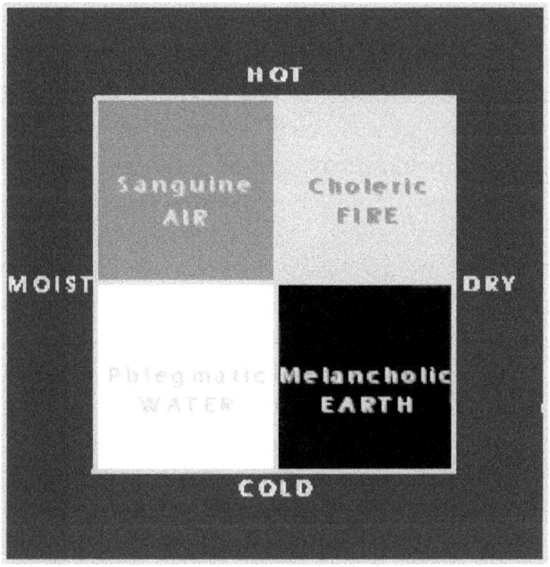

Figure 5.1: The temperatures of each humour

In health the Sanguine humour prevails. Its hot and moist nature, which is referred to as the "natural heat", thereby provides the starting point against which the temperatures of herbs are contrasted. Nicholas Culpeper, who translated Galen's *Art of Physic*, refers to the temperatures as the *"manifest virtues of medicines"* and goes on to explain that they are *"obvious to the senses, especially to the taste and smell"*.

The Manifest Virtues are in contrast to the Hidden Virtues, which employ the Planetary symbolism to perceive them. In practice the Manifest Virtues are based upon taste, for in savouring the herb on the tongue, the relative qualities of hot, cold, dry and moist are ascertained. Visualising how the herb acts upon the tongue gives insight as to how the herb acts elsewhere in the body. If you imagine the taste of ginger, for example, it not hard to understand how it will confer heat and stimulation throughout the body. By contrast, if you imagine the taste of cucumber, its cooling and moistening effect on the body is readily apparent.

Temperatures of herbs should not be considered as fixed; they will of course vary in temperature with different habitats and growing conditions. The lists should only serve as a guide, and part of the skill of physic is in knowing just how differences in growing conditions affect the manifest virtues of plants. A key part of the training of herbalists therefore was getting to know the temperatures of herbs by direct experience.

The Manifest Virtue can be different from the Hidden Virtue (covered in Chapter 17); it may diverge or even be contrary. For example, the willow has a Lunar rulership. From this it might be expected that since the Moon is cold and moist, and connected to the Water Element, so too the temperature of the willow might be thought to be cold and moist. In fact, from the taste the temperature is considered to be cold and dry to the 2nd degree.

Understanding these divergences between the Hidden and Manifest Virtues leads to very specific uses of herbs being identified. In the case of willow, its Lunar rulership confers an affinity with the Phlegmatic humour in the lungs, but the temperature being cold and dry means that it has a drying influence on the mucus secretions in the lung.

In Galen's schemata herbs and plants are classified into hot, cold, dry and moist. Of these four qualities hot and cold are considered to be the active primary qualities, in contrast to dry and moist, which are seen as passive secondary qualities. The primary qualities are further categorised into four degrees of heat or coldness.

Therapeutically, hot herbs are used to counteract cold conditions and vice versa, but skill lies in knowing the exact degree of heat or coldness to employ to restore the temper of the humours and bring it back to its natural heat. Today Galen's concepts may sound simplistic, but there is a lot of physiological wisdom encapsulated in these ideas, and the importance placed on selecting herbs suit the temper/distemper of the body does ring true. Normal body temp is 37°C; it is the optimum temperature for the physiology of the body. Below 32.5°C the body is considered to be hypothermic, and once below 26°C metabolic processes are seriously compromised and become life-threatening, with loss of consciousness. Conversely when the body reaches 41.1°C in an excessive fever it also becomes life-threatening.

The effect of the ambient temperature can have a marked bearing on the functioning of the body. Temperature extremes can place the body under considerable stress in order to preserve its optimum temperature. Once the external temperature is in excess of 37°C, sweating ceases to be able to cool the body down. Excessive sweating leads to rapid fluid loss from the body, which will quickly become life-threatening in a matter of hours if it is not replenished.

Conversely, when external temperature falls below freezing, then the heat lost from the body may exceed its capacity to generate heat. The result is the body falling into hypothermia and loss of consciousness. If no rescue occurs the bodily fluids will ultimately freeze, and death will result.

The role of heat and cold in influencing pain is frequently used in various types of injury and inflammation. For example, ice packs are very useful in helping relieve the pressure of swelling of physical trauma and easing the pain. By contrast, heat packs are helpful in relieving the pain of muscular spasm, especially arising from inflammation of the internal organs. Temperature therefore is a critical factor in health and disease.

Of Medicines Temperate

The first category are the temperate herbs, which on tasting have no perceivable heat or coldness. Culpeper explains:

> *Medicines are called temperate for being added to medicines, change not their qualities, they make them neither hotter nor colder.*

Culpeper says they are used in diseases where there is

> *no manifest distemper of heat and cold, for example; in obstruction of the bowels, where cold medicines might make the obstruction greater, and hot medicines cause a fever.*

Alternatively, he suggests,

> *In fevers of phlegm, where the cause is cold and moist, and the effect hot and dry; in such, use temperate medicines which may neither increase the fever by their heat, nor condensate the phlegm by their coldness.*

He adds,

> *they are of great use, to preserve the constitution of the body temperate, and the body itself in strength and vigour, and may be used without danger, by considering which part of the body is weak, and using such temperate medicines as are appropriated to that part.*

Temperate Herbs

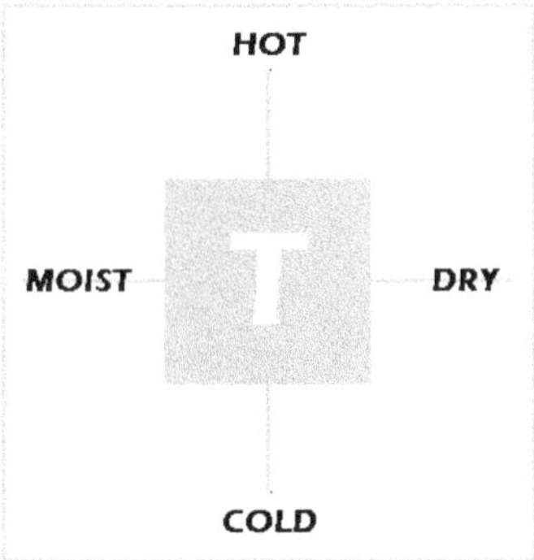

Figure 5.2: Herbs considered to be temperate and also lack moisture and dryness

Examples of herbs considered to be temperate and also to lack moisture or dryness include asparagus (*Asparagus officinalis*), cinquefoil (*Potentilla reptans*), cowslips (*Primula veris*), couch or dog's grass (*Agropyron repens*) and liquorice (*Glycyrrhiza glabra*).

Of the herbs in this list, asparagus and couch grass are well known as herbs that work on the urinary tract. Asparagus is a powerful diuretic, and within half an hour of eating it, the distinctive smell of asparagine is found in the urine. Couch or dog's grass, with its temperate nature, is particularly soothing of inflammation within the urinary tract, making it useful in passage of gravel and inflammation of the bladder. The tonic action of liquorice on the Vital Force is enhanced by it having a temperate nature.

Temperate and Moist Herbs

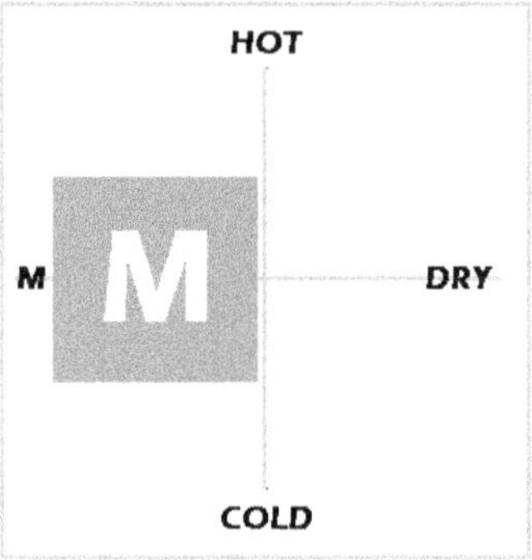

Figure 5.3: Herbs considered to be temperate and moist

Herbs considered to be temperate and moist include wild carrot (*Daucus carota*) = t M1, mallow species (*Althaea officinalis* and *Malva sylvestris*) = t M1;

borage (*Borago officinalis*) = t M2;

and houseleek (*Sempervivium tectorum*) = t M4. Some of these will be discussed under moist herbs.

Temperate and Dry Herbs

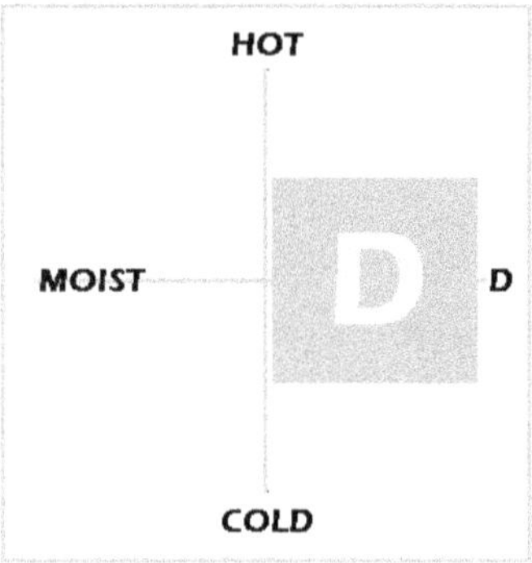

Figure 5.4: Herbs considered to be temperate and dry

Herbs considered to be temperate and dry include burnet (*Sanguisorba major*) = t D1, dandelion (*Taraxacum officinale*) = t D1, mullein (*Verbascum thapsus*) = t D1;

hyssop (*Hyssopus officinalis*) = t D2, lime flowers (*Tilea europaea*) = t D2, roses (*Rosa damascena*) = t D2, vervain (*Verbena officinalis*) = t D2;

bistort (*Polygonum bistorta*) = t D3, docks (*Rumex* spp.) = t D3 and flixweed (*Descuraninia sophia*) = t D3. Some of these will be discussed under drying herbs.

Of Medicines Hot

Culpeper begins his explanation of Hot Medicines by stressing the importance of correctly understanding the degrees of temperature, otherwise more harm can be done rather than good:

> *The care of the ancient Physicians was such that they did not labour to hide from, but impart to posterity, not only the temperature of medicines in general, but also their degrees in temperature, that so the distempered part may be brought to its temperature, and no further; for all things which are of a contrary temperature, conduce not to cure, but the strength of the contrariety must be observed, that so the medicine may be neither weaker nor stronger, than just to take away the distemper; for if the distemper be but meanly hot, and you apply a medicine cold in the fourth degree, it is true, you may soon remove that distemper of heat, and bring another of cold twice as bad.* [Galen, de simp. med. facul. lib. 3. cap. 126]

He continues the point:

> *Secondly, not only the distemper itself, but also the part of the body distempered must be heeded; for if the head be distempered by heat, and you give such medicines as cool the heart or liver, you will bring another disease, and not cure the former.*

Of Medicines Hot in the 1st Degree

Herbs hot in the 1st degree induce a moderate heat to the body and its organs either cold by nature or cooled by accident. By these herbs the natural heat is restored when weak or deficient. Their modest heat restores the body to its natural heat, just as *"a fire doth the external parts in cold weather"*.

A second effect of using hot in the 1st degree herbs is that they mitigate pain arising from a cold distemper. Furthermore, Culpeper also states that

> *It should be noted that the anodyne effects are found in other medicines, cold or hotter than the 1st degree, when they are appropriately to the degree of heat or cold of the distemper.*

This indicates that within humoral physiology pain is seen to arise as the balance or temper of the blood is lost. Depending on whether the distemper is hot or cold and the degree to which it is disrupted, so all the herbs, hot or cold, when they are appropriately used in restoring the natural heat to the blood have their roles in alleviating pain.

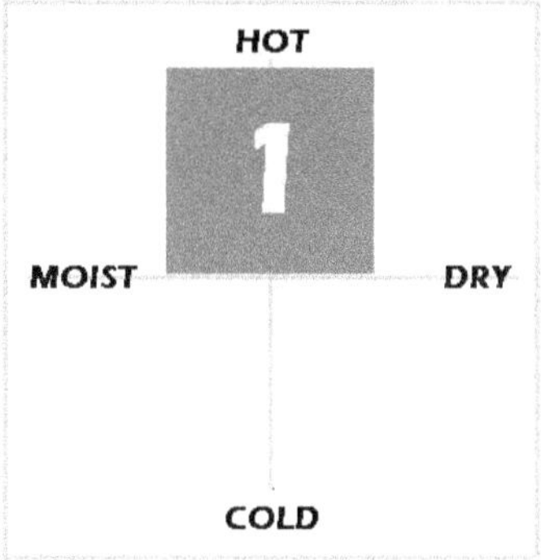

Figure 5.5: Medicines hot in 1st degree

Returning to Culpeper,

> *Medicines hot in the 1st degree make the offending humours thin and expel them by sweat, or insensible transpiration, and these of all others are most congruous or agreeable to the body of man, for there is no such equal temperature of heat and cold in a sound man, but heat exceeds, for we live by heat and moisture, and not by cold.*

Of herbs hot in the 1st degree generally, Culpeper quotes Galen saying that they

> *cherish heat in the internal parts, help concoction, breed good blood, and keep it good in temper, being bred.*

Herbs hot in the 1st degree just correspond to the natural heat of the body. Those herbs that are hotter or colder have the potential to disrupt the balance of the humours if used unskilfully. Culpeper then describes another effect of these herbs being used topically in a fever where they

> *take away weariness, and help fevers, being outwardly applied, because they open the pores of the skin, and by their gentle heat prepare the humours, and take away those fuliginous* [sooty] *vapours that are caused by fevers.*

This makes sense since in the first part of a fever, through vasoconstriction, blood is concentrated in the internal organs where it heats up. In so doing blood is removed from the surface of the skin, which becomes cold and sticky. The heat from the herbs will warm the skin, encouraging the blood flow to return, which brings out the heat from within the body and promotes sweating, cooling the patient down and thereby making them more comfortable.

Culpeper provides the caution, even with these moderately hot herbs, that

> *Too much use of them, to consume not only what is inimical in the body, but also the substance itself, and the strength of the spirits whence comes faintings, and sometimes death: besides, by applying them to the parts of the body they are not appropriated to, or by not heeding well the complexion of the patient, or the natural temper of the part of the body afflicted, for the heart is hot, but the brain temperate.*

Excessive or prolonged stimulation does have the danger to exhaust the body's resources, in a similar way that a prolonged fever can ravage the body.

Herbs Hot in the 1st Degree

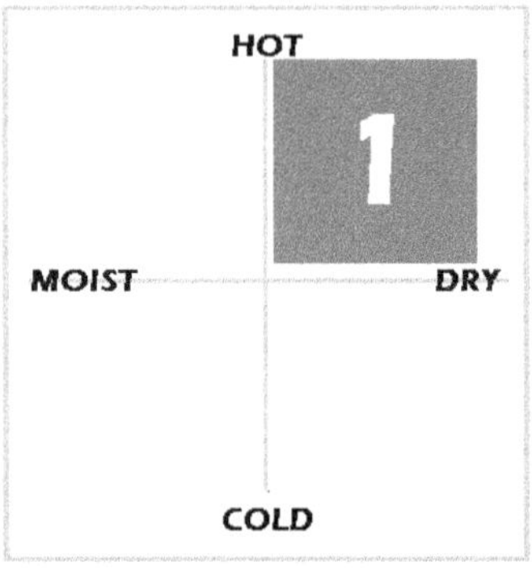

Figure 5.6: Examples of herbs considered to be hot and dry in the 1st degree

Examples of herbs considered to be hot and dry in the 1st degree include barberry (*Berberis vulgaris*) = H1D1, bilberries (*Vaccinium myrtillus*) = H1D1, burdock (*Arctium lappa*) = H1D1, elder (*Sambucus nigra*) = H1D1, ground ivy (*Glechoma hederacea*) = H1D1, black horehound (*Ballota nigra*) = H1D1, chicory (*Chicorium intybus*) = H1D1, lovage (*Ligusticum levisticum*) = H1D1, marigold (*Calendula officinalis*) = H1D1, melilot (*Melilotus officinalis*) = H1D1, self-heal (*Prunella vulgaris*) = H1D1 and wormwood (*Artemisia absinthium*) = H1D1.

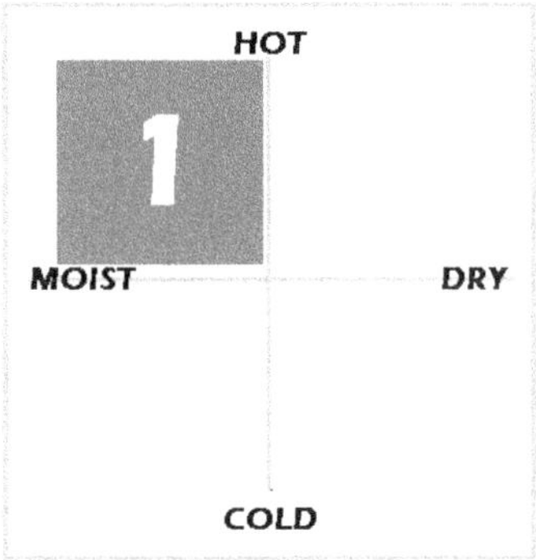

Figure 5.7: Examples of herbs considered to be hot and moist in the 1st degree

Examples of herbs considered to be hot and moist in the 1st degree include bugle (*Ajuga reptans*) = H1M1 and coltsfoot (*Tussilago farfara*) = H1M1. The expectorant action of coltsfoot is enhanced by the hot and moist nature of the herb, for the moisture will help lubricate consolidated phlegm and assist its expulsion by the lungs.

Of Medicines Hot in the 2nd Degree

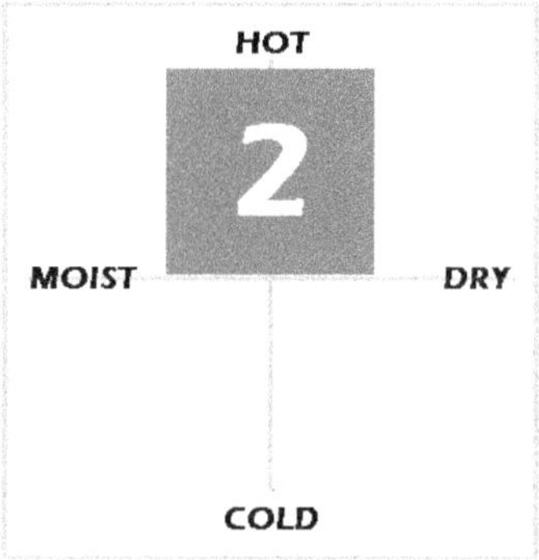

Figure 5.8: Medicines hot in 2nd degree

Herbs hot in the 2nd degree are slightly hotter than the natural temper of a man. Culpeper describes *"Their use for such whose stomachs are filled with moisture, because their faculty is too hot and dry."* This describes a hyper-acidic stomach that typically causes acid reflux and heartburn.

Culpeper carries on:

> *they take away obstructions or stoppings, open the pores of the skin (not in the same manner as* [herbs hot in the 1st degree] *for they do it without force by a gentle heat concocting, and expelling the humours, by strengthening and helping nature in the work) by cutting tough humours, and scatter them by their own force and power when nature cannot.*

Herbs Hot in the 2nd Degree

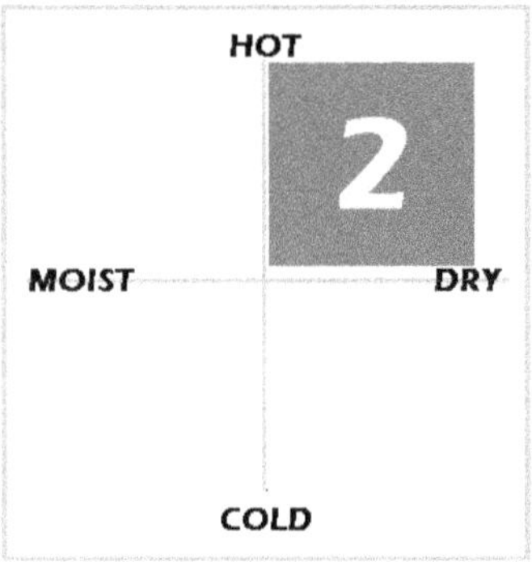

Figure 5.9: Examples of herbs considered to be hot and dry in the 2nd degree

Examples of herbs considered to be hot and dry in the 2nd degree include fennel (*Foeniculum vulgare*) = H2D1, fenugreek (*Trigonella foenum-graecum*) = H2D1 and periwinkle (*Vinca major*) = H2D1;

agrimony (*Agrimonia eupatoria*) = H2D2, anemone (*Anemone pulsatilla*) = H2D2, angelica (*Angelica archangelica*) = H2D2, avens (*Geum urbanum*) = H2D2, lemon balm (*Melissa officinalis*) = H2D2, betony (*Stachys betonica*) = H2D2, chamomile (*Matricaria chamomilla*) = H2D2, blessed thistle (*Carbenia benedicta*) = H2D2, lesser celandine (*Ranunculus ficaria*) = H2D2, ginger (*Zingiber officinale*) = H2D2, hops (*Humulus lupulus*) = H2D2, lady's mantle (*Alchemilla vulgaris*) = H2D2, lady's thistle (*Carduus marianus*) = H2D2, meadowsweet (*Filipendula ulmaria*) = H2D2, mistletoe (*Viscum album*) = H2D2, motherwort (*Leonurus cardiaca*) = H2D2, nettle (*Urtica dioica*) = H2D2, pellitory of the wall (*Parietaria diffusa*) = H2D2, sea squill (*Urginea maritima*) = H2D2, St John's wort (*Hypericum perfoliatum*) = H2D2, walnut (*Juglans regia*) = H2D2, wild marjoram (*Origanum vulgare*) = H2D2, wild thyme (*Thymus serpyllum*) = H2D2, valerian (*Valeriana officinalis*) = H2D2;

aloes (*Aloe vera*) = H2D3, bogbean (*Menyanthes trifoliata*) = H2D3, feverfew (*Chrysanthemum parthenium*) = H2D3, garden thyme (*Thymus vulgaris*) = H2D3, sage (*Salvia officinalis*) = H2D3, sanicle (*Sanicula europaea*) = H2D3, tansy (*Tanacetum vulgare*) = H2D3 and white horehound (*Marrubium vulgare*) = H2D3.

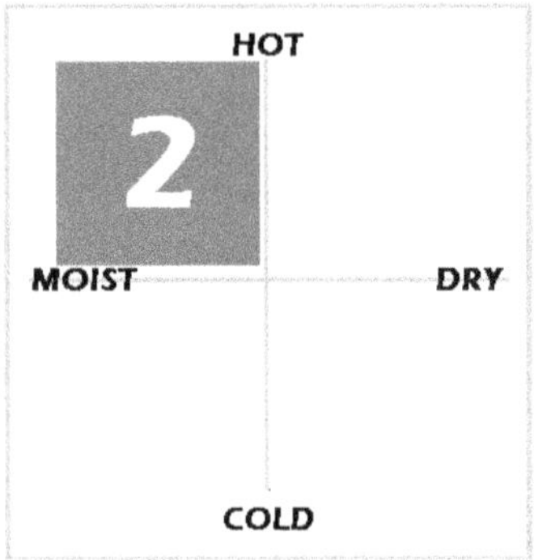

Figure 5.10: Examples of herbs considered to be hot and moist in the 2nd degree

Examples of herbs considered to be hot and moist in the 2nd degree include artichoke (*Cynara scolymus*) = H2M2, marsh cudweed (*Gnaphalium uliginosum*) = H2M2, goldenrod (*Solidago virgaurea*) = H2M2, herb Robert (*Geranium robertianum*) = H2M2, samphire (*Crithmum maritimum*) = H2M2 and sea holly (*Eryngium maritimum*) = H2M2.

The heating effect of these herbs cutting phlegm in the chest is particularly evident in angelica, sea squill, thyme, marsh cudweed and goldenrod. Meadowsweet is well known for countering a hyper-acidic stomach. The stimulating effects of these herbs on digestion are familiar in such herbs as thyme, artichoke and samphire.

Of Medicines Hot in the 3rd Degree

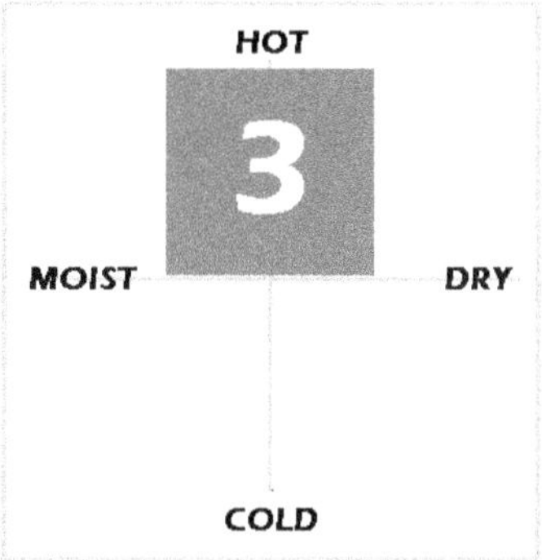

Figure 5.11: Medicines hot in 3rd degree

Herbs hot in the 3rd degree are definitely hotter than the natural temper of a man. They all have the same properties as those herbs hot in the 2nd degree; but because they are hotter, they are more powerful in heating and cutting. Caution is given that they can cause fevers. Culpeper describes their use: *"to cut tough and compacted humours, to provoke sweat abundantly; hence it comes to pass they all of them* [help the body] *resist poison"*.

Herbs Hot in the 3rd Degree

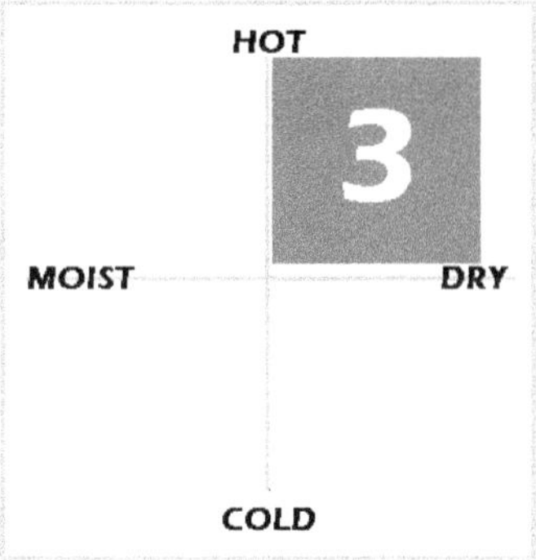

Figure 5.12: Examples of herbs considered to be hot and dry in the 3rd degree

Examples of herbs considered to be hot and dry in the 3rd degree include dill (*Anethum graveolens*) = H3D2, gentian (*Gentiana amarella*) = H3D2, parsley (*Petroselinum crispum*) = H3D2 and radish (*Raphanus sativus*) = H3D2;

alexanders (*Smyrnium olusatrum*) = H3D3, aniseed (*Pimpinella anisum*) = H3D3, bay (*Laurus nobilis*) = H3D3, calamint (*Calamintha ascendens*) = H3D3, caraway (*Carum carvi*) = H3D3, greater celandine (*Chelidonium majus*) = H3D3, small centaury (*Erythraea centaurium*) = H3D3, watercress (*Nasturtium officinale*) = H3D3, elecampane (*Inula helenium*) = H3D3, eyebright (*Euphrasia officinalis*) = H3D3, hawthorn (*Crataegus oxycantha*) = H3D3, juniper (*Juniperus communis*) = H3D3, lady's smock (*Cardamine pratensis*) = H3D3, lavender (*Lavandula officinalis*) = H3D3, peppermint (*Mentha* x *piperita*) = H3D3, pennyroyal (*Mentha pelegium*) = H3D3, rosemary (*Salvia rosmarinus*) = H3D3, scurvy grass (*Cochlearia officinalis*) = H3D3, sweet marjoram (*Origanum majorana*) = H3D3, tormentil (*Potentilla erecta*) = H3D3 and walnut tree (*Juglans regia*) = H3D3;

garden rue (*Ruta graveolens*) = H3D4.

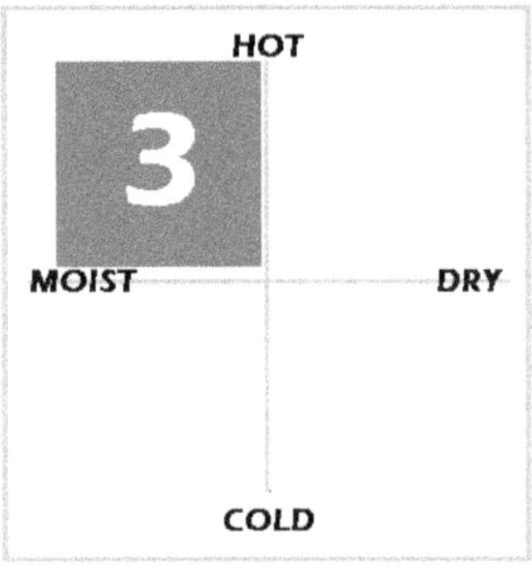

Figure 5.13: Example of a herb considered to be hot in the 3rd degree

Historically scurvy grass, as its name suggests, has been used since Roman times for treating scurvy, long before the role of vitamin C was discovered. Its Jupitarian rulership linked the herb to the liver and restoring the balance of the humours in the blood, while its hot and dry temperature would have countered the cold and moist condition of scurvy. In modern terms the herb is a source of ascorbic acid, which would have made it successful in countering scurvy.

The hot and dry temperature of lady's smock would have made it useful for improving digestion of those patients, *"such whose stomachs are filled with moisture"*. The main symptom of stomach acid is pain felt over the heart, giving rise to the term "heartburn". This former use of this Lunar herb to counter the acidity of the stomach is preserved in its generic name *Cardiamicus*, since it is derived from the Latin meaning "friend of the heart".

The extremely hot and drying nature of garden rue is well known since it can cause in susceptible people blistering of the skin from just the slightest contact.

Example of a herb considered to be hot and moist in the 3rd degree is garden basil (*Ocimum basilicum*) = H3M3.

Of Medicines Hot in the 4th Degree

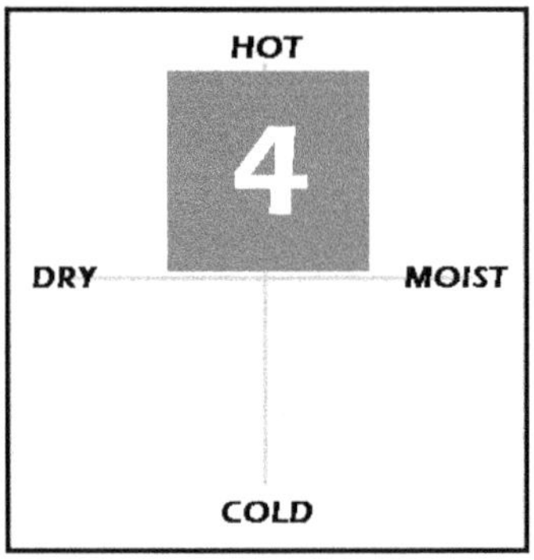

Figure 5.14: Medicines hot in 4th degree

Herbs hot in the 4th degree *"are markedly hotter than the natural temper of a man. These herbs obtain the highest degree of heat, so much so that they burn body of a man, being outwardly applied to it, and cause inflammations, or raise blister."* These herbs are known as rubifacient remedies. Consequently, they need to be used judiciously, in moderate doses, for as short a time as possible. They can be added in a small amount to boost the absorption of other herbs.

Herbs Hot in the 4th Degree

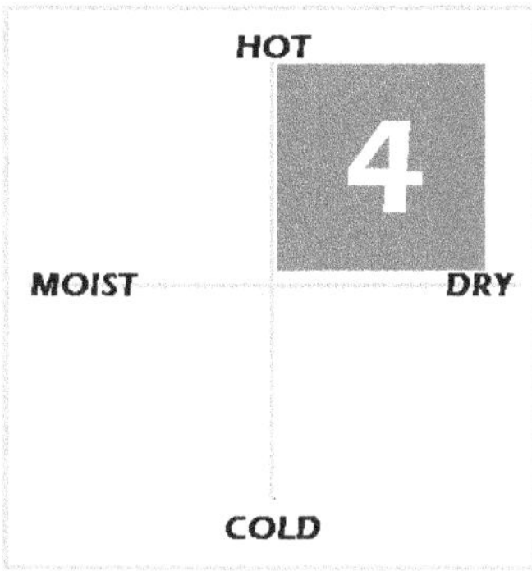

Figure 5.15: Examples of herbs considered to be hot and dry in the 4th degree

Examples of herbs considered to be hot and dry in the 4th degree include arsesmart (*Polygonum hydropiper*) = H4D4, capsicum (*Capsicum minimum*) = H4D4, chives (*Allium schoenoprasum*) = H4D4, dragons (*Dracunculus vulgaris*) = H4D4, figwort (*Scrophularia nodosa*) = H4D4, garlic (*Allium sativum*) = H4D4, horseradish (*Armoracia rusticana*) = H4D4, onions (*Allium cepa*) = H4D4, sundew or rosa solis (*Drosera rotundifolia*) = H4D4, and jack by the hedge or sauce alone (*Alliaria petiolata*) = H4D4.

Of these herbs arsesmart, or water pepper, is probably the hottest and most pungent. Many of the herbs in this list are spicy, digestive remedies and are often used, like horseradish on beef, to make foods more easily digested.

There is no category of hot and moist in the 4th degree, since the extreme heat of the herb dries out any remaining moisture.

Of Cooling Medicines

In contrast to the four degrees of heat there are also four observed degrees of coldness.

Of Medicines Cold in the 1st Degree

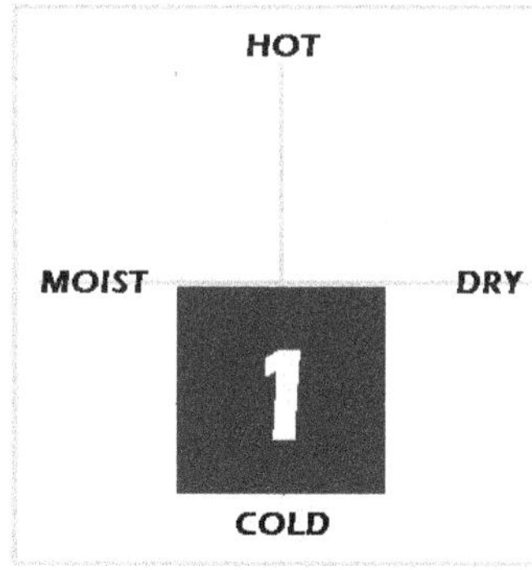

Figure 5.16: Medicines cold in 1st degree

Herbs cold in the 1st degree are the least cold of all since our bodies are nourished and live by heat, for, as Culpeper says,

> *therefore no cold medicines are friendly to the body, but what good they do our bodies, they do it by removing an unnatural heat, or the body heated above its natural temper.*

He continues,

> *The giving then of cold medicines to a man in his natural temper, the season of the year also being but moderately hot, extinguishes natural heat in the body of man.*

Of their uses firstly Culpeper mentions *"in nourishment, that so the heat of food may be qualified, and made for a weak stomach to digest"*. A simple example would be frying onions with coriander powder to make them easier to digest. Onion, according to Galen's classification, are hot and dry to the 4th degree. Similarly, as coriander is classified as cold and dry in the 1st degree, it moderates the heat of the onions, making them less injurious to the natural temper of the body.

Their second use is

> *to restrain and assuage the heat of the bowels, and to cool the blood in fevers. Therefore, if the distemper of heat be but gentle, herbs cold in the 1st degree will suffice; also children, and such people whose stomachs are weak, are easily hurt by cold medicines.*

Herbs Cold in the 1st Degree

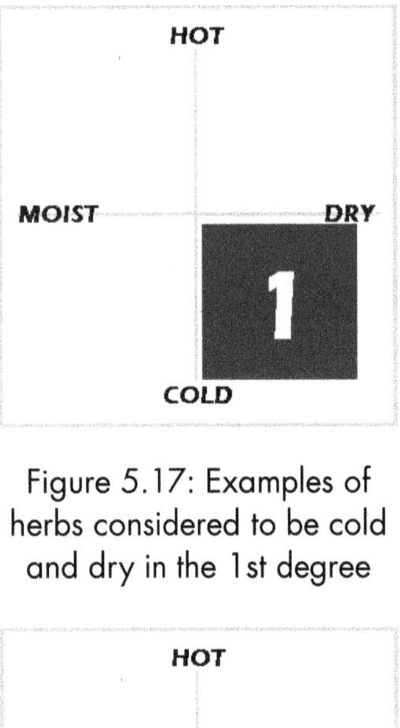

Figure 5.17: Examples of herbs considered to be cold and dry in the 1st degree

Examples of herbs considered to be cold and dry in the 1st degree include barley (*Hordeum vulgare*) = C1D1, broad bean (*Vicia faba*) = C1D1, French bean (*Vicia vulgaris*) = C1D1, bladderwrack (*Fucus vesiculosus*) = C1D1, coriander (*Coriandrum sativum*) = C1D1, fumitory (*Fumaria officinalis*) = C1D1, loosestrifes (*Lythrum salicaria* and *Lysimachia vulgaris*) = C1D1, oats (*Avena sativa*) = C1D1, olive (*Olea europaea*) = C1D1 and rye (*Secale cereale*) = C1D1;

rupturewort (*Herniaria glabra*) = C1D2 and yarrow (*Achillea millefolium*) = C1D2;

wild campion (*Silene dioica*) = C1D3, oak (*Quercus robur*) = C1D3 and vine (*Vitis vinifera*) = C1D3.

Examples of herbs considered to be cold and moist in the 1st degree include archangels (Red = *Lamium purpureum*, White = *L. album* and Yellow = *Lamiastrum galeobdolon*) = C1M1, garden clary (*Salvia sclarea*) = C1M1, wild clary (*Salvia verbenaca*) = C1M1, cleavers (*Galium aparine*) = C1M1, strawberry (*Fragaria vesca*) = C1M1 and violet (*Viola odorata*) = C1M1;

cucumber (*Cucumis sativus*) = C1M2, daisy (*Bellis perennis*) = C1M2 and heartsease (*Viola tricolor*) = C1M2.

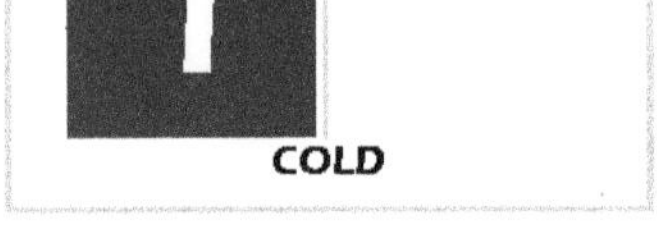

Figure 5.18: Examples of herbs considered to be cold and moist in the 1st degree

Of Medicines Cold in the 2nd and 3rd Degree

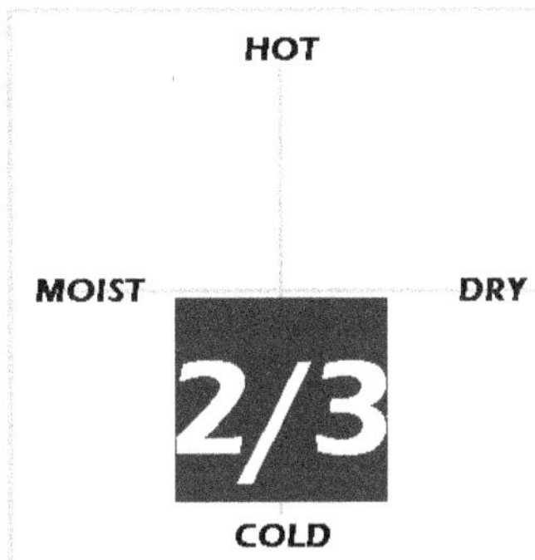

Figure 5.19: Medicines cold in 2nd and 3rd degree

Of the uses of herbs cold in the 2nd degree Culpeper firstly describes, *"Such whose stomachs are strong and livers hot, may easily bear cold in the second degree medicines, and in cases of extremity find much help by them."*

Similar uses are for herbs cold in the 3rd degree: *"the extremity of the disease, considered, for by both these the unbridled heat of choler is assuaged".*

The second use of these herbs, Culpeper says: *"outwardly applied to hot swellings, due consideration being had, that if the inflammation be not great, use those that are less* [that is] *herbs cold in the 2nd degree; if the inflammation be vehement, make use of herbs cold in the 3rd degree."* Again, Culpeper stresses the caution: *"In the second or third degree, always let the remedy correspond to the just proportion of the affliction."*

A more significant third use in fevers is described by Culpeper,

> *sometimes the spirits are moved inordinately through heat, thence follows immoderate watchings, if not deprivation of the senses, this also must be remedied with cold medicines, for cold stops the pores of the skin, makes the humours thick, represses sweat, and keeps up the spirits from fainting.*

Herbs Cold in the 2nd Degree

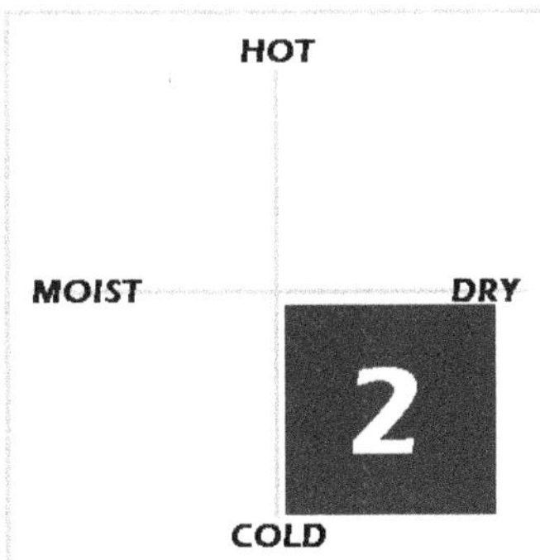

Examples of herbs considered to be cold and dry in the 2nd degree include love lies bleeding (*Amaranthus hybridus*) = C2D2, cornflower or blue bottle (*Centaurea cyanus*) = C2D2, buckshorn plantain (*Plantago coronopus*) = C2D2, clown's woundwort (*Stachys palustris*) = C2D2, crosswort (*Galium cruciata*) = C2D2, hawkweed (*Hieracium murorum*) = C2D2, horsetail (*Equisetum arvense*) = C2D2,

Figure 5.20: Examples of herbs considered to be cold and dry in the 2nd degree

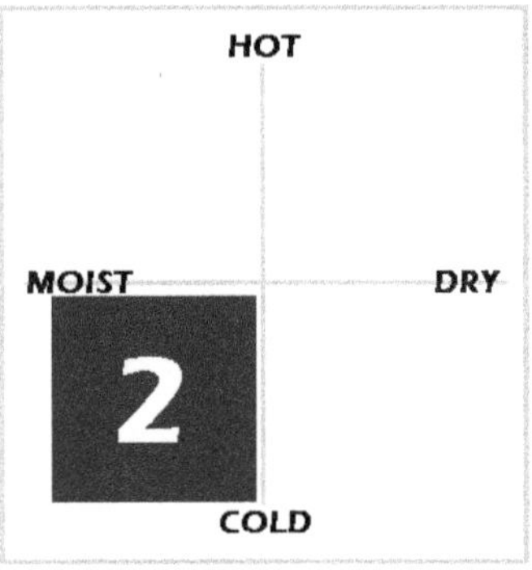

Figure 5.21: Examples of herbs considered to be cold and moist in the 2nd degree

hound's tongue (*Cyanoglossum officinale*) = C2D2, orpine (*Sedum telephium*) = C2D2, plantains (*Plantago major* and *P. lanceolata*) = C2D2, smallage or celery (*Apium graveolens*) = C2D2 and willow tree (*Salix alba*) = C2D2.

Examples of herbs considered to be cold and moist in the 2nd degree include bears breeches (*Acanthus spinosus*) = C2M2, birch tree (*Betula alba*) = C2M2 and white lily (*Lilium candidum*) = C2M2.

Herbs Cold in the 3rd Degree

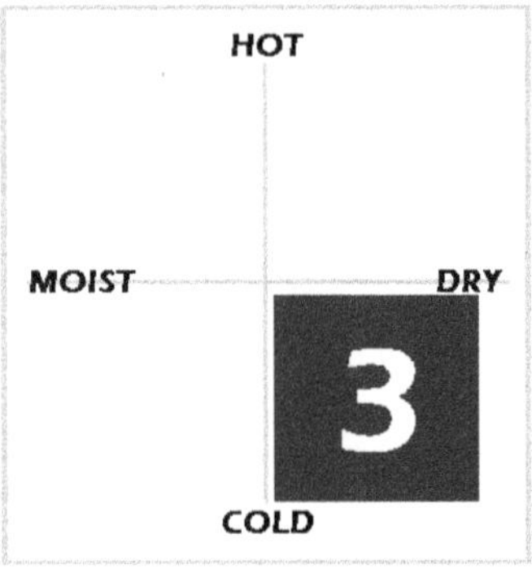

Figure 5.22: Examples of herbs considered to be cold and dry in the 3rd degree

Examples of herbs considered to be cold and dry in the 3rd degree include lettuce (*Lactuca virosa*) = C3D1;

comfrey (*Symphytum officinale*) = C3D3, shepherd's purse (*Capsella bursa-pastoris*) = C3D3 and water lily (*Nymphaea odorata*) = C3D3.

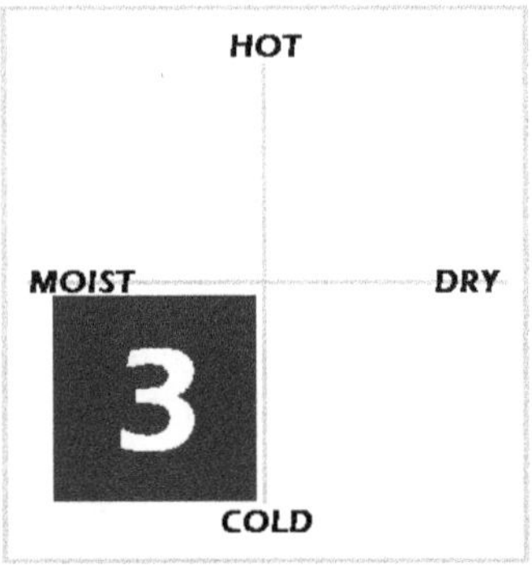

Figure 5.23: Examples of herbs considered to be cold and moist in the 3rd degree

Examples of herbs considered to be cold and moist in the 3rd degree include purslane (*Portulaca oleracea*) = C3M2 and chickweed (*Stellaria media*) = C3M3.

Of Medicines Cold in the 4th Degree

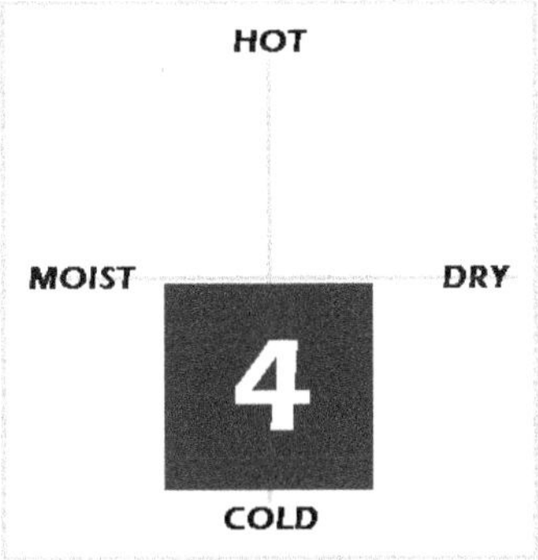

Figure 5.24: Medicines cold in 4th degree

Following on from the previous degrees of cold, Culpeper says,

> *Lastly, herbs cold in the 4th degree mitigate desperate and vehement pains, stupifying the senses, when no other course can be taken to save life.*

This category contains a number of the most poisonous herbs of the Western tradition. For the lay person they are best left well alone. For herbalists they are restricted schedule 20 herbs that have strict dosage guidelines.

Herbs Cold in the 4th Degree

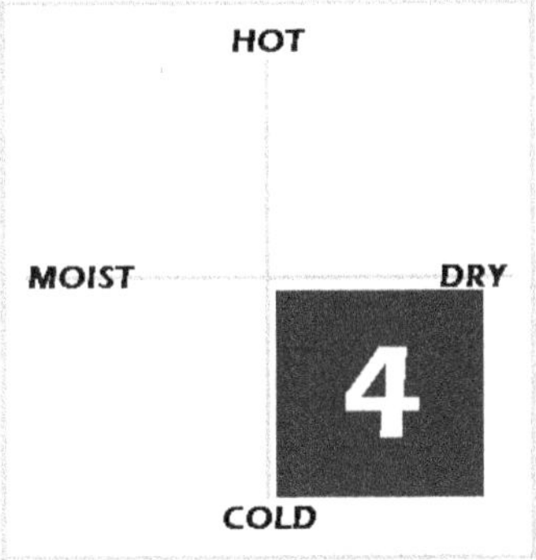

Figure 5.25: Examples of herbs considered to be cold in the 4th degree

Examples of herbs considered to be cold in the 4th degree include henbane (*Hyoscyamus niger*) = C4D1, black hellebore (*Helleborus foetidius*) = C4D2, hemlock (*Conium maculatum*) = C4D3, deadly nightshade (*Atropa belladonna*) = C4D4 and opium poppy (*Papaver somniferum*) = C4M2.

What is particularly interesting is that within Galen's classification these highly poisonous herbs were so clearly identified thousands of years ago and recognised by their extremely cold temperature to be lethally damaging to the Vital Force.

Of Moistening Medicines

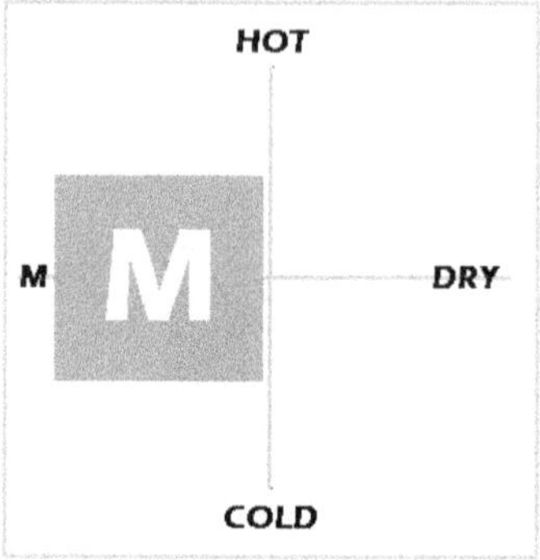

Figure 5.26: Of moistening medicines

Of the passive qualities dry and moist the classification into degrees is not practical, despite the listings showing to the contrary, for, as Culpeper says,

> *There can be no such difference found amongst moistening medicines, that they should surpass the second degree. For seeing all medicines are either hot or cold, neither heat nor cold, seeing they are extremes, can consist with moisture, for the one dries it up, the other condensates it.*

Culpeper describes generally that

> *moist medicines lenifies and make slippery, ease the cough, and help the roughness of the throat. These operations are proper to moist in the 1st degree medicines.*

Herbs moist in the 2nd degree or higher,

> *take away natural strength, help the sharpness of humours, make both blood and spirits thicker, looses the belly, and fits it for purgation.*

Of the herbs classified as being temperate and moist, the mallows and borage fall into the category of demulcent remedies. Demulcents are herbs that generally contain mucilage, which can lubricate and soothe inflammation in different part of the body it makes contact with. Of the mallows, marshmallow is particularly noted as being soothing to the digestive and urinary tracts. The common mallow has a similar action but it not as mucilaginous as the marshmallow. The demulcent action of borage is focused on the lungs where it helps ease the inflammation of bronchitis and pneumonia.

Similarly, the moistening temperature of wild carrot makes the herb helpful in the elimination of kidney stones. Also, the moistening temperature of the juice of the houseleek made it useful for relieving hot fevers, inflammations, burns and scalds to the skin, shingles, fretting ulcers and stings.

However, Culpeper cautions against the excessive use of moist herbs: *"The immoderate or indiscreet use of them dulls the body, and makes it unfit for action."* This latter description perhaps most fits the effects of the opium poppy (*Papaver somniferum*) = C4M2.

Of Drying Medicines

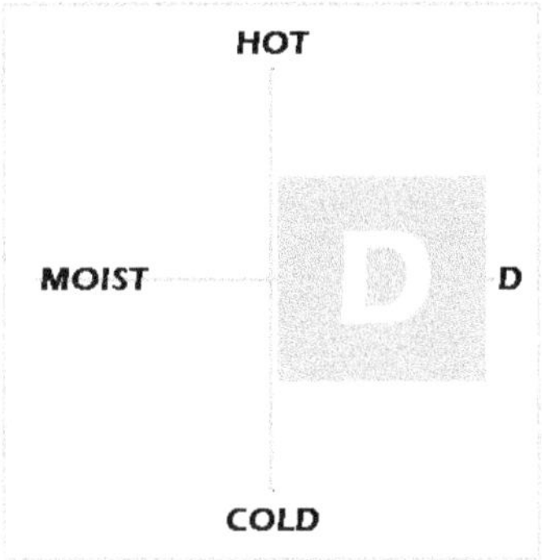

Figure 5.27: Of drying medicines

Of drying medicines Culpeper says they

> *consume moisture, stop fluxes, and make such parts dry as are slippery, they make the body and members firm, when they are weakened by too much moisture, that so they may perform their proper functions.*

Essentially these are astringent herbs.

Culpeper cautions against the excessive use of drying medicine, for while different part of the body may be strengthened by a herb's astringent action, he is concerned that they do not dry out their radical moisture and become devitalised.

> *If then this moisture be consumed by using, or rather over use of drying medicines, the members can neither be nourished, nor yet perform their proper actions.*

Furthermore, he says that herbs drying in the 3rd degree or higher,

> *unadvisedly given, hinder the parts of the body they are appropriated to, of their nourishment and by that means brings them into consumption.*

Culpeper, in response to Galen's concerns for herbs drying in the 4th degree, provides the following rules for drying medicines:

1 *"If the moisture be not extreme, let not the medicine be extremely drying."*
2 *"Let it be proper to the part of the body afflicted, for if the liver be afflicted by moisture, and you go about to dry the brain or heart, you may sooner kill than cure."*

Of the herbs listed as being temperate and dry the greater burnet (*Sanguisorba major*) has enjoyed considerable reputation as a vulnerary that rapidly dries up the blood. The generic name *Sanguisorba* literally means "absorbing the blood". Its flowerhead even has a signature of looking like a blood clot.

Historically the humble flixweed is also worth mention. The herb derives its name from treating the bloody flux. The bloody flux was the name given to the passage of blood and diarrhoea as found in dysentery and cholera. Here the astringent action of the herb would have been valuable for reducing inflammation in the digestive tract.

CHAPTER SIX

Salerno

Salerno lies at the heart of the Italian Amalfi coast and grew rich as a major centre of trade, linking the eastern and western Mediterranean, thereby fusing a number of cultures, including Greek, Latin, Persian, Jewish and Arabic. In this cultural melting pot, a School of Medicine was founded by a group of physicians in the 9th century, which was to become a major centre of medicine in the medieval world.

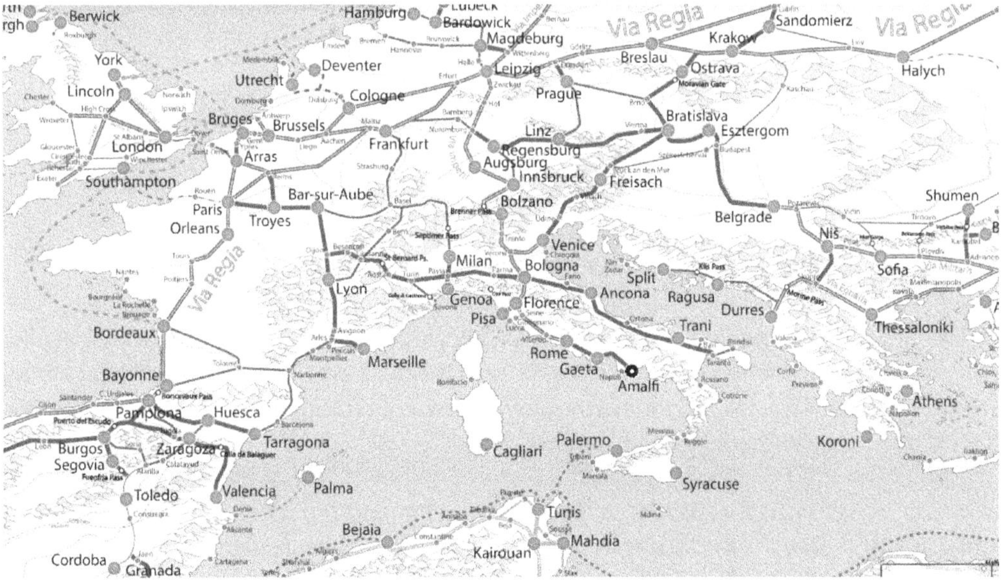

Figure 6.1: Map of medieval trade routes: Amalfi was the epicentre of Mediterranean trade

According to legend, a Greek pilgrim called Pontus visited Salerno when a thunderstorm struck. Needing shelter for the night he took refuge under the arches of the Arcino aqueduct. He was soon joined by an injured Italian runner, called Salernus, who also needed to escape the downpour. Pontus was curious about the dressing on Salernus' leg used to dress his wound. Pontus' curiosity attracted the interest of two more travelling physicians seeking shelter: Helinus, who was Jewish and Abdela, an Arab. When they realised that they were all physicians from different cultural traditions, they decided to pool their collective knowledge and skills, and start a medical school.

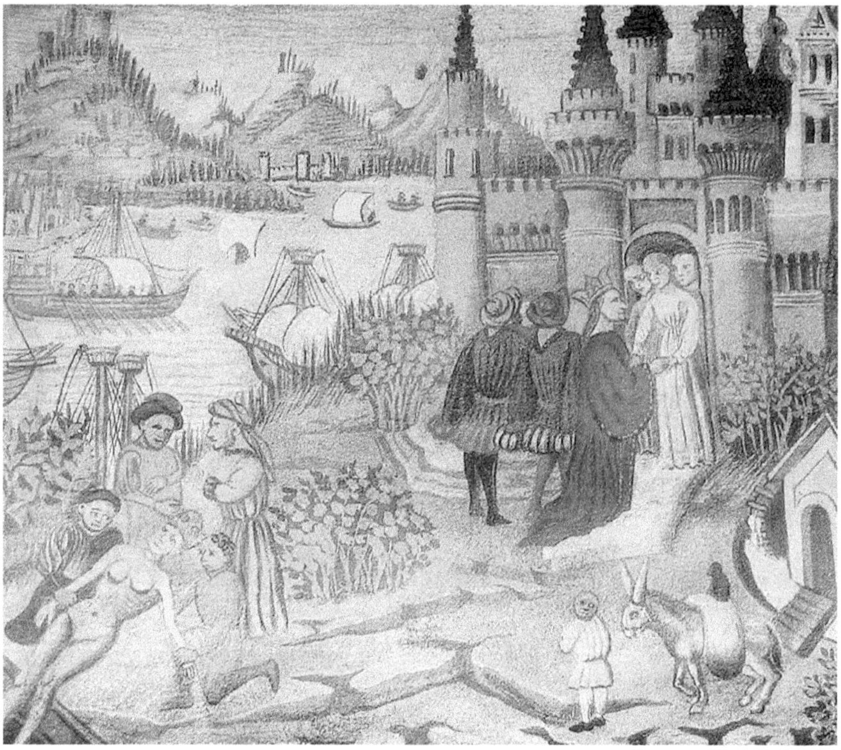

Figure 6.2: The Schola Medica Salernitana in a miniature from Avicenna's Canon. Public domain

This school was known as Schola Medica Salernitana, and it was destined to become the most important centre of medical learning in the medieval world. The medical school started from the dispensary of the monastery in Salerno, where the local populace would have come to collect herbs for their ailments.

The location of the monastery, in the picture, is shown by following the line of sight from the gangway in the marina to the buildings beyond the harbour, where the tower and Cathedral of Santa Maria degli Angeli can be seen. The inset shows the Cathedral of Santa Maria degli Angeli in more clarity.

Amazingly, the medical school lasted more than a thousand years, only closing in 1976. As significant a development as this school was, its fame happened several decades after its founding when, in 1077, a physician called Constantine of Carthage arrived.

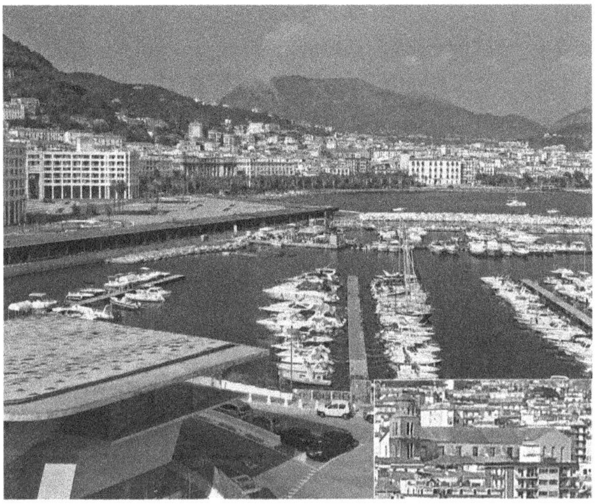

Figure 6.3: The city of Salerno viewed from the International Passenger Terminal. Inset: Cathedral of Santa Maria degli Angeli

Constantine brought with him Arabic texts of Hippocrates, Galen and Dioscorides, as well as medical texts by other Arabic physicians. Soon after his arrival, he started translating these texts from Arabic to Latin. Constantine, having been a physician in Tunisia, would have translated these texts with the experience of having using the principles in practice.

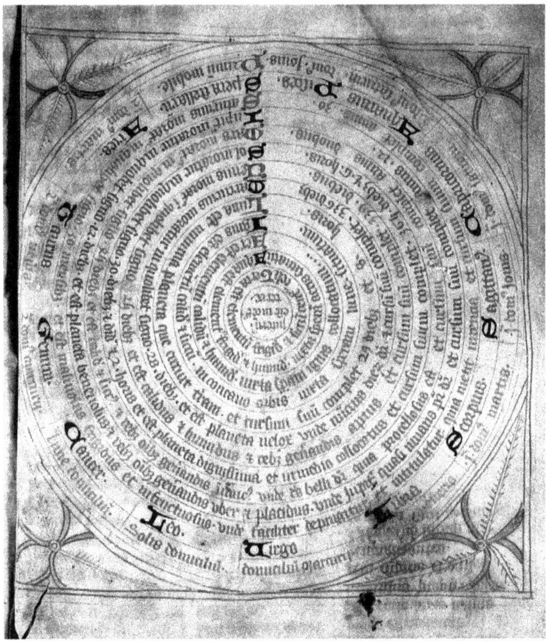

Figure 6.4: A page from the manuscript "Miscellanea medica". Wellcome Institute Library

This page from the manuscript "Miscellanea medica" from the Wellcome's collection of Salernitan medical works reveals the nature of the Hermetic cosmology that Galen incorporated into his writings, being taught at Salerno.

The Zodiacal signs, Planetary spheres and Elements comprising the Hermetic Three World view can be seen within the concentric circles.

- Starting at the outer ring is Primum Mobile—the Universum or first motion.
- The next circle contains the Sphere of the Stars, in which the names of the Zodiacal Signs are listed: Aries, Taurus, Gemini. Cancer, Leo, Virgo, Libra, Scorpio, Sagittarius, Capricorn, Aquarius and Pisces.
- Within, the next seven circles comprise the Planetary spheres of Saturn, Jupiter, Mars, Sun, Venus, Mercury and Moon.
- Finally, the last four inner circles comprise the four manifest Elements of Fire, Air, Water and Earth, along with *terra firma* in the centre. It is also noteworthy that the Planets are listed with their Aristotelian primary qualities: hot, cold, wet and dry.

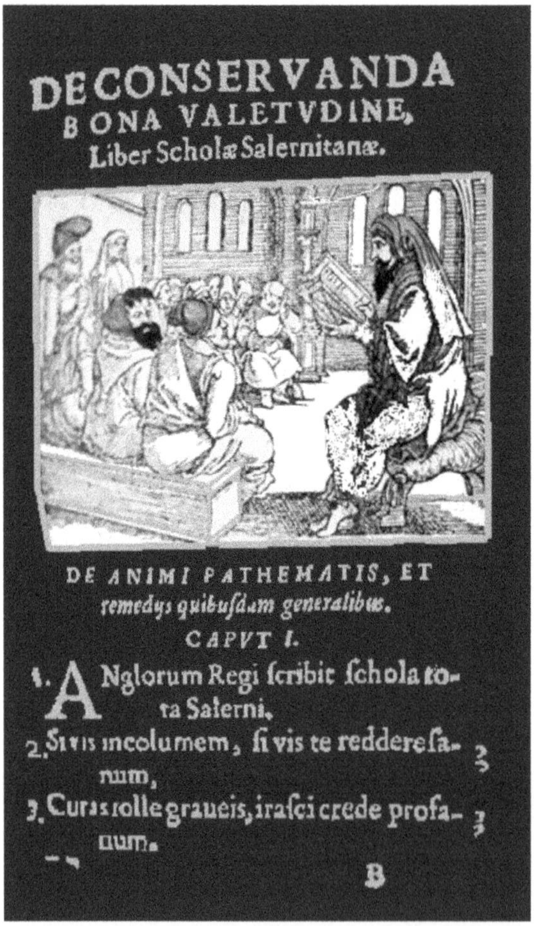

Figure 6.5: The cover of *De Conservanda Bona Valetudine* (Of the Conservation of Good Health) showing Constantine teaching his students. Wellcome Institute Library

In 1231, the authority of the school was sanctioned by Emperor Federico II. In the Emperor's constitution (legal code) of Melfi it was established that the activity of a doctor could only be carried out by doctors holding a diploma issued by the Schola Medica Salernitana.

The news of Constantine's teaching spread rapidly throughout Europe. This was in part due to Salerno being such an important mercantile centre.

The success of the school meant that new Latin manuscripts were much valued, while the reawakening of the principles of physic led to an increasingly lucrative international trade in herbs, roots and seeds.

With the fame of the medical school, increasing numbers of students arrived wanting to study medicine at Salerno, along with many patients seeking a cure from their ailments. The school's endorsement by Alfano I, the Archbishop of Salerno, later Pope Pius lll, gave it the Catholic seal of approval.

Constantine also has come to be known as Constantine of Monte Cassino, for when he retired from his teaching at Salerno, he became a monk at the Benedictine monastery at Monte Cassino, about 100 miles away.

The monastery at Monte Cassino was famous for its collection of manuscripts, including the works of Galen and Hippocrates. Access to this collection must have been part of Constantine's decision to spend the rest of his life there.

The success of the school coincided with the Cluniac reforms, which emphasised and intensified the monastic discipline of St Benedict, along with encouraging the study of the Seven Liberal Arts.

Though the Cluniac reforms were a big boost in the momentum for Benedictine and Augustinian orders, arguably it was the Cistercian order that most benefited from them. It was established soon after the reforms were announced, so never had to change "old ways".

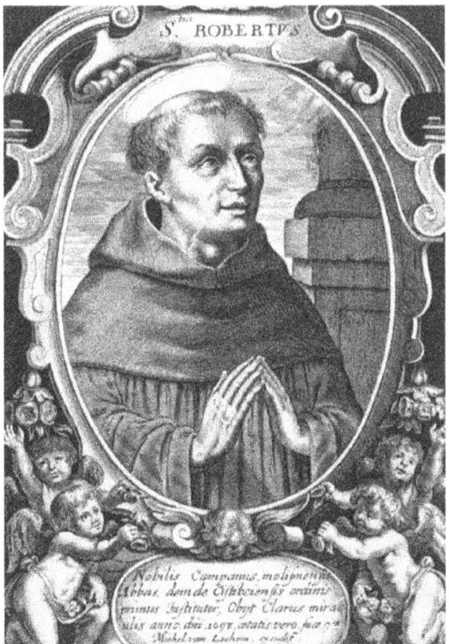

Figure 6.6: St Robert of Moleme. Public domain

Inspired by Saint Robert of Molesme, the order was actually founded by Saint Bernard of Clairvaux, who left the abbey to form a new foundation at Citeaux, from which the Cistercian order derived its name. The Cistercian order was well supported financially, since Bernard's uncle was one of the founding fathers of the Knights Templars. The Templars were the warrior monks who protected pilgrims travelling to the Holy Land. They also founded the first European banking network, entrusted by kings and emperors to exchange and transfer monies.

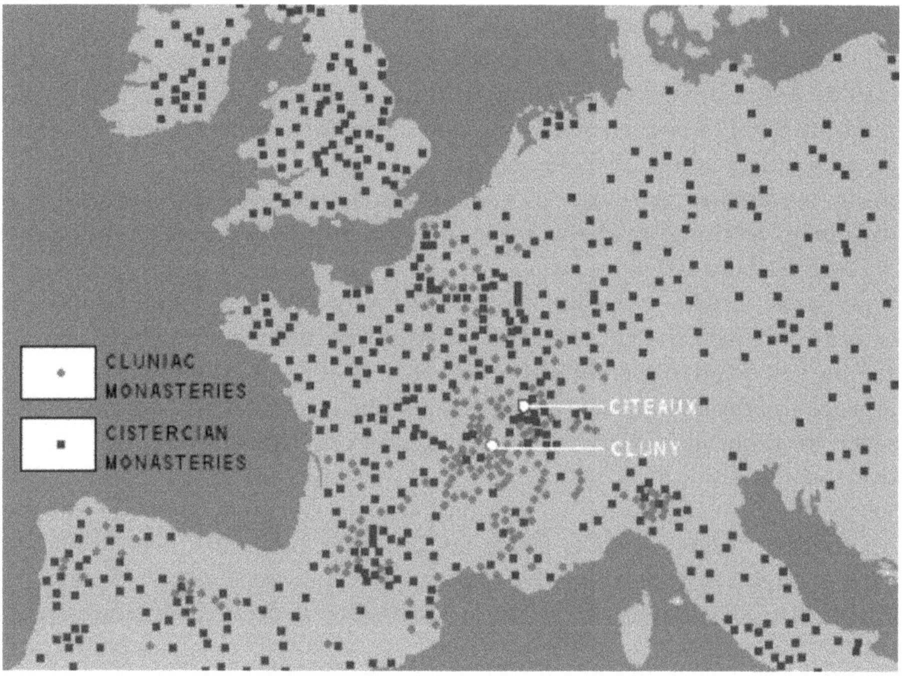

Figure 6.7: The spread of Cluniac and Cistercian monasteries between the 12th and 13th centuries

The speed and extent of the spread of the Cistercian foundations throughout France, Spain, Portugal, Italy, Britain and Ireland within its first century is impressive. Each foundation was instrumental in setting up two daughter foundations. The order grew exponentially using this mechanism, and in so doing also established strong trade and communication links throughout their network. Pilgrims journeying to their chosen religious destinations could take advantage of the hospitality of the monasteries along the way.

With the Cistercian order encouraging new learning, especially in service of the community, the resurrection of Hippocratic and Galenic humoral medical ideas at Salerno, some 1,500 years after Hippocrates first expounded them, would have been enthusiastically absorbed into the movement.

This illustration from a medical manuscript made at the Cistercian Abbaye d'Ourscamp, located roughly 100 miles northeast of Paris, shows the Centaur Chiron, who in Greek myth taught the Art of Medicine to Apollo.

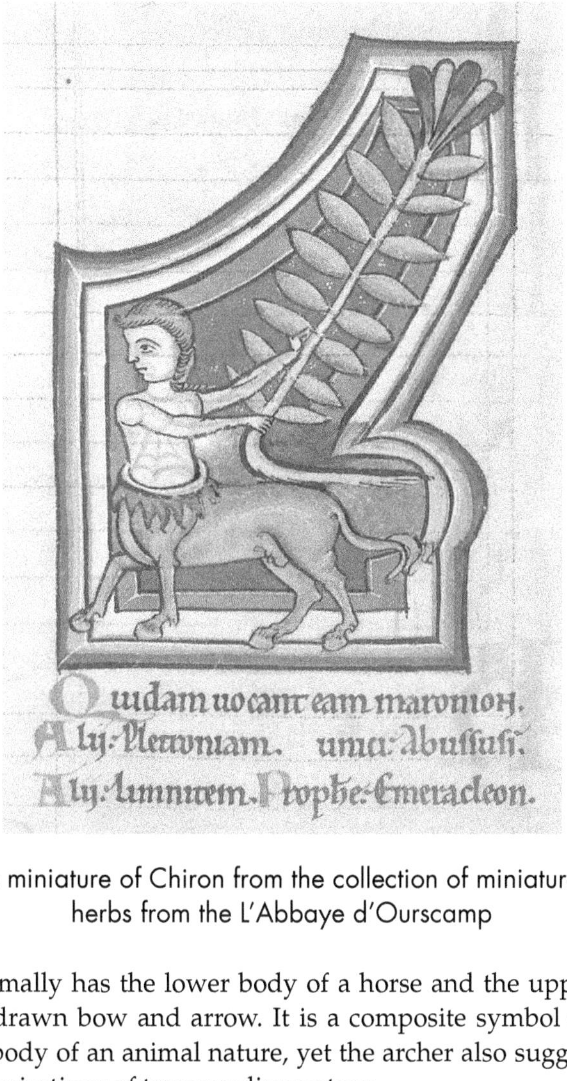

Figure 6.8: The miniature of Chiron from the collection of miniatures of medicinal herbs from the L'Abbaye d'Ourscamp

The centaur normally has the lower body of a horse and the upper torso of a man, usually bearing a drawn bow and arrow. It is a composite symbol showing Mankind having a physical body of an animal nature, yet the archer also suggests a higher mind that has spiritual aspirations of transcending nature.

Here the more typical portrayal of Chiron as an archer is very specifically changed to holding the stem of a herb. The herb has leaves arranged in eight pairs, ascending the stem. At the top a flower is depicted with five petals.

Thus, symbolically the d'Ourscamp Chiron is displaying the Hermetic cosmology that has been seen in the Salerno manuscript. The four horse legs correspond to the four Elements, while the eight pairs of leaves on the plant correspond to the seven Planetary spheres and the eighth the Zodiacal signs. When it is recalled that the name Hippocrates means the "power of the horse", then this Chiron image is a homage to the Father of Medicine.

The ladder-like leaf configuration of the leaves and five-petalled flower resemble a species of gentian. As has been explained in Chapter 2, the common gentian is particularly associated with Chiron.

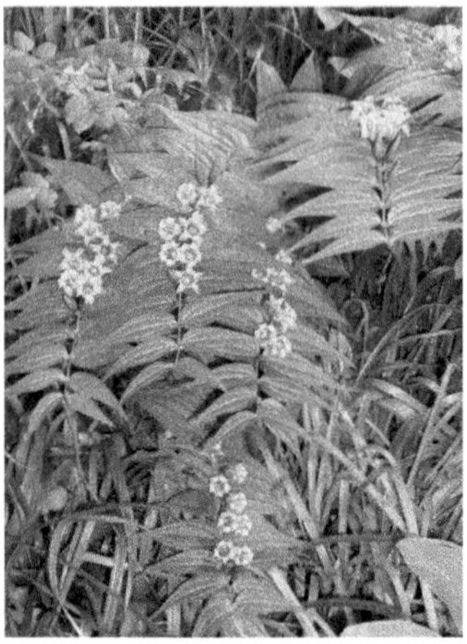

Figure 6.9: The willow gentian (*Gentiana asclepiadea*)

However, in the Eastern Mediterranean, where the cult of Asclepius flourished, another species, the willow gentian, grows with leaves arranged in pairs along a slender stem with blue, five-petalled, trumpet-shaped flowers. Most interestingly Linnaeus gave willow gentian the Latin name *Gentiana asclepiadea*, for this species of gentian too has been linked to Asclepius the Greek god of medicine.

The centaur is a composite symbol, half man and half horse. It embodies the struggle of mankind to transcend its bestial nature. The four legs of the horse are linked to the four Elements of the natural world, while the upper torso man is free to reach to the heavens. Thus, with Chiron holding this gentian, it shows the role of the physician in connecting to the spiritual world, and thus the practice of physic involves understanding about the seven Planets and how they describe the virtues of herbs. This figure of Chiron in the L'Abbaye d'Ourscamp manuscript is clear evidence of the spread of Hippocratic and Galenic teachings within the Cistercian order.

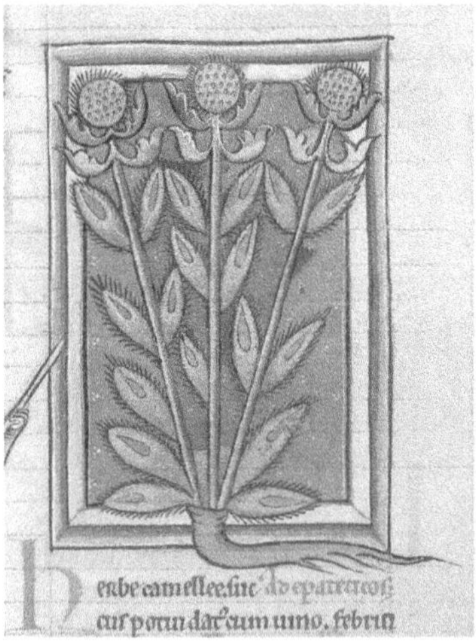

Figure 6.10: The miniature of *Herba melancholia* from the L'Abbaye d'Ourscamp

Another illustration revealing the spread of this knowledge is *Herba melancholia* or melancholy thistle. As its name implies, the thistle was used for treating an excess of the Melancholic humour.

Thistles generally are ruled by Mars through the multitude of their spines. The melancholy thistle is notable for the marked lack of spines, and instead has a strong central stem and flat, sandpaper-like leaves, though the leaf edges have small, sharp serrations, like a hack-saw blade.

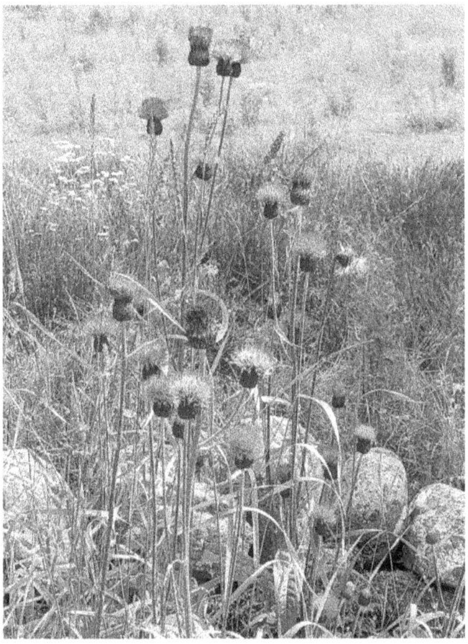

Figure 6.11: Melancholy thistle (*Cirsium heterophyllum*)

Here, the general Martian signature is muted and more benign. The use of a Zodiacal sign in its rulership generally describes the habitat that the herb likes to grow in.

Of the thistle's rulership Culpeper says, *"It is under Capricorn, and therefore under Saturn and Mars."* As the picture shows, the melancholy thistle flourishes in poor soils in the crevices between rocks, terrain that is associated with the Earth sign of Capricorn. Since the Zodiacal sign of Capricorn is ruled by Saturn, it is where Mars is exalted. In other words, Mars' energy is expressed well in the sign of Capricorn.

Culpeper states,

> *Their virtues are but few, but those to be despised: for the decoction of the thistle in wine being drunk, expels superfluous melancholy out of the body, and makes a man as merry as a cricket.*

Thus, Culpeper visualised the Saturnine virtue of the herb having a specifically powerful affinity with the Melancholic humour, where the heat of Mars warms, expands and dissolves the stagnant energy of the humour, thereby lifting the spirits. Galen describes the temperature of melancholy thistle as being hot and dry in the 2nd degree, confirming this action of the herb as ameliorating melancholy. Dioscorides too stated that the herb *"removes all diseases of melancholy"*.

The Ourscamp Miniatures Collection has other interesting details that give insight into the spread of herbal knowledge through the monasteries. Many of the illustrations are deliberately stylised as a means of illustrating the energetic virtue of the herb. A good example is "Herba betonica" (*Stachys betonica*), a much-valued medical herb and one of the sacred herbs of the Celts. This very stylised image is striking, for it looks distinctly different from the betony herb in real life. In fact, if the illustration did not have the name written underneath, it would not be easy to identify it.

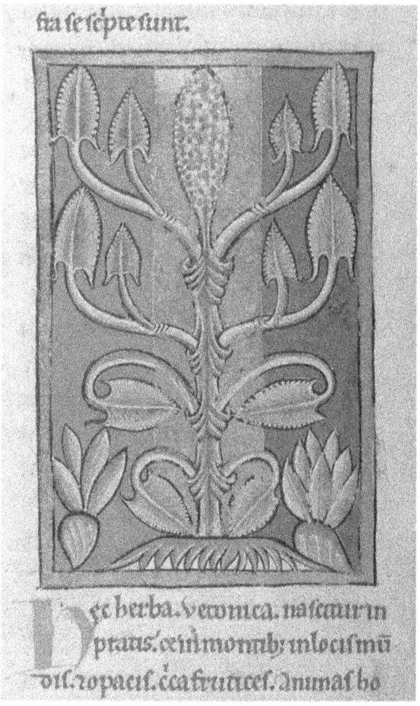

Figure 6.12: The miniature of *Herba betonica* from the L'Abbaye d'Ourscamp

Why was betony herb depicted in this way? It is easy to dismiss its morphological inaccuracy as artistic licence, such as when its creator has not actually seen the herb, but this is a well-known medicinal herb and most likely would have even been cultivated in the Abbey's physic gardens at Ourscamp. Consider too the use of gold leaf, a very expensive material in medieval times, which was obviously very deliberately incorporated into this depiction of the herb.

On closer inspection, the image was in fact a sort of "mandala" of the herb, depicting an energetic perspective of its herbal use. This was an image for monks and nuns to contemplate, thereby enhancing their understanding of the "virtues" of the herb and its influence on the body. It also reveals the degree of sophistication of the herbal knowledge in the monasteries of the 12th century.

The traditional rulership of betony is Jupiter in Aries. The zodiacal sign of Aries, the ram is ruled by Mars, the god of war. This Martian signature can easily be seen in the miniature from the pointed "arrowhead"-like leaves. This theme too can be seen at the leaf nodes, where the leaves are shown growing out of the stem depicted by the artists as a series of "plates" such as you find in a medieval suit of armour to protect the armpits.

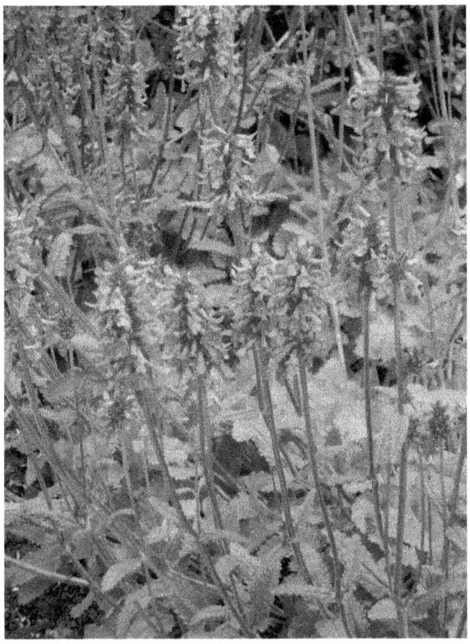

Figure 6.13: Wood betony (*Stachys betonica*)

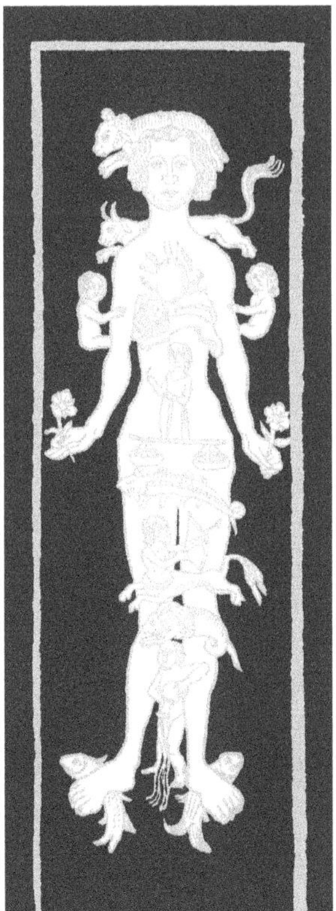

Figure 6.14: Woodcut of Zodiacal Man

The sign of Aries is traditionally linked to the head, as seen in this representation of Zodiacal Man where a ram is shown lying across the head, while the other Zodiacal signs are ascribed to different parts of the body, as they descend.

The arrowhead-like leaves in the upper half of the "herba betonica" image clearly point upwards to the flowerhead. This indicates the healing energy or virtue of the herb, shown as directing energy upwards to the head.

The Jovial rulership symbolically connects the virtue of the herb to the Sanguine humour, which, as has been shown, in humoral physiology was the principal humour of the blood, embodying the other Choleric, Phlegmatic and Melancholic humours in a state of balance. The influence of Jovial herbs thus helps restore the balance to the humours, thereby enhancing the flow of vital energy through the blood. Just as a thunderstorm relieves tension and clears the air, so too was betony, with its Jupiter in Aries rulership, visualised in releasing the tension of a headache and clearing the mind. The name betony is said to come from the Celtic "bew", meaning "head" and ton, "good", indicating the herb has long been recognised as good for complaints of the head.

This idea of balance is further conveyed by the striped background to the image. The tripartite components reflect the three alchemical principles of Salt, Sulphur and Mercury used to evaluate the functioning of the Vital Force. These will be fully explained in Chapter 17.

In the miniature, the three colours connect with the alchemical principles, with further symbolic correspondences. The colour red of the left-hand stripe is connected to Mars, which links it to the masculine Sulphur principle. The colour blue of the right-hand stripe is connected to Venus, which links it to the feminine Salt principle. The central gold stripe is linked to the Mercury principle. The symmetry of how the betony plant is centrally placed clearly shows how the herb has a balancing and harmonising influence on the Vital Force.

Gold is the metal and colour of the Sun. In humoral physiology the Sun was seen symbolically to be linked to the generation of the Vital Force in the body. Just as a border defines a picture, so too the gold frame symbolically defines betony as a truly healing herb and indicates just how much it was venerated at the time.

The most curious detail of the miniature is the representation of the flower spike, which totally lacks the definition such as you can see in the woodcut found in Gerard's *Herball*. If you can pardon the anachronism, the flowering spike is just a pixelated blur! However, considering the use of the herb for treating headaches, naturally betony would have been the herb of choice for treating migraines, which in medieval times were referred to by the more expressive, subjective name of "me-grims". One of the classic prodromal symptoms of the onset of a migraine is vision splintering into specks of colour and light. It suggests that the artist who depicted this herb suffered from me-grims and, realising that the flowerhead was analogous to the head in the body, wished to convey visually the use of betony for treating them.

CHAPTER SEVEN

The Seven Liberal Arts

Henry de Blois had been educated at Cluny Abbey, which initiated the principles of the Cluniac reform. This movement encouraged intellectual freedom of the Seven Liberal Arts, in conjunction with the high standards of devotion within monastic discipline. Henry was keen to promote these in Britain after his posting as Bishop of Winchester.

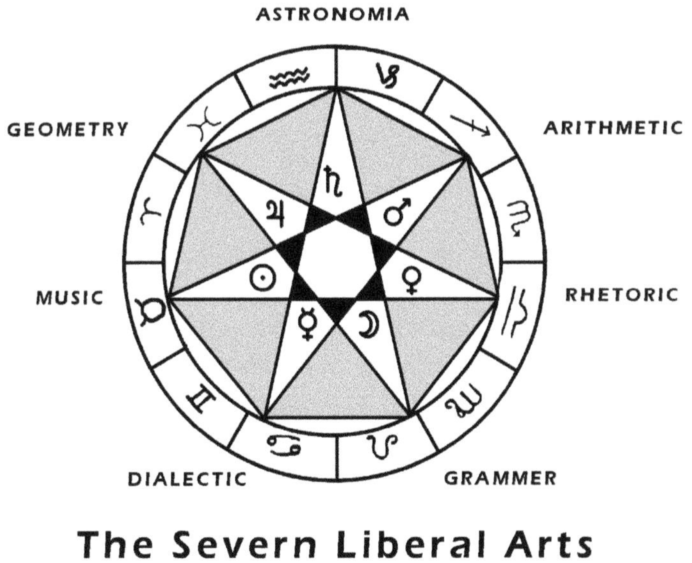

Figure 7.1: Depiction of the Seven Liberal Arts

The Seven Liberal Arts corresponded to the seven planetary spheres of the Celestial World. The subjects constituting the arts were deliberately sequenced to facilitate the development of the soul, enabling it ultimately to complete its journey through planetary spheres. The seven topics were arranged in two sections: the *trivium* and *quadrivium* respectively. The three subjects constituting the *trivium* were essentially preparatory for the more important four principal subjects of the *quadrivium*.

Trivium

The first liberal art was **grammar**, which in reality meant the study of Latin, with its inherent often-complex grammatical rules. Latin was the common tongue used by scholars and academics across Europe. Thus, the study of Latin not only facilitated access to learning the texts of diverse topics but also enabled the freedom to communicate with scholars from other countries.

The first planetary sphere is symbolically linked to the Moon. With the Moon representing imagination, this sphere is all about developing imagination and places importance upon using imagination to access intuitive faculties and so start the inner journey.

The second liberal art was **didactic**. The sphere of Mercury is where the soul gains the ability to express and communicate what it thinks and feels. As above alludes to the teachings of the twelve Apostles; likewise, students were encouraged to give instruction to others. The teaching of knowledge was recognised as not only important for communicating it to others, but also enhancing the student's understanding of the subject, through explanation. In the sphere of Mercury, the soul develops a symbolic perception of life, understanding the inner world reflected in the outer.

The third liberal art was **rhetoric**. The sphere of Venus is where the soul experiences love. Rhetoric is the cultivation of the art of speech, for the purpose of influencing others. To this end words are selected carefully to express harmony and so inspire others to the selflessness of the spirit.

Quadrivium

The fourth liberal art was **music**. The sphere of the Sun gives power to the senses and imagination, which enriches the aesthetic appreciation of beauty and harmony. At this sphere, the soul understands its link to creation. Music has the power to lift the spirits and enrich the soul. The medieval practice of plainsong, which linked the harmony of music with sacred texts, was more than an aide-memoire, it was done to deliberately encourage the soul and elevate it on its journey through the spheres. The seven notes constituting the musical octave were also seen as symbolically parallel to the seven planetary spheres.

The fifth liberal art was **arithmetic**. In medieval times arithmetic or *mathemata* was synonymous with astrology. In the sphere of Mars the soul learns how to use power well. Knowing the right moment to act not only leads to a precision of action but also to economy of energy. Astrology provided the knowledge to find and understand the right moment. Consequently, at the sphere of Mars the soul creates order, discipline and purpose. In an era before clocks, knowledge of the movements of the Planets and the Zodiacal signs in the heavens was very important to the timing of events in the Church calendar and holding daily services.

The sixth liberal art was **geometry**. The sphere of Jupiter facilitates receptivity of the soul to inspiration from the spiritual world. The patterns and shapes of geometry were used to elevate the spirit beyond the physical form. Consequently, sacred geometry was employed extensively in the building of cathedrals and palaces to elevate the mind as well as communicating and preserving spiritual knowledge.

The seventh liberal art was **astronomia**. *Astronomia* was the recognition of the constellational patterns of the Zodiac. The sphere of Saturn is where the soul learns a clear sense of right from wrong, light from darkness, and thus gains the power of reason and logic. The study of *astronomia* was quite literally the study of the light of the stars from the darkness of the heavens. In medieval times, before electric light, the study of the night skies was naturally highly significant.

The *quadrivium* was also seen as corresponding to the symbolism of the Five Elements. Geometry, literally meaning "measurement of the earth", corresponds to the Earth Element. Water is symbolically the Element of connection, which corresponds to music as a medium of emotional expression. Setting sacred texts to music enhances their memory, while the harmonies lift the spirits. Air corresponds to astronomy, the observation of the spatial relationship of the Planets in the Zodiacal signs, while finally Fire corresponds to the calculations necessary to do an astrological chart. The balance of these elements enabled the student to correctly observe the relationship between heaven and earth, to do on earth what is in accordance with the heavens.

Once a student had perfected each of these four component stages, symbolic of their elemental balance, he became rewarded as a Master of the Arts, as a recognition of his quintessential achievement. This mastery of the arts was the foundation point for further studies of medicine, theology and law.

> *The character of the liberal arts curriculum was derived from the convenient relationship between two meanings of the Latin word* liber, *the root of such modern terms as library and liberate: to read was the attribute of the classical freeman, to the medieval mind to read was to set oneself free—the twelfth century was to be one of philosophical liberation.* [N. Campion, "History of Western Astrology", vol. II, p. 44]

At a deeper level, it was to be preparatory for setting the soul free on its journey back to the light.

A particularly fascinating illustration of the Seven Liberal Arts and how they were incorporated into the teachings of the Catholic Church is found in the important illuminated manuscript of the *Hortus deliciarum*, authored by Herrad of Landsberg, who was the Abbess of the convent of Hohenburg on Mount St Odile in Alsace. The original manuscript was dated to roughly 1180, but sadly it was destroyed during the bombing of Strasbourg in the Franco-Prussian War of 1870.

Herrad described the manuscript as "the nectar of the various flowers plucked from Holy Scripture and philosophical works". It was clearly compiled for the education of the nuns at Hohenburg. Its importance is reflected in the fact that a number of copies had been made, typical of the monastic tradition, so that its wisdom was disseminated to other convents. Fortunately, these have survived, enabling the appreciation of her magnum opus.

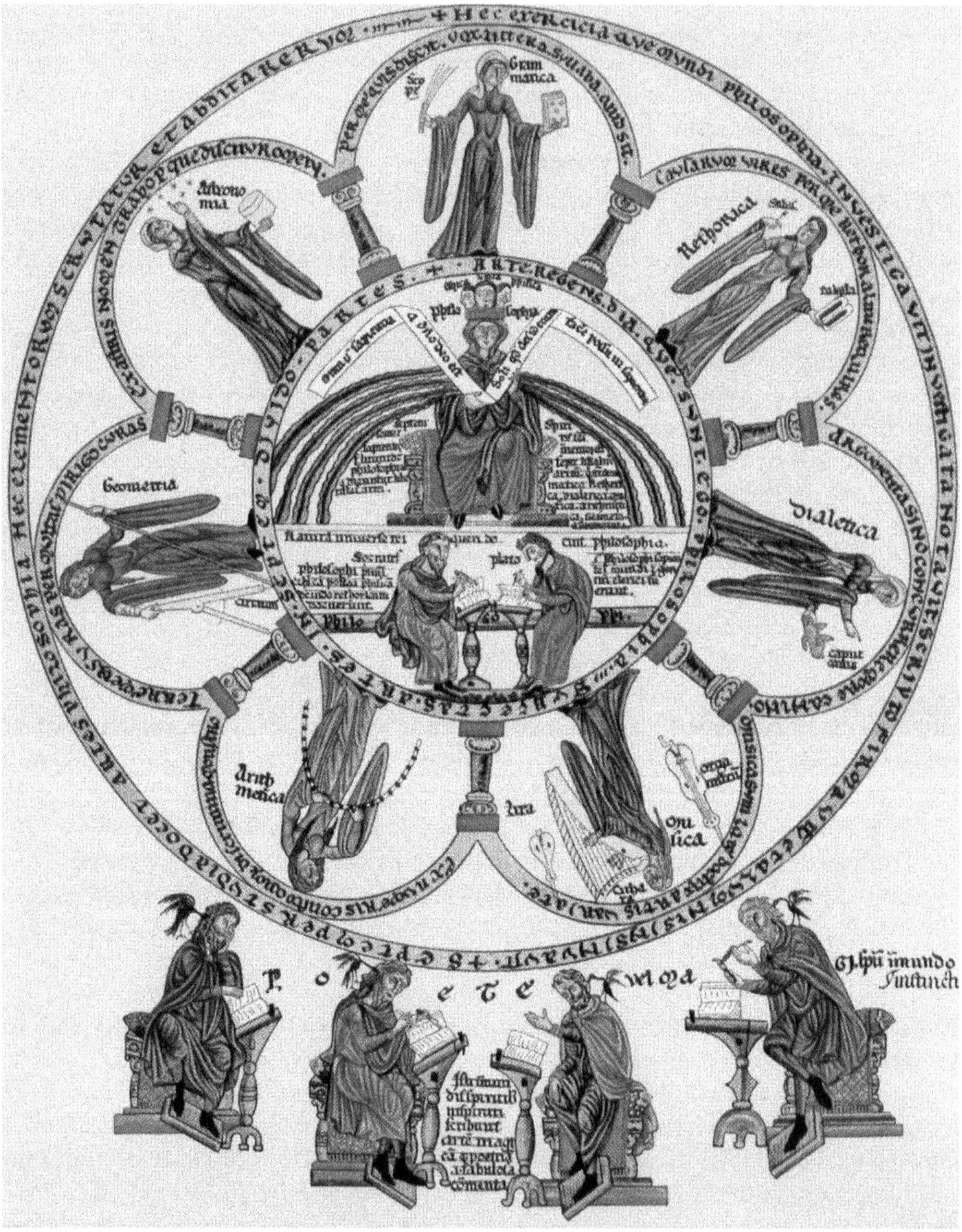

Figure 7.2: Illumination from *Hortus deliciarum*, by Herrad of Landsberg, Abbess of Hohenburg, c. 1180

The main structure of this illustration is based upon the Solar glyph (☉), composed of the Circle of the Soul encapsulating the central dot, representing the seed of light within the soul. The word "philosophy" literally means "the love of Sophia", the Greek goddess of wisdom. Philosophy here is represented as a Queen, sitting on a throne, at the centre of the circle. Her crown has three heads: these are identifiable as *ethica*, *logica* and *physica*, the tripartite division of Platonic philosophy.

She wears blue robes that symbolically link Philosophy with Venus the goddess of love, and, within Christian iconography, to the Virgin Mary. She holds a scroll which reads, "All wisdom comes from the Lord God; the wise alone achieve what they desire." To her right is an inscription which reads: "seven streams of wisdom, called the Liberal Arts, flow from Philosophy". To her left the inscription reads: "the Holy Spirit inspired seven liberal arts: grammatica, rhetorica, dialectica, musica, arithmetica, geometria, and astronomia". The seven streams of the liberal arts are depicted flowing from her heart. The heart is symbolically ruled by the Sun. Thus, by loving the inner light of the soul the essence of philosophy is created.

The circumference of the inner circle reads: "I, Godlike Philosophy lay out seven arts which are subordinate to me; by them I control all things with wisdom." Below Philosophy seated on her throne are the Greek philosophers, Plato and his teacher, Socrates, depicted sitting at desks.

Between the outer and inner circles are seven arches corresponding to the Seven Liberal Arts. Starting at top and proceeding clockwise, the first arch encloses the figure of Grammar holding a book and a whip. The inscription within the arch reads: *"Through me all can learn what are the words, the syllables, and the letters."*

The second arch encloses the figure of Rhetoric holding a tablet and stylus. The inscription reads: *"Thanks to me, proud speaker, your speeches will be able to take strength."*

The third arch encloses the figure of Dialectic who points with a one hand and holds a barking dog's head in the other. The inscription reads: *"I allow arguments to join, dog-like, in battle."* Grammar, rhetoric and dialectic make up the three streams of the *trivium*. Dialectic, or learning through argument and debate, is an alternative to didactic, which is learning through teaching and explaining to others. The sequence too of the *trivium* topics in this illustration is slightly different from the more usual sequence of the Seven Liberal Arts: grammar, didactic/dialectic and rhetoric. It may have been a mistake of the scribe who copied this illustration or possibly was peculiar to Herrad's teaching of philosophy at Hohenburg.

The fourth arch encloses the figure of Music holding a harp, with a lute and another medieval stringed instrument. The inscription reads: *"I teach my art using a variety of instruments."*

The fifth arch encloses the figure of Arithmetic holding a cord with threaded beads—a simple counting aid. The inscription reads: *"I base myself on the numbers and show the proportions between them."*

The sixth arch encloses the figure of Geometry holding a staff and compass. The inscription reads: *"It is with exactness that I survey the ground."*

The seventh arch encloses the figure of Astronomy who points to the stars and holds a mirror or some sort of receptacle. The inscription reads: *"I hold the names of the celestial bodies and predict the future."*

Music, Arithmetic, Geometry and Astronomy make up the four streams of the *quadrivium*. As was discussed in the *trivium*, the arts of arithmetic and geometry are normally found reversed.

The outer ring contains four philosophical aphorisms: *"What it discovers is remembered;" "Philosophy investigates the secrets of the elements and all things;" "Philosophy teaches arts by seven branches;" "It puts it in writing, in order to convey it to the students."*

Underneath the circle are four men seated at desks, described as "poets and magicians", located outside the ring and symbolically unable to be reached by the spirit of Philosophy. Their minds are guided and taught by impure spirits, hence they can only produce tales, fables, frivolous poetry or magic spells. The illustration shows black birds, representing evil spirits, whispering into their ears.

CHAPTER EIGHT

Monastic culture

> *To every thing there is a season, and a time to every purpose under the heaven: A time to be born, and a time to die; a time to plant, and a time to pluck up that which is planted; A time to kill, and a time to heal; a time to break down, and a time to build up; A time to weep, and a time to laugh; a time to mourn, and a time to dance; A time to cast away stones, and a time to gather stones together; a time to embrace, and a time to refrain from embracing; A time to get, and a time to lose; a time to keep, and a time to cast away; A time to rend, and a time to sew; a time to keep silence, and a time to speak; A time to love, and a time to hate; a time of war, and a time of peace.*
>
> Ecclesiastes Ch3, v1–8 [King James translation]

Completion of the Seven Liberal Arts essentially trained the student to obtain the Hermetic vision of the heavens above being reflected on Earth below, in order to understand God's will. This astrological frame work underpinned Catholic theology.

The sowing illustration from this famous book of hours, called *Les Très Riches Heures du Duc de Berry*, reveals the sky in October, with the constellations of Libra, the scales and Scorpio, the scorpion clearly visible.

This gives us a glimpse of the importance that astrology had for understanding the annual cycle within the Christian calendar. Similarly, before clocks were widely available, observations of the stars were used to time the daily monastic services, especially those held during the night. The setting of the date for Easter remains to this day based on the formula, as being held on the first Sunday following the full Moon, after the Sun has entered the sign of Aries, at the Spring Equinox.

Theological thinking within the cathedral schools encouraged five levels of learning, corresponding to the Five Elements. These five levels were symbolised by depictions of Christ, surrounded by representations of the Four Evangelists: Matthew, Mark, Luke and John.

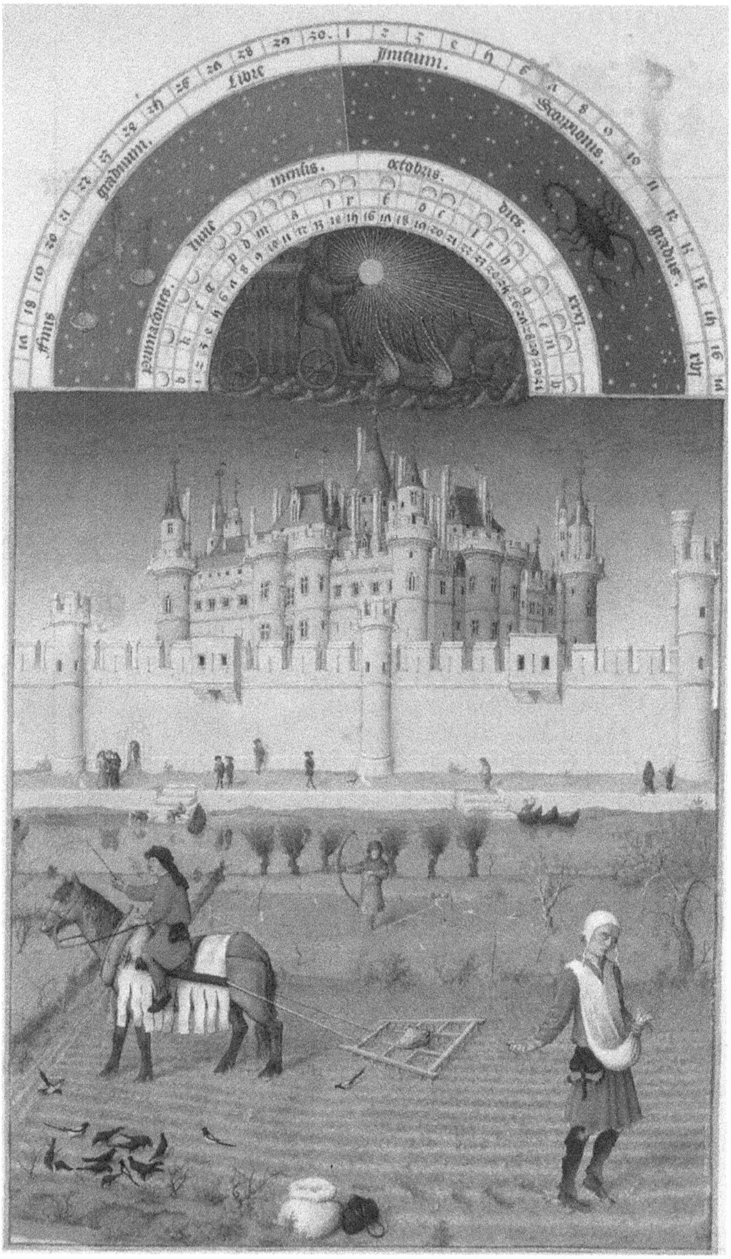

Figure 8.1: "A time to sow." October from *Très Riches Heures du Duc de Berry*, 1416, by the Limbourg brothers/Barthélemy d'Eyck. R.M.N./R.-G. Ojéda. Public domain

Matthew is represented by an Angel, Mark by a Lion, Luke by a Bull, and John by an Eagle, as in the Vision of Ezekiel. These correspond to the four fixed signs of the Zodiac: the Angel to the Air sign of Aquarius (♒), the Lion to the Fire sign of Leo (♌), the Bull to the Earth sign of Taurus (♉), and the Eagle to the Water sign of Scorpio (♏). Christ represents the Ether Element.

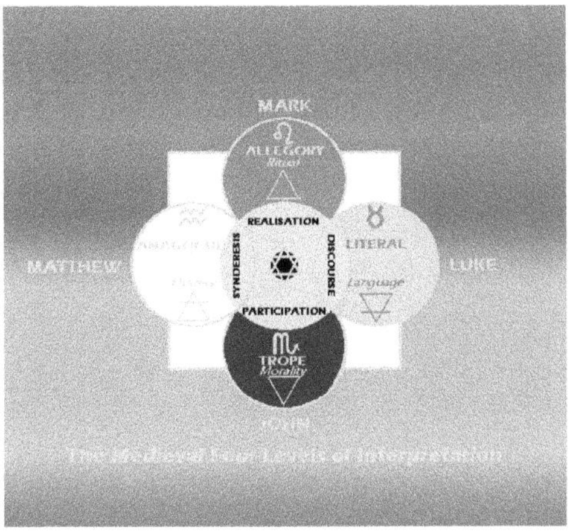

Figure 8.2: The Four Elemental levels of learning

The illustration shows the Four Elemental spheres of learning, arranged in a cross, united by the circular glyph of the Sun at the centre, representing the transcendent Element Ether.

The Four Vesica so formed by the overlapping spheres represent the assimilation of knowledge from these Elemental spheres into the Soul (☉). Illuminated by the Light of the Soul, this symbolic perspective of the spheres of learning—the literal, tropological, anagogical and allegorical—becomes much clearer to understand.

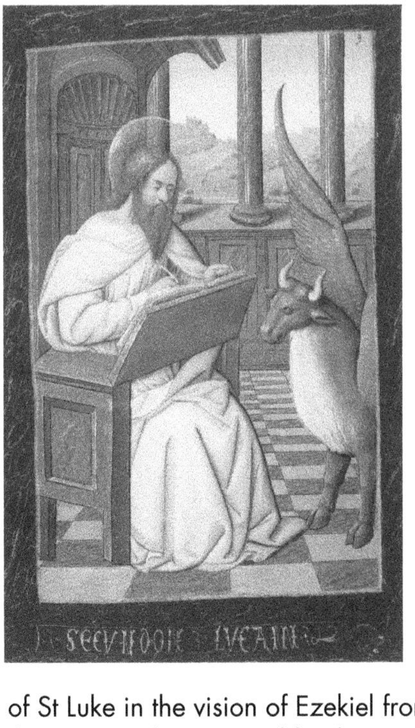

Figure 8.3: Depiction of St Luke in the vision of Ezekiel from *The Book of Hours of Henry IV of France*. Public domain

The **literal sphere** is represented by the Bull of St Luke. Taurus (♉) an Earth sign that is associated with the written word of scripture, accepting the text of the New Testament at face value as being true account of the historical life of Jesus. However, discourse describes the degree to which the student is able to transcend the literal word and see the inner meaning of the scripture, thereby enriching their soul with it.

The parable of the "Sower and the Seed" in Matthew 13 is particularly illuminating in this respect. Jesus explained many things in parables to his disciples, saying, in a modern translation:

> *A farmer went out to sow his seed. As he was scattering the seed, some fell along the path, and the birds came and ate it up. Some fell on rocky places, where it did not have much soil. It sprang up quickly, because the soil was shallow. But when the sun came up, the plants were scorched, and they withered because they had no root. Other seed fell among thorns, which grew up and choked the plants. Still other seed fell on good soil, where it produced a crop—a hundred, sixty or thirty times what was sown. Whoever has ears, let them hear.*

The parable reflects the Five Elements: in order for the seed (Ether) to germinate and flourish, it needs the balance of the Elements. The first instance of the birds concerns the Air Element, describing a mind that is distracted and does not listen to or value the teachings. The second instance concerns the rocky dry soil (Earth), where the seeds lack moisture, and describes a mind that lacks the imagination to understand the teachings. The third instance of the thorns (Fire) symbolises a mind overcome with too many desires to be receptive to the teachings. Finally, the seed that lands on fertile ground, with adequate moisture (Water), is highly productive. It is symbolic of the receptive mind, blessed with a good imagination, which becomes rewarded with spiritual wisdom.

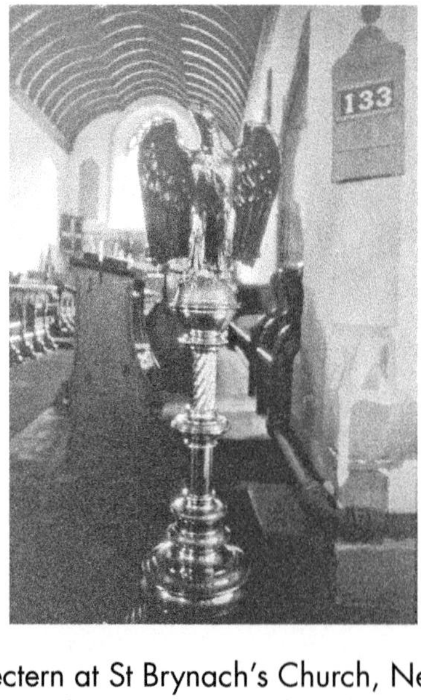

Figure 8.4: The Eagle Lectern at St Brynach's Church, Nevern, Wales. The Eagle, in soaring high up in the heavens, holding the Bible, is symbolic of having brought the word of God down to Earth

The **tropological sphere** is represented by the Eagle of St John. Scorpio (♏), the fixed Water sign, is connected to the realm of emotions. Water also relates to the Hermetic Celestial World. When Water is still, it becomes calm and reflective. Similarly, when the emotions are still, as in quiet meditation, this gives the student the opportunity to reflect on what their emotions are telling them. Rather than be caught up in conflict and suffering, it provides the opportunity to learn from their mistakes, so they can be "turned" into inner wisdom. Quietening the emotions allows the Soul to participate in a rich inner life.

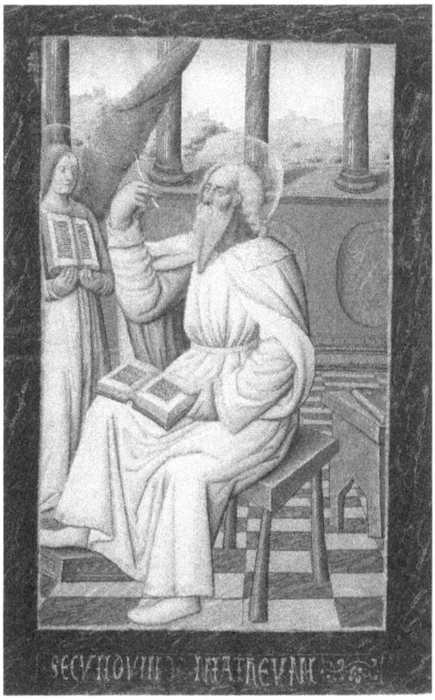

Figure 8.5: Depiction of St Matthew in the vision of Ezekiel from *The Book of Hours of Henry IV of France*. Public domain

The **anagogical sphere** is represented by the Angel of St Matthew. Aquarius (♒), the fixed Air sign, is connected to the realm of ideas. Air is the Element of the mind and, in the Hermetic cosmology, together with the Angel is symbolic of the Angelic realm of the Intellectual World. The Air Element provides the connection for the mystical or anagogical experience. In the presence of a Saint, the mind of the student becomes overpowered by the inner Light of their holiness, is swept clean of all emotional dross as their attention focuses upon their Soul. In this state, ideas are readily communicated or transmitted without words. The word "mysticism" is derived from the Latin verb *mysterio*, meaning "to be silent".

When the Soul is thus open and receptive, it will absorb far more knowledge than that which is physically spoken. This inner connection confers "synderesis", that is, the innate ability to understand moral principles and to spontaneous act accordingly.

The **allegorical sphere** is represented by the Lion of St Mark. Leo (♌) is the fixed Fire sign, which is connected to action and ritual. For most Christians, the central ritual is taking the communion of the bread and wine at the altar, symbolic of the flesh and blood of Christ.

However, the ritual starts with entering the church or abbey through the West Door, being symbolic of entering your own inner temple.

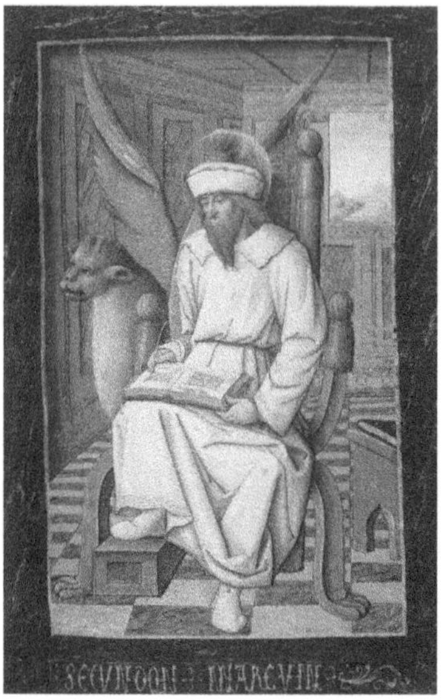

Figure 8.6: Depiction of St Mark in the vision of Ezekiel from *The Book of Hours of Henry IV of France*. Public domain

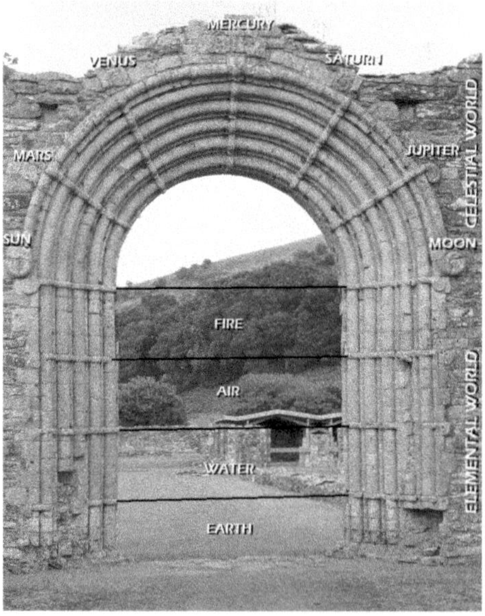

Figure 8.7: The West Gate of Strata Florida Abbey, Tregaron, Wales, symbolic of entering the Hermetic Cosmology of the Three World view

This is why in the Gothic era the architecture of abbeys was infused with sacred geometry, reflecting the symbolic principles of creation. Participation in the rituals of the allegorical sphere led to the realisation of the inner world reflected in the outer world.

For example, the monks entering through this archway at Strata Florida Abbey was a daily ritual of immersion into the Hermetic cosmology of the Three World view.

You can see the Four Elements of the Elemental World arising vertically up the columns, while the Romanesque archway has seven radial lines, with their bosses corresponding to the Seven Planets of the Celestial World. The vertical columns or labia, which correspond to the Orders of Angels in the Intellectual World, are incomplete. The main sponsor of Strata Florida Abbey, the Lord Rhys, died twenty years into construction of the Abbey, before the masons were able to carve angelic figures into the stonework, such as can be found at Reims Cathedral.

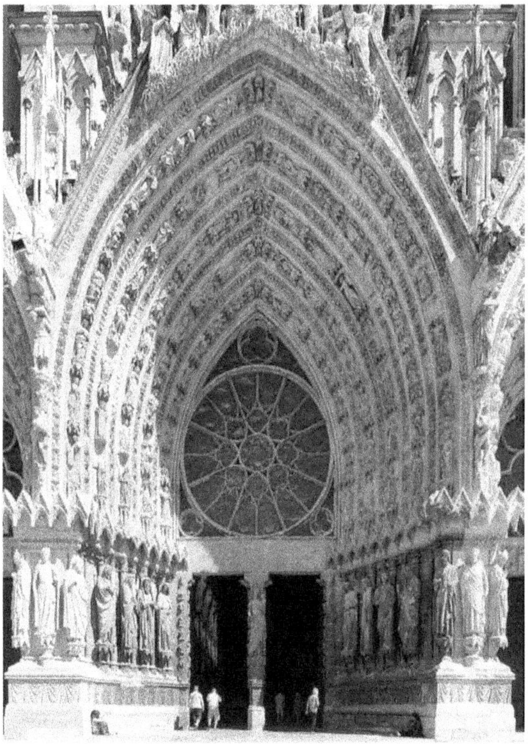

Figure 8.8: The magnificent West Door of Reims Cathedral

With the new learning encouraged by the Cluniac Reforms, the figure of Zodiacal Man started to appear among the manuscripts of their scriptoriums. Most likely this was in response to the newly available translation of works by Hippocrates and Galen. It was an expression of Man being made in the image of the heavens. The progression of the Zodiacal signs, starting with Aries, was projected onto the human body:

- Aries (♈) rules the head.
- Taurus (♉) rules the neck, throat and shoulders.

- Gemini (♊) rules the arms and hands.
- Cancer (♋) rules the chest and stomach.
- Leo (♌) rules the heart.
- Virgo (♍) rules the intestines.
- Libra (♎) rules the kidneys.
- Scorpio (♏) rules the sexual organs.
- Sagittarius (♐) rules the hips and thighs.
- Capricorn (♑) rules the knees.
- Aquarius (♒) rules the calves and ankles.
- Pisces (♓) rules the feet.

Images of Zodiacal Man evolved through the Gothic era, so that by the 15th century a much more sophisticated depiction of Zodiacal Man can be found in *Très Riches Heures du Duc de Berry*, 1416. Its design now incorporates several key Hermetic ideas.

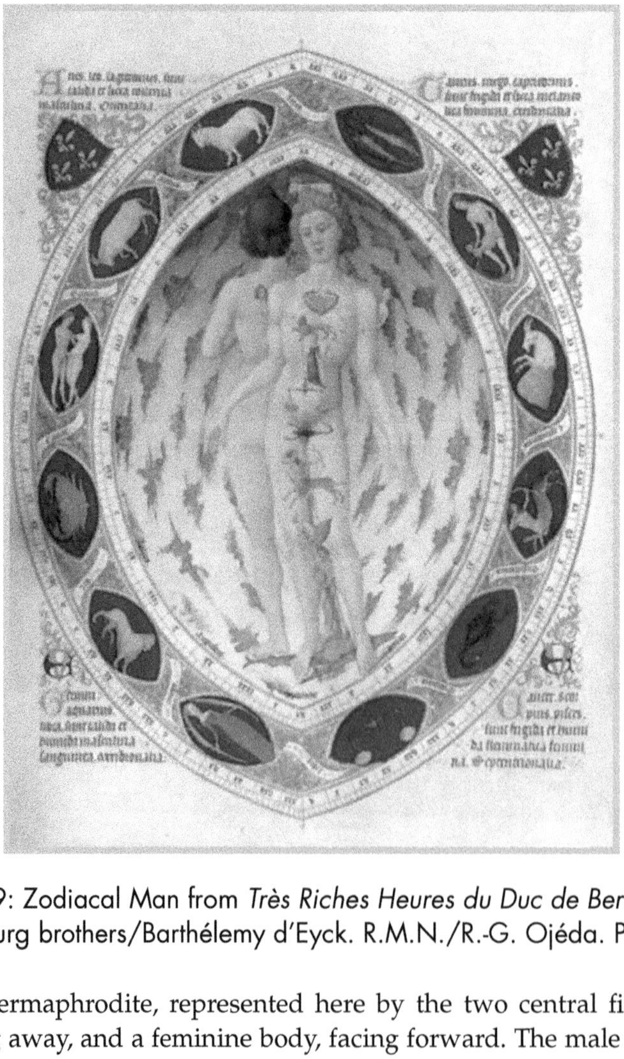

Figure 8.9: Zodiacal Man from *Très Riches Heures du Duc de Berry*, 1416, by the Limbourg brothers/Barthélemy d'Eyck. R.M.N./R.-G. Ojéda. Public domain

Mercury is hermaphrodite, represented here by the two central figures: a masculine body, facing away, and a feminine body, facing forward. The male body represents the physical body, while the female body, with the Zodiacal symbols running down it, represents the vital or etheric body.

Both bodies are surrounded by a large Vesica Piscis, which contains all the Zodiacal constellation in the labia. It symbolises the body being born or made in the image of the heavens, with the constellations above, reflected along the length of the body below. The illustration also contains Plato's Elemental symbolism, with the four corners containing descriptions of Zodiacal signs with their qualities of hot, cold, wet and dry, along their matching humour:

- In the top left corner, the Fire signs are listed: Aries (♈), Leo (♌) and Sagittarius (♐) as being hot and dry, linking them to the Choleric humour.
- In the bottom left corner, the Air signs are listed: Gemini (♊), Libra (♎) and Aquarius (♒) as being hot and moist, linking them to the Sanguine humour.
- In the top right corner, the Earth signs are listed: Taurus (♉), Virgo (♍) and Capricorn (♑) as being cold and dry, linking them to the Melancholic humour.
- In the bottom right corner, the Water signs are listed: Cancer (♋), Scorpio (♏) and Pisces (♓) as being cold and moist, linking them to the Phlegmatic humour. This makes the hermaphrodite figures correspond to the Fifth Element, Ether.

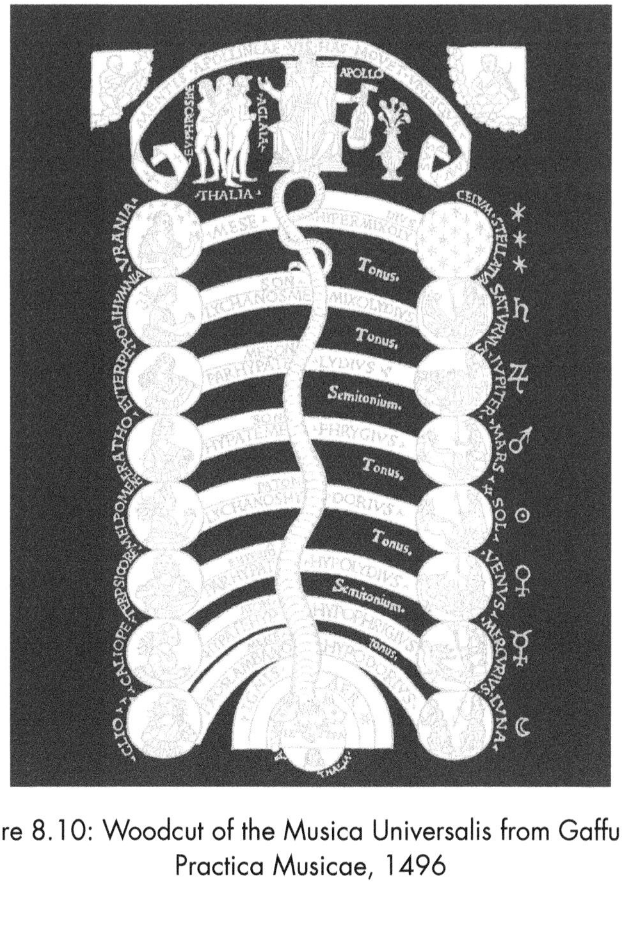

Figure 8.10: Woodcut of the Musica Universalis from Gaffurius' Practica Musicae, 1496

The two masculine sets of Zodiacal signs are on the left-hand side, corresponding to the masculine figure in the middle, while the two feminine sets of Zodiacal signs are on the right-hand side, corresponding to the feminine figure.

In the womb the Soul incarnates through the Four Elements, acquiring a physical body. Thus, the Hermetic Three Worlds can be seen with the Intellectual World corresponding to the labia of the Vesica Piscis. The Celestial World corresponds to the feminine figure with the Zodiacal symbols. The Elemental World corresponds to the masculine figure. Mankind was essentially seen in relation to the heavens.

Within the scriptoriums of the monasteries and nunneries a massive fusion of knowledge from different metaphysical traditions happened during the Gothic era. A particularly fascinating example is this illustration of the *Musica Universalis* from Gaffurius' *Practica Musicae*, 1496.

Here Apollo, ruling music and art, is shown presiding over the Muses and Tones on the left, along with the modes and Planetary Spheres on the right. To the left of Apollo are the Three Graces: Euphrosine (Mirth), Aglaea (Splendour) and Thalia (Comedy).

They stand over the Muses: in descending order, Urania (Astronomy), Polyhymnia (Hymns), Euterpe (Music, song and elegiac poetry), Erato (Lyric poetry), Melpomene (Tragedy), Terpischore (Dance), Calliope (Epic poetry) and Clio (History).

To the right of Apollo is a vase of five flowers, which is a reminder of the Apollonian connection to Five Elements of humoral medicine and the practice of physic. Below the vase are the Planetary spheres, which in Galen's writings are linked to the hidden virtues of herbs.

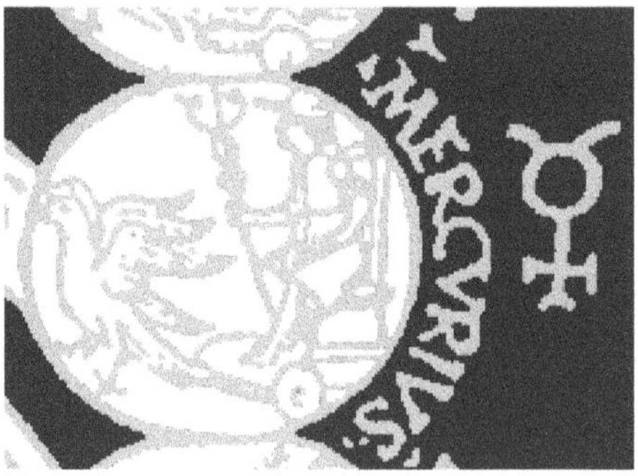

Figure 8.11: Detail of the Caduceus in the *Musica Universalis*

The central snake hanging down alludes to the python of Asclepius and his healing power. The snake has three heads, which would allude to the Caduceus (the insert of Mercury shows him holding a Caduceus) and the Three Alchemical Principles of Sulphur, Salt and Mercury.

A curious detail is Thalia's unhappy face sharing the same sphere of Earth, being confronted by the three heads of the snake. When Thalia is translated as humour rather than comedy, then her second location under the Four Elements is a reference to Hippocrates' humoral physiology.

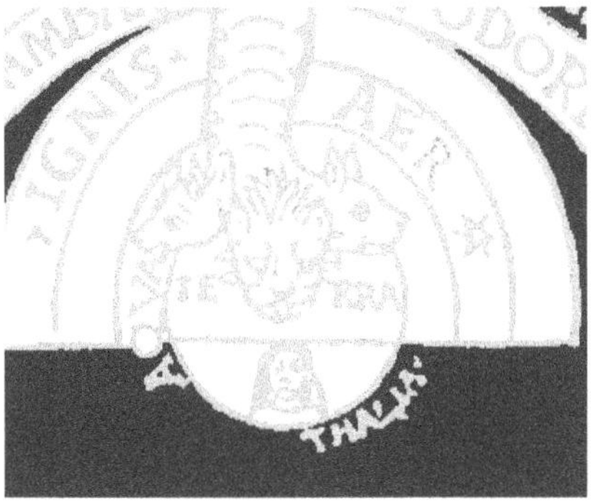

Figure 8.12: Detail of the Snake's Head in the *Musica Universalis*

But as one of the Three Graces that has fallen to Earth, this also symbolically alludes to the Christian idea of the Original Sin and the Fall from Grace resulting from Eve's temptation to eat of the fruits of the Tree of Knowledge in the Garden of Eden, described in the book of Genesis.

The Snake thus combines the Caduceus of Hermes with Snake of Satan in the Garden of Eden and the Python of Asclepius. Thus, this illustration shows the synthesis of Hermetic, Cabalistic and Apollonian teachings all within the Catholic umbrella. It also shows how readily Constantine's translations of Galen and Hippocrates at Salerno were incorporated into the monastic teachings in the Gothic era.

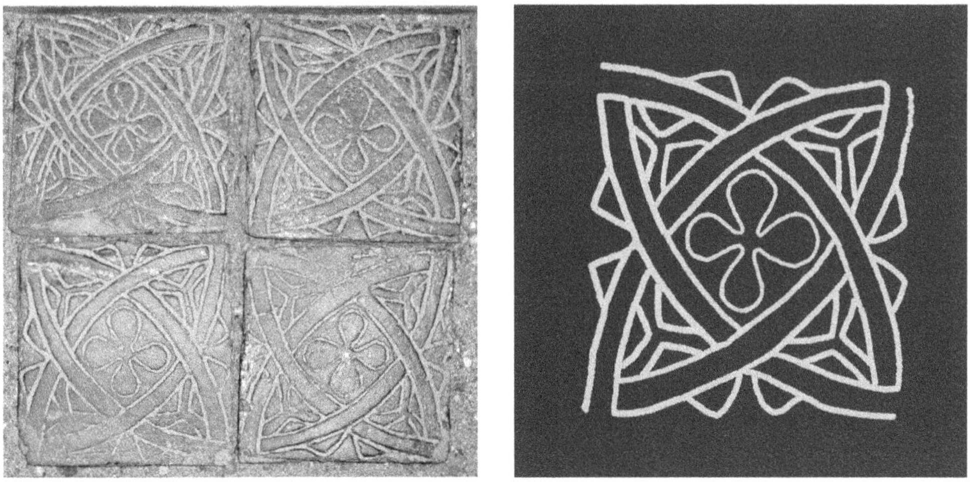

Figure 8.13: Tiles rescued from the floor of Strata Florida Abbey, their surface charred by fire, most likely from when the Abbey was dissolved. Right shows the pattern digitally enhanced

Floral symbolism was commonly used in the decoration of abbeys, cathedrals and churches. This tile motif is one of a number of different floral tile patterns combining geometric symbolism that have been found in the floor of Strata Florida Abbey, a Cistercian foundation, near Tregaron, in west Wales. It consists of two interwoven Vesica Pisces, representing the two pairs of compatible Elements: Fire and Air, and Water and Earth, forming a diagonal cross. Essentially the Vesica are giving birth to the Fifth Element, Ether, represented by the four-petalled flower, within a slightly curved, square space. The flower symbolises the unfolding inner awareness that comes about through the balancing of the Elements within.

In Christian symbolism the Vesica was associated with the Virgin Mary, while the Solar glyph is the Light of Christ. But the magic really happens when several tiles are observed placed side by side.

From walking in prayer or meditation across this section of the floor, monks would have symbolically seen a dynamic interplay of the Solar glyphs with the Vesica Pisces, giving birth to the Five Elements. It is also possible to see the vision the monks had for the herbal kingdom and the interconnection of life.

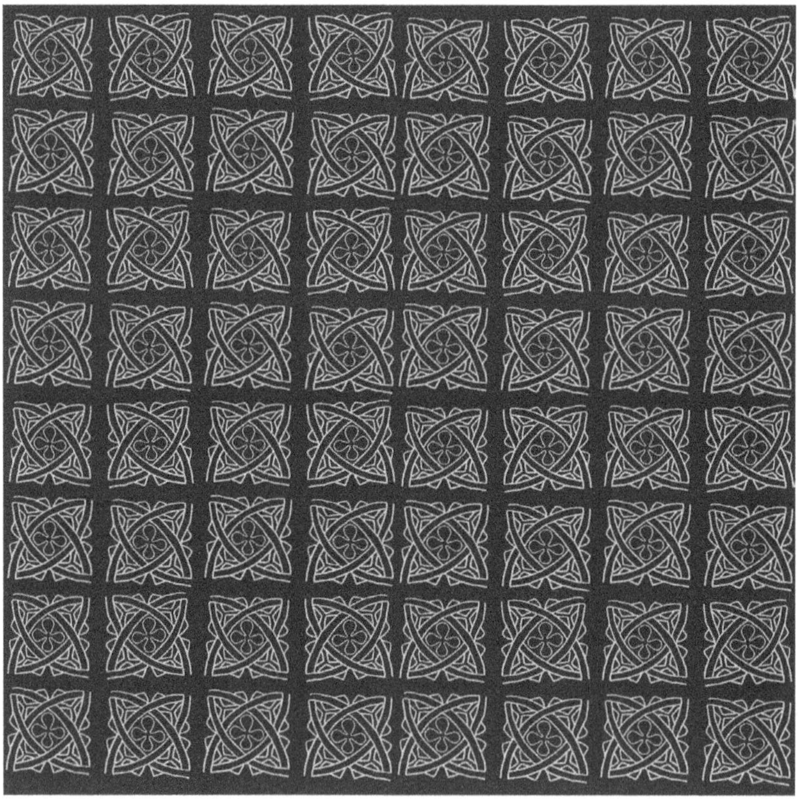

Figure 8.14: Digital projection of the motif from the tiles found in Strata Florida Abbey

This may be why this Abbey derives its name Strata Florida, from the Latin meaning "Layers of Flowers", implying the Elemental layers of awareness and understanding symbolised by the growth and interaction of flowers and herbs. In time the Abbey became the epicentre of Welsh herbal medicine from the quality of the physicians who were trained here. Some of them were rewarded for their skills by being given lands surrounding the Carmarthenshire village of Myddfai. In time they came to be known as the legendary Physicians of Myddfai.

Figure 8.15: Digitally reconstructed motif from the floor of Tintern Abbey

By contrast, another tile motif, from the floor of Tintern Abbey, a Cistercian foundation in the Wye valley, emphasises an inner germination of spiritual awareness. Taking the Solar glyph (☉) as its template, the motif shows that its central dot has multiplied into four seeds, from which four stems have sprouted into a cross pattern, with their apical stellate flowers having penetrated through the circumference of the Circle of the Soul.

At the centre, a cross of trilobed clover-shaped leaves, an emblem of the Trinity, also emerges from the cluster of seeds. Halfway up each flowering stem is found a pair of leaves arranged like the glyph for Aries (♈). Aries being the sign where the Sun is exalted. When it is recalled that Jesus was referred to as Agnus Dei or lamb of God, then the motif shows the transformation of the Soul through the light of Christ, to connect with the light of heaven—in other words, finding the kingdom of heaven within.

CHAPTER NINE

Monastic herbs

Herbs of our lady

Plants that have "lady" in their common name, like lady's mantle (*Alchemilla vulgaris*), lady's smock (*Cardamine pratensis*), lady's bedstraw (*Galium verum*) and lady's thistle (*Carduus marianum*), all refer to Our Lady or the Virgin Mary.

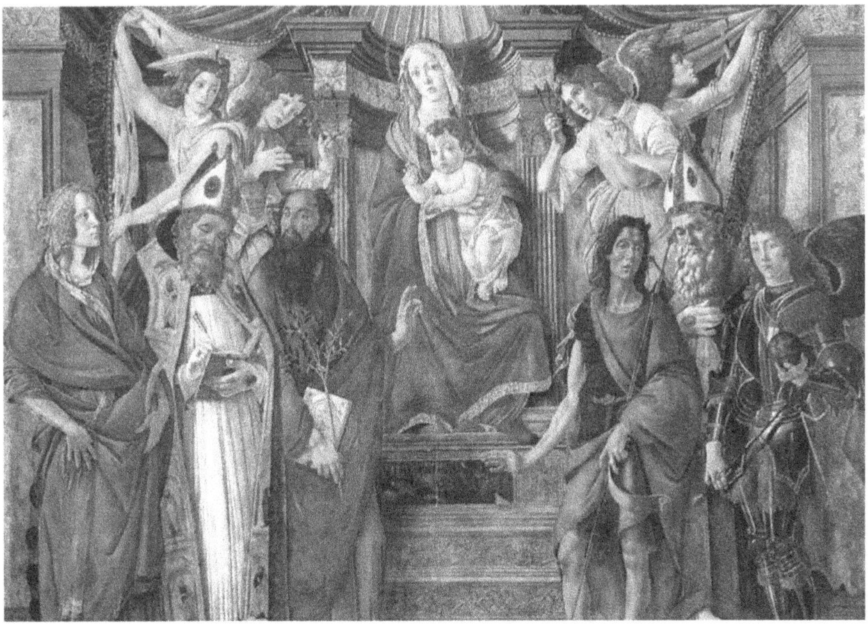

Figure 9.1: Sandro Botticelli's "Virgin and Child with Saints" from the altarpiece of San Barnabas, 1488. Public domain

As has been shown, much of the symbolism of the Virgin Mary was borrowed from the goddess Venus. This is particularly highlighted in Sandro Botticelli's painting "Virgin and Child with Saints". Blue is the colour associated with Venus, and here the Virgin Mary is depicted wearing a blue robe. Venus is born from the waves. In his work "Birth of Venus", Botticelli most famously portrays Venus emerging from a scallop shell. The opening of the scallop shell is symbolic of the opening of the heart to express love. Here Botticelli places the scallop shell above her head, forming her mantle, which is thereby symbolic of her wisdom. Furthermore, the face of the female figure on the left-hand side of the altarpiece is identical to his portrayal of Venus in "Birth of Venus", who gazes adoringly at the Virgin Mary.

In the case of lady's mantle (*Alchemilla vulgaris*), its leaf has seven lobes in the structure. This species is distinct from the garden variety, commonly used as a bedding plant (*Alchemilla mollis*), which has eight to ten lobes in its leaf. The number seven is important, for it connects the virtue of the herb to Venus, which is reflected in the herb being used as a uterine tonic.

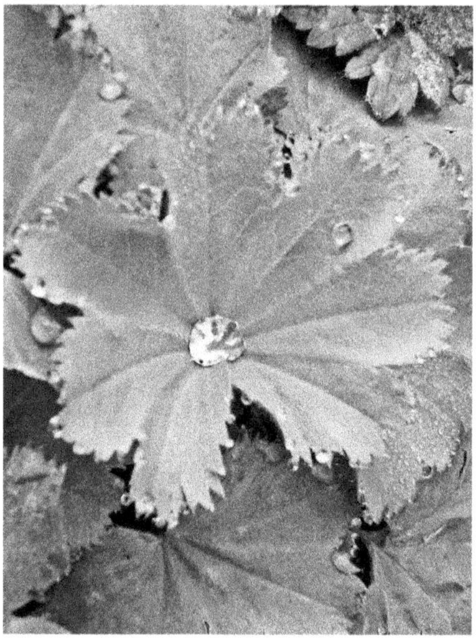

Figure 9.2: Leaves of lady's mantle (*Alchemilla vulgaris*)

The shape of the leaf clearly alludes to the mantle of the Virgin Mary, who, as shown in the "Illumination from Hortus Deliciarum", was the font of the seven streams of wisdom. This herb has long been regarded as magical, for in the cool of the night it becomes bejewelled with dew drops. In the morning, long after the sun has dried out the leaves of other herbs, those on lady's mantle linger and glisten in the sunlight. The water droplets, ducted by the seven veins, collect at the centre of the leaves and were thought as having magical healing powers, imbued with the wisdom of the heavens. Thus, the herb demonstrates the "seven streams of wisdom" being united as one. Hence, the plant was visualised as performing its own alchemy, leading to the Latin name *Alchemilla*.

Plant physiology describes the collection of "dew" in the leaves of lady's mantle as being caused by a phenomenon called guttation. This happens when the water pressure from the roots is too high, and the excess water is forced up through the plant and out through the stomata of the leaves. The tiny droplets collect and coalesce in the channels of the veins, which drain to the central point at the leaf base. This phenomenon, combined with the sevenfold structure of the leaf, becomes the very embodiment of the "seven springs of wisdom".

Lady's mantle is traditionally ruled by Venus, who in myth emerges from the oceans in a shell. The leaf shape of lady's mantle is clearly analogous to Venus' shell, where each lobe can be seen as a mnemonic for the Seven Liberal Arts of grammar, didactic/dialectic, rhetoric, music, geometry, astronomy and arithmetic. At a time when few people were literate, a simple aid like the shape of this leaf would have been very useful to explain the relationship of the seven arts.

Another example of geometry being applied to herbs is found in Solomon's seal (*Polygonum multiflorum*). How does it get such a name?

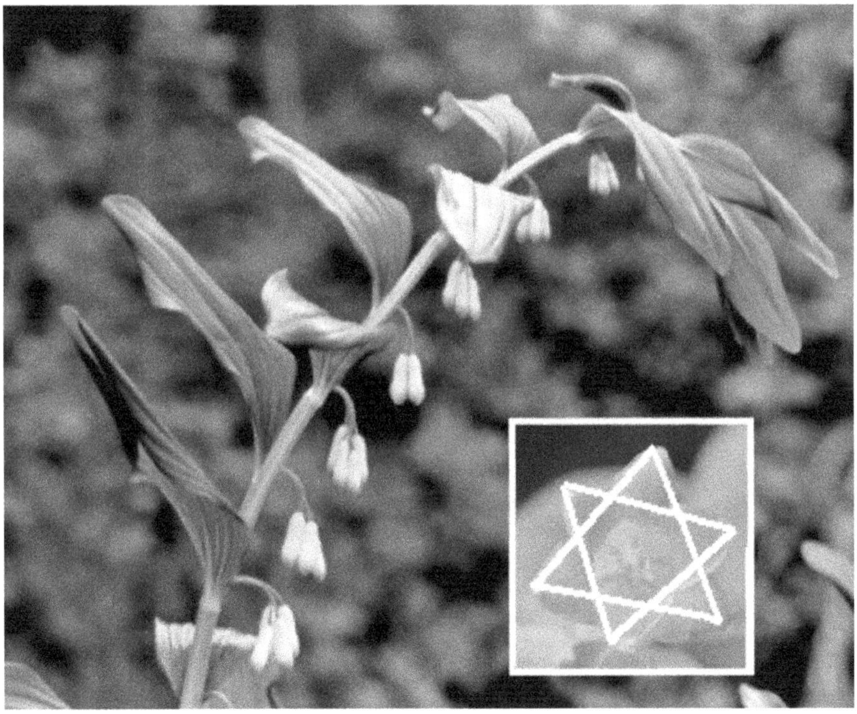

Figure 9.3: Solomon's seal (*Polygonum multiflorum*). Insert: close-up of the flower showing the six-pointed star of Ether

If you read old herbals, it is thought that the plant derives its name from the prominent scars on its rhizome, formed from previous year's flowering, which resembles the imprint of a ring in molten wax. While that would explain the seal part of the name, it does not explain the association with Solomon.

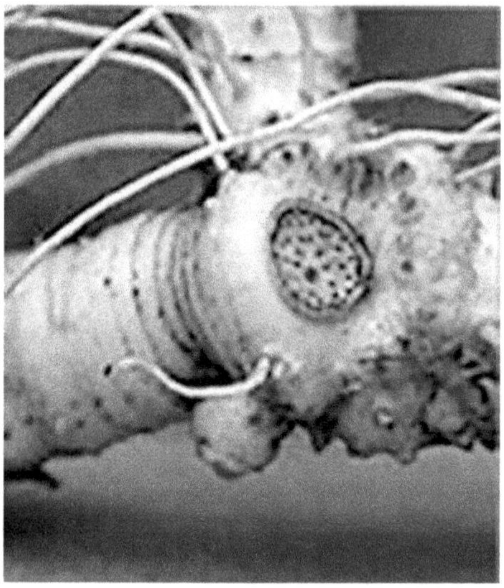

Figure 9.4: The root scar of solomon's seal

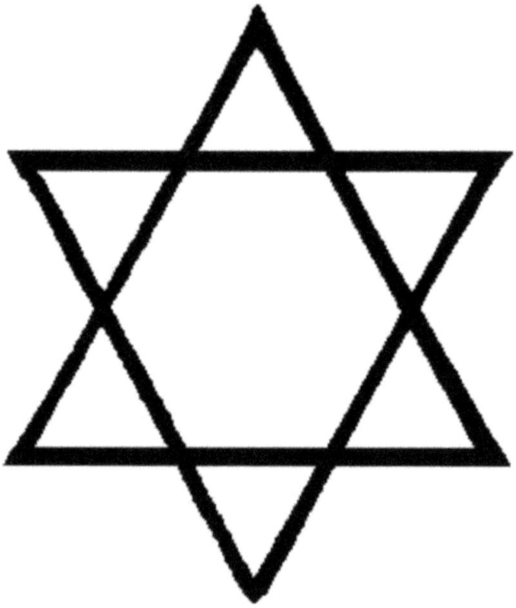

Figure 9.5: The six-pointed star of Ether

The name solomon's seal is in fact another name for the six-pointed star that represents the Ether Element. The enigma is resolved when you look closely at the shape of the flower, for in the arrangement of the petals the lips form a green six-pointed star.

The biblical King Solomon was renowned for his wisdom. So, what wisdom does solomon's seal bring to the practice of physic? As we have already seen in Chapter 1, Ether embodies the four material Elements that were used by Hippocrates to define the four humours within the blood. But there is more to the symbolism of the Elements.

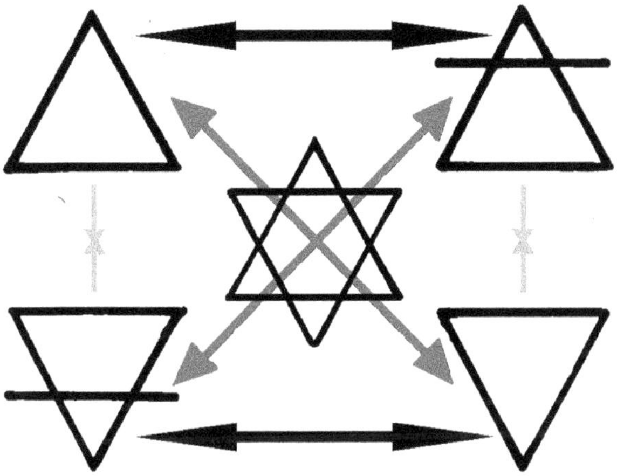

Figure 9.6: The compatibilities and incompatibilities of the Four Elements

There is a whole set of interactions between the Elements, ranging from harmonious to conflictive. The two Masculine Elements, Fire and Air, are compatible, since they are the Elements of combustion. Likewise, the two Feminine Elements, Earth and Water, are compatible, since they are the Elements of fertility and nurturing.

Fire and Water are the least compatible and therefore the most reactive. An excess of Fire evaporates Water, while an excess of Water extinguishes Fire.

Air and Earth are also incompatible but the least reactive. They make contact but remain inert. Inspiring as a mountain peak is to look at, as it soars into the heavens, very little can flourish there. It is a barren combination.

Air and Water are immiscible. Water evaporates into Air, creating mist, fog and mirages. Air ruffles Water, creating bubbles and waves. Fire and Earth are mutually unsustainable: Fire scorches Earth, while Earth does not support Fire.

Similarly, it is possible to see the compatibilities of the Elements in the humours. The Elemental compatibility of the Sanguine and Choleric humours is reflected in the physiological importance of the dynamism of the circulation in transporting oxygen from the lungs to the tissues of the body, whereby the body derives energy. The Elemental compatibility of the Melancholic and Phlegmatic humours is reflected in the maintenance of optimal blood viscosity and the nutritional function.

By contrast, the Elemental incompatibility of the Choleric and Phlegmatic humours is reflected in the heat of a fever and the maintenance of bodily hydration. The Elemental incompatibility of the Sanguine and Melancholic humours is reflected in the thrombotic occlusion of the blood vessels and the causing of anoxia. The incompatibility of the Sanguine and Phlegmatic humours is reflected in the congestion of the lungs by excessive mucus. The incompatibility of the Choleric and Melancholic humours is reflected in the wasting of the resources of the body by a prolonged fever.

You can see how the herb solomon's seal can be used as a mnemonic to explain the Elemental principles of physic. Its drooping flowers are literally bringing this knowledge down to Earth.

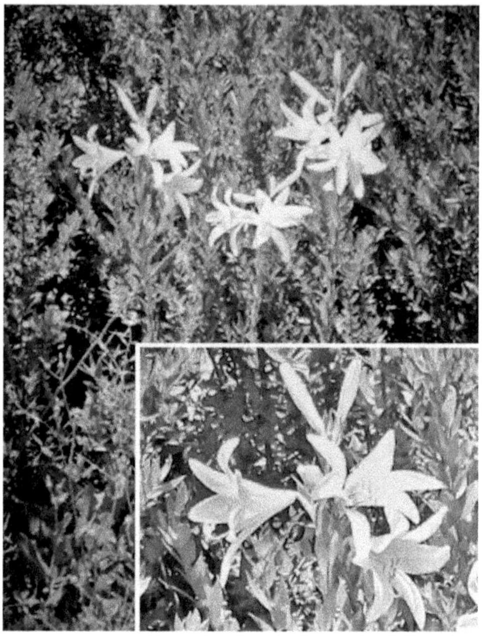

Figure 9.7: Madonna lily (*Lilium candidum*)

The symbolism of the six-pointed flower is taken further with the Madonna lily (*Lilium candidum*), which has been used by artists in their paintings of the Annunciation to depict the Immaculate Conception.

In Christian symbolism Ether is known as the Holy Spirit. Paintings of the Annunciation generally depict the angel Gabriel appearing, bearing a stem of a Madonna lily. The trumpet shape of the flower alludes to the vagina, thus the gift of the lily to the Virgin Mary symbolises her "insemination" by the Holy Spirit. Afterwards the lily is placed beside the Virgin Mary in a vase, which is deliberately shaped like a womb, symbolising that the Immaculate Conception has taken place.

It is noteworthy here that in astrology the Planet Mercury, connected with Ether, is exalted in the sign of Virgo—The Virgin. The sign is traditionally described as the "Joy of Mercury".

Fra Lippi's depiction of the Annunciation, painted around 1450, is particularly interesting in this respect, for when some simple geometric lines are added, more significance become apparent. Geometry and symmetry were often used by medieval and Renaissance artists as the foundation of their compositions. Firstly, in taking a central vertical division, the line separating the painting into two halves links God above at the apex to a Cross of Matter in the tiles of the floor below. The right-hand section depicts the Virgin Mary bathed in Light, while the left-hand section shows the angel Gabriel in shadow, which emphasises the white lily flowers. Gabriel bears a lily stem in his left hand in an analogous way to Mercury bearing the Caduceus, as he announces her conception to Mary.

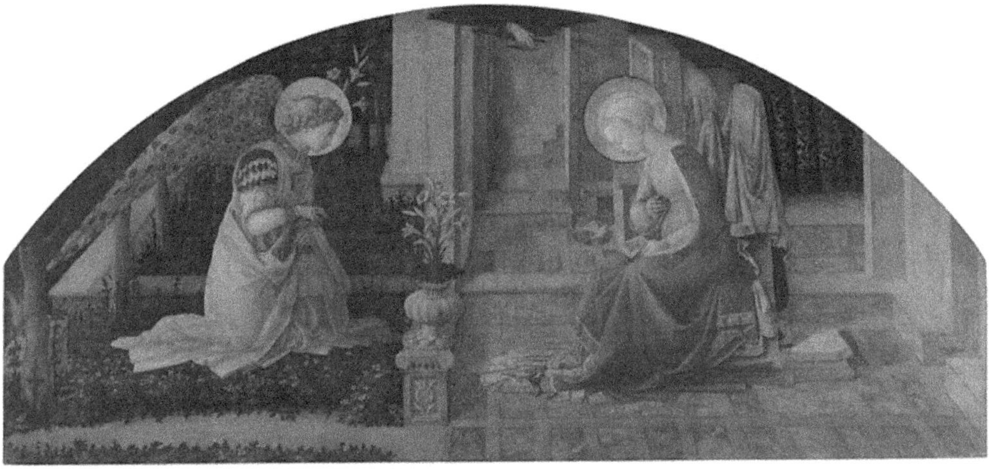

Figure 9.8: Fra Lippi's "Annunciation"

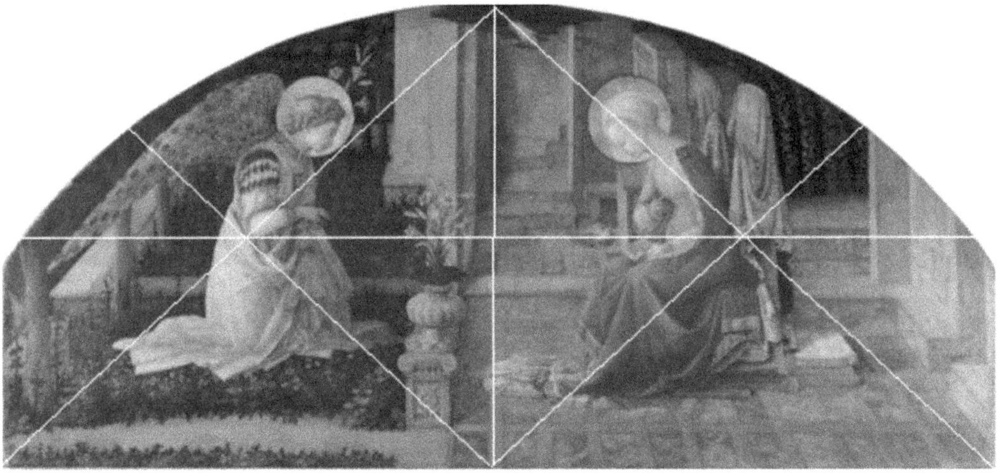

Figure 9.9: The geometry found in Fra Lippi's "Annunciation"

When the diagonal lines are drawn in the squares of each section, the two triangular shapes generated reflect the Hermetic maxim "as above, so below", essentially forming a diamond shape in the middle. Along the diagonal line that leads from the central point at the top, to the bottom right-hand corner, the Hand of God can clearly be seen pointing to the Virgin Mary as the chosen one to be the mother of Jesus.

A horizontal line running through the painting clearly links the lily that has been placed in the vase to the dove of the Holy Spirit, which hovers in the vicinity of Mary's womb in anticipation of its future incarnation of Jesus. It is a visual device that symbolically unites the sixfold shape of the lily to the dove of the Holy Spirit.

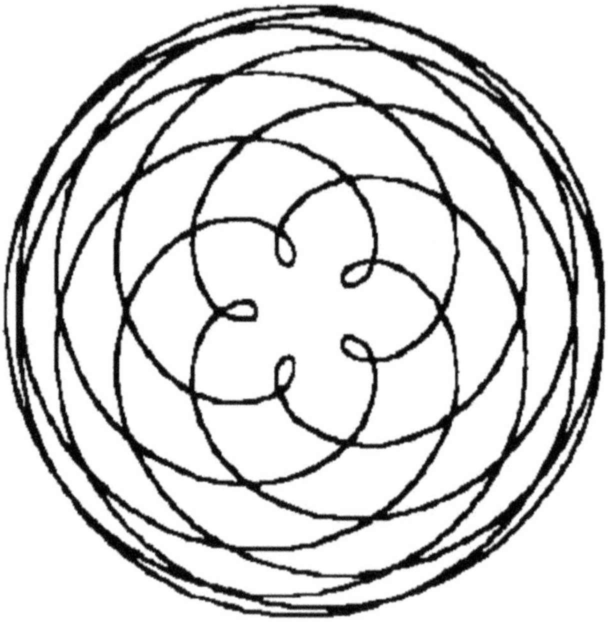

Figure 9.10: The rose pattern of Venus' orbit around the Sun

The rose pattern of Venus' orbit around the Sun is an example of geometry being projected into the heavens. Venus is the brightest Planet in our solar system, and its orbit around the Sun has been observed and held in reverence by astrologers since ancient times.

Every eight years the orbit of Venus, when viewed from Earth, traces a stunningly beautiful pentangular rose-like pattern, known as the "Rose of Venus".

Venus is located inside Earth's orbit around the Sun, and consequently is never observed to be more than 47° away from the centre of the Sun.

The blue planet is only ever visible in the night sky shortly before the Sun rises at dawn or at dusk shortly after the Sun sets. From this phenomenon, Venus is known as Phosphorus, the morning star and Hesperus, the evening star respectively. As Venus' orbit moves closer to the centre of the Sun, its rays obscure her visibility.

In astrology, when a Planet is within 18° of the Sun it is described as "under sunbeams", where symbolically its influence is significantly diminished. Closer still, within 8°, it is described as "being combust", where symbolically its influence is completely overpowered by the light of the Sun.

The one exception to this is the phenomenon of "cazimi", where a Planet is within a degree of being conjunct the Sun, when the light of the Sun symbolically magnifies and radiates the influence of the Planet. This is visible on Earth as Venus' transit across the face of the Sun.

Venus makes two exact conjunctions with the Sun. First is a "superior conjunction", where she is furthest away from the Earth, behind the Sun, making her completely invisible on Earth. Second is an "inferior conjunction", where she is closest to Earth and her silhouette can be observed passing across the face of the Sun. The inferior conjunctions correspond to the inner "loops" seen in the rose pattern of her orbit.

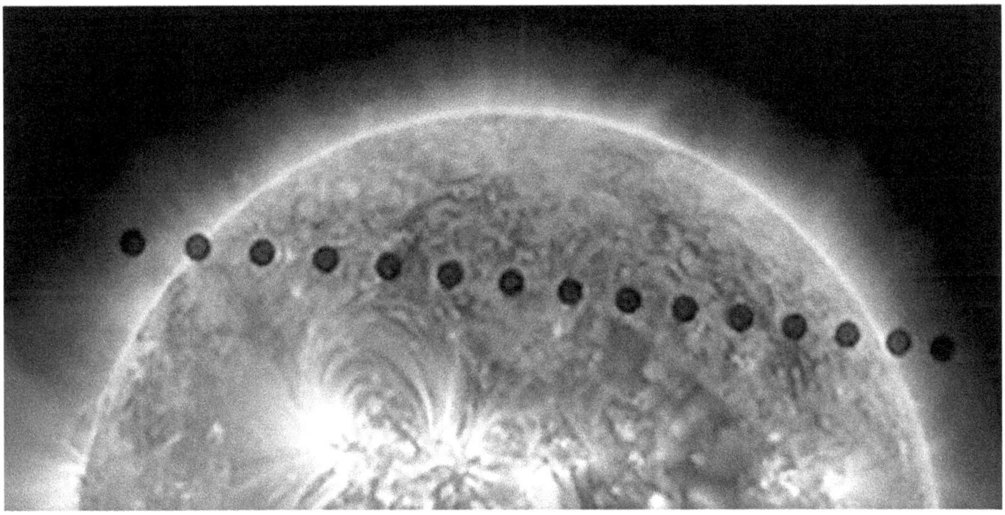

Figure 9.11: The time lapse Transit of Venus across the Sun. NASA

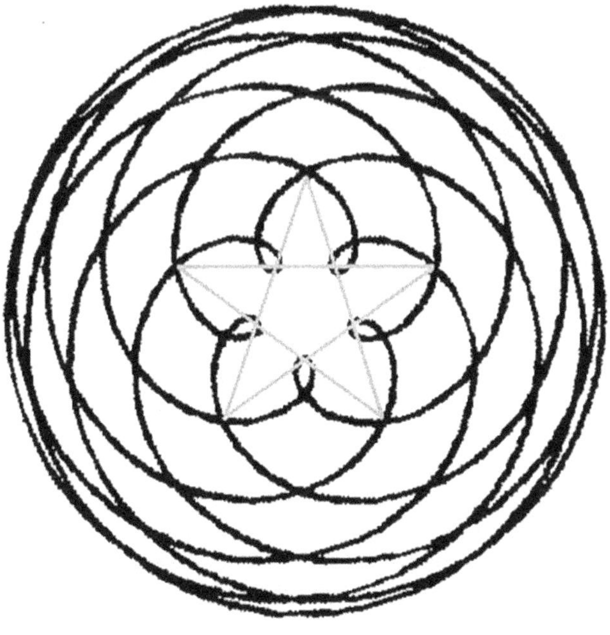

Figure 9.12: The Pentacle generated by the Inferior Conjunction of Venus

The cazimi phenomena of inferior conjunctions were seen to be especially significant, for when Venus, the Planet of love, passes across the heart of the Sun, representing the light of the Soul, it symbolises a transcendent love beyond the constraints of physical existence. Five of these cazimi moments occur within Venus' eight-year cycle, forming an inner pentangular pattern, which has been transposed onto the floral arrangement of herbs. Hence it is linked to the illuminated lives of saints, with their love of humanity.

You can see the Pentacle of Venus reflected in the little five-petalled yellow flowers of wood avens (*Geum urbanum*), which, with its distinctive pointed calyxes, is well known in woodlands at springtime and early summer.

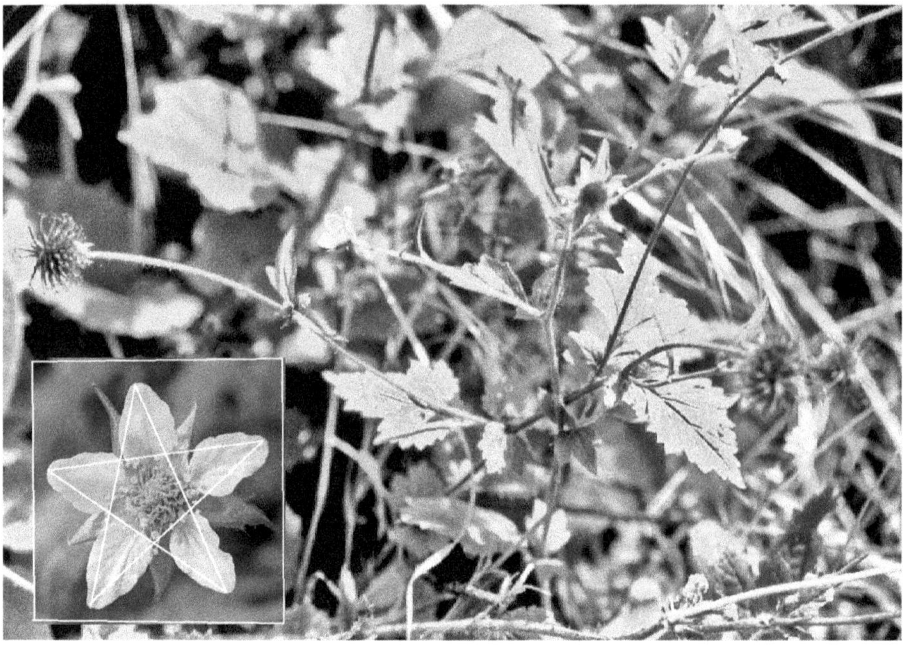

Figure 9.13: Herb bennet or wood avens (*Geum urbanum*)

Far less well known is its alternative common name herb bennet. Even fewer people might recognise that name Bennet was a truncation of the 6th-century Italian monk and mystic, St Benedict from Nursia (c. AD 480–550).

Benedict eventually became the abbot of the monastery at Monte Cassino. History credits St Benedict as being the "Father of Western Monasticism", for he wrote the monastic rules for monks living together under the authority of an abbot, in a work entitled *The Rule of Saint Benedict*.

His instructions became the foundation of the Benedictine Order. It is very appropriate that St Benedict should have become remembered by this humble pentangular-flowered herb.

His monastery at Monte Cassino became famous for acquiring a large number of medical manuscripts. This was the same monastery to which Constantine, several centuries later, retired after his teaching and translation work in Salerno.

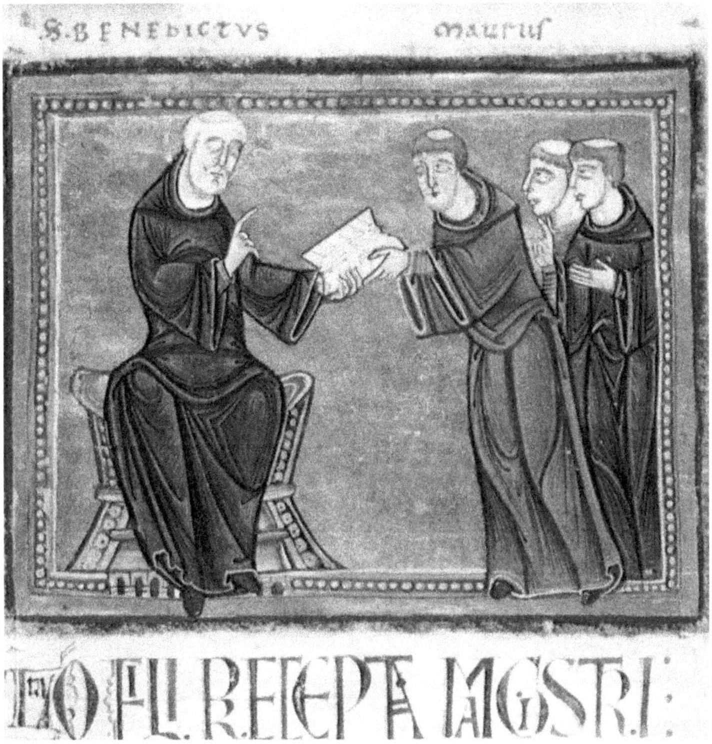

Figure 9.14: St Benedict teaching his disciples. Public domain

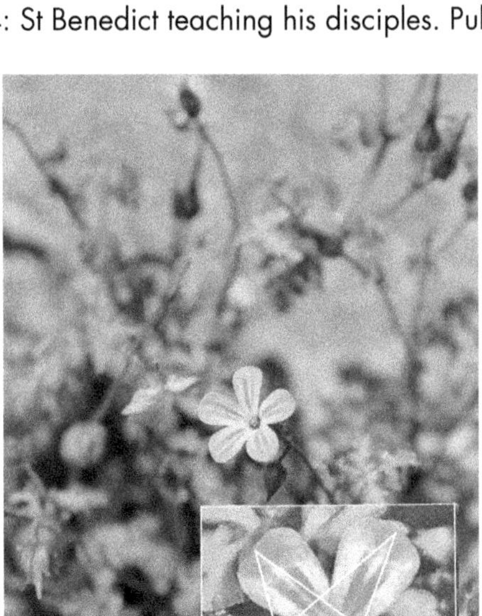

Figure 9.15: Herb robert (*Geranium robertianum*)

Similarly, the little pink pentangular flowers of herb robert are often connected to Saint Robert of Molesme, whose life inspired the birth of the Cistercian order.

Robert was born c. 1028. At the age of 15 he entered the Benedictine abbey of Montier-la-Celle, near Troyes in France, where he became an exemplary monk, and consequently its abbot.

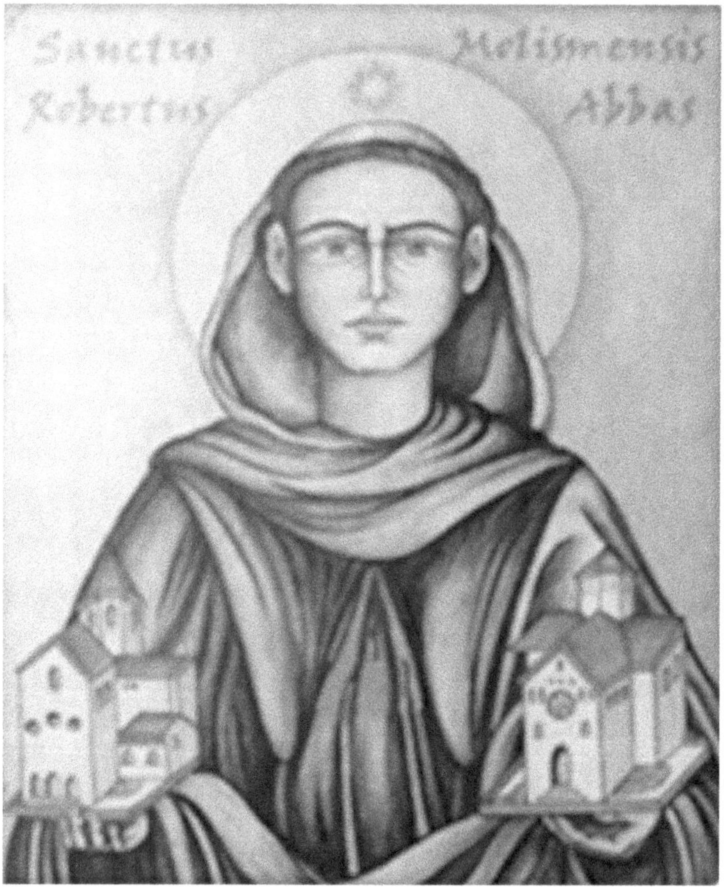

Figure 9.16: Saint Robert of Molesme

In 1070 Robert was asked to become the abbot of St Michel-de-Tonnerre, specifically charged with instilling discipline into the resident monks. However, after two years of trying, he admitted failure in this task, and took the opportunity to move on to become prior of Saint-Aiyoul. In 1075, a number of hermits from Collan persuaded Robert to leave Saint-Aiyoul to found a new monastery at Molesme in the Burgundian valley of Langres.

Under Robert's instructions, the abbey at Molesme quickly became known for its piety and sanctity, and Robert's reputation as a saintly man grew. A group of monks from Molesme went on to found Cîteaux Abbey (Latin: "Cistercium") appropriately on St Benedict's Day, 21 March 1098, determined to follow more closely the Rule of

St Benedict as well as include the principles of the Cluniac reforms. St Robert of Molesme became the first abbot at Cîteaux and remained so until his death on 17 April 1111. Though he did not found founded the Cistercian order, he was revered as being the inspiration behind it.

2 *Roſa rubra.*
The red Roſe.

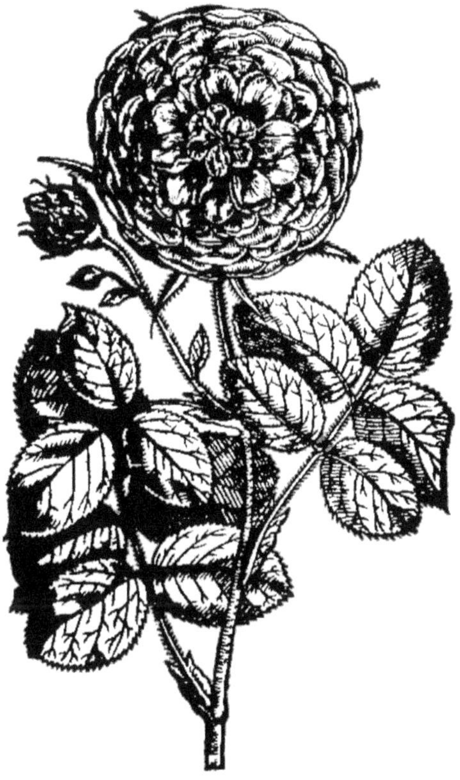

Figure 9.17: Red rose woodcut from *The Herball* by John Gerard, 1633 Edition

The beauty and fragrance of the rose has been synonymous with the Planet Venus for centuries. With love being such an important part of the Christian message, the rose is often seen in Christian artwork and imagery, from ornamentation of illuminated manuscripts and paintings to the geometric complexity of rose windows.

Furthermore, prayer beads are traditionally made from rose leaves, leading to the name "rosary". Clearly these were a key part of the ritual of cultivating divine love.

The opening of the rose is synonymous with the unfolding of the heart, homologous to the lotus flower in Oriental religions. The beauty of the flower arises from its thorny stems, symbolising the power of love to transcend the pain and suffering of worldly experience. The complete opening of the rose resembles the orbital pattern of Venus, thus symbolises the transcendent love of humanity.

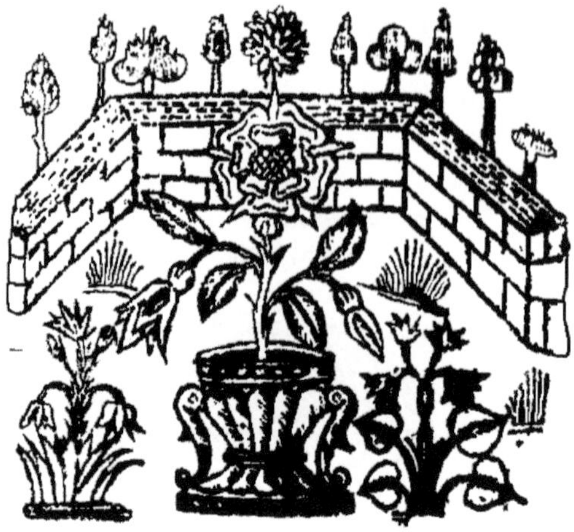

Figure 9.18: Woodcut illustration of a *hortus* or secluded garden

The accompanying woodcut illustration of a *hortus* or secluded garden demonstrates how the rose has been used to describe inner growth. The location of the rose inside an external wall suggests the whole scene is referring to the cultivation of love within the heart.

The rose, with its five-pointed calyx, which corresponds to the Five Elements, is growing out of a pot with two fishes forming its handles.

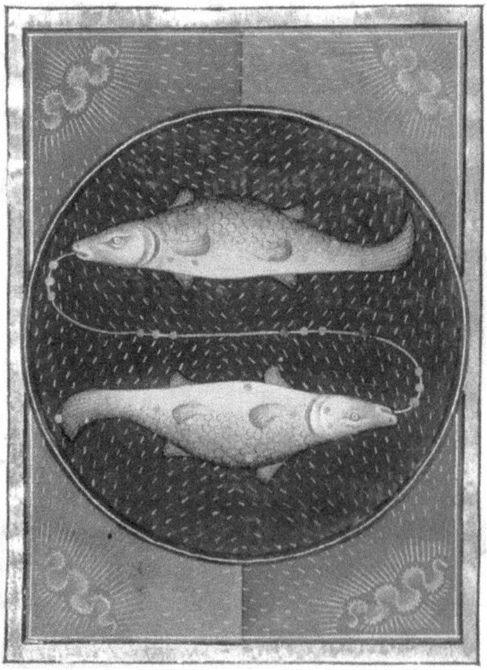

Figure 9.19: Depiction of the two fishes of Pisces linked by a silver thread

The two fishes represent the Zodiacal sign of Pisces (♓), where Venus has her exaltation. The fishes are united by a sacred cord, which shows the struggle in the Soul between sensual indulgence, represented by the lower fish, and spiritual aspiration, represented by the upper fish.

The lilies represent rebirth into Christian teachings, the optimal conditions for enhancing inner growth. The central tree behind the wall is most likely a bay tree, deliberately stylised into an orb, representing the Sun, and the Light of Christ—see Chapter 1. The flowering rose, through cultivating love within the heart, creates inner balance and harmony of the Elements by which a person is able to receive the light of Christ and unfold their spiritual potential. The vase shows both the fish of Pisces pointing upwards, hence the resolution to this struggle.

CHAPTER TEN

The physic garden

In the Gothic era, many monastic institutions had physic gardens, which at the most basic level was a convenient location for the harvesting of herbs utilised by the monks and nuns. However, the design and planting were deliberately created to provide a teaching aid of herbal principles and ultimately a mnemonic of the individual properties of herbs, from their locations in the garden. So, when a physician left the confines of the monastery to practise physic in the community, they simply had to visualise where in the physic garden the herb was growing to recall its medicinal properties.

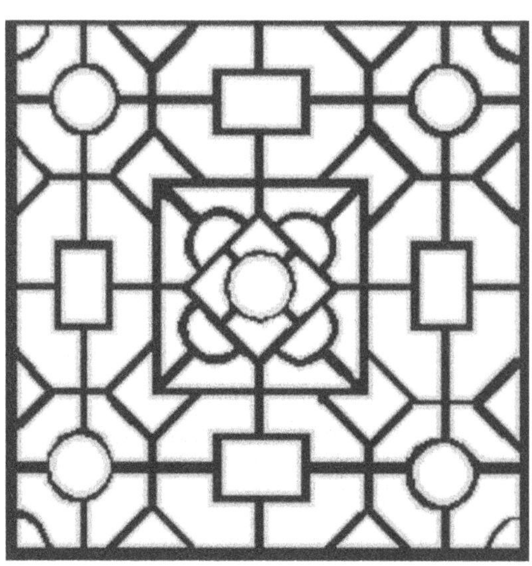

Figure 10.1: A typical layout of a cloistered physic garden

To this purpose the orientation, design and geometry of the garden were carefully considered to enhance its educational role. In essence the physic garden was a mandala of Elemental, Humoral and seasonal correspondences, which symbolically connected with the Hippocratic and Galenic teachings, the basis of medieval medicine. According to the wealth of the institution, the design of the ranged from a simple cross shape within a circular circumference to layouts of highly sophisticated geometric construction, reflecting the cosmology of the medieval Three World view. The planting of herbs within the garden was done in accordance with their Planetary virtues and temperatures.

The spread of the monasteries in the 12th century across Europe became a catalyst for a wave of new learning within their libraries and scriptoriums. The ideas of Hippocrates and Galen were dovetailed into the synthesis of all this new learning and applied in the community, as the monks and nuns tended to the needs of the sick. The physic garden was the embodiment of all this knowledge, forming layers of herbal understanding.

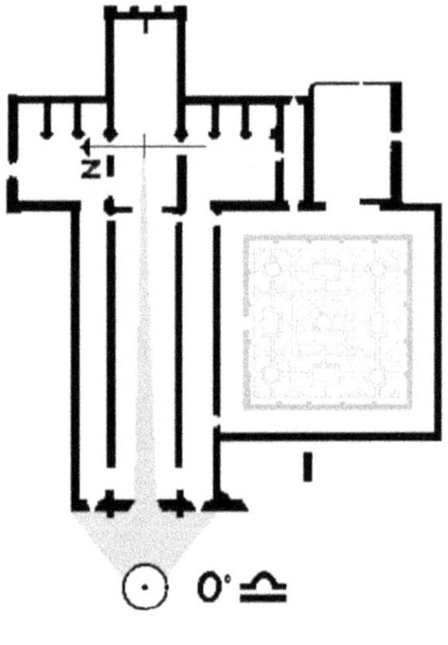

Figure 10.2: The typical location of the physic garden within a monastery

Within the monastery, the physic garden was generally given pride of place at the centre of the cloisters. The cloistered quadrangle was typically adjacent to the abbey on the south side of the nave, with its orientation taking advantage of the East/West alignment of its nave. Cistercian abbeys were all founded at sunset on the Autumnal Equinox, so that the last rays of the Sun shone through the aperture of the West Door along the main nave, creating a perfect East/West axis. The Autumnal Equinox is when the Sun enters the Zodiacal sign of Libra, containing the stars making up the constellation of Virgo—the Virgin, prominent in the Western sky. With the walls of the Church representing the body of the Virgin Mary, and the West Door being stylised as a vulva, the penetration of the sunlight into the nave can be seen to be symbolic of the Immaculate Conception.

The West Door of St David's Cathedral, for example, even shows the stylised representation of the glyph for Libra (♎), alternating through the ornamentation in the stonework of the fourth arch surrounding the door, alluding to the time of the year when the Cathedral was founded. See detail, in bottom right, for greater clarity.

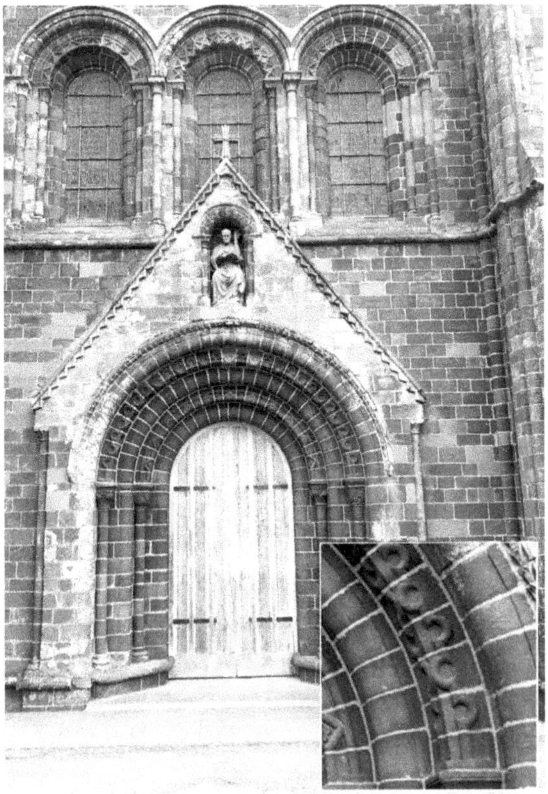

Figure 10.3: The West Door of St David's Cathedral

The physic garden was generally laid out along the axes of the compass, so that the four quadrants symbolically connect with the Four Elements, Humours and Seasons, respectively. At the centre, the central circle represents the Sun, which was often further emphasised by the planting of a bay tree—a Solar tree dedicated to Apollo, which connected to the Hippocratic tradition. In order to keep the tree to a manageable size, it was regularly pruned to preserve a spherical shape as a further reminder of the celestial orb it represents.

With the Sun at the centre of the quadrants, the southeast square is connected to Spring, the Air Element and Sanguine humour. The southwest square is connected to Summer, the Fire Element and Choleric humour. The northwest square is linked to Autumn, the Earth Element and the Melancholic humour. Finally, the northeast square to Winter, the Water Element and the Phlegmatic humour.

In turn, the four squares to the physic garden would correspond to Galen's Elemental progression through the seasons, as shown in the diagram. In the days following the Spring Equinox, the increasing elevation of the Sun daily creates more heat, which dries out the moisture left over from the Winter (Phlegmatic) season.

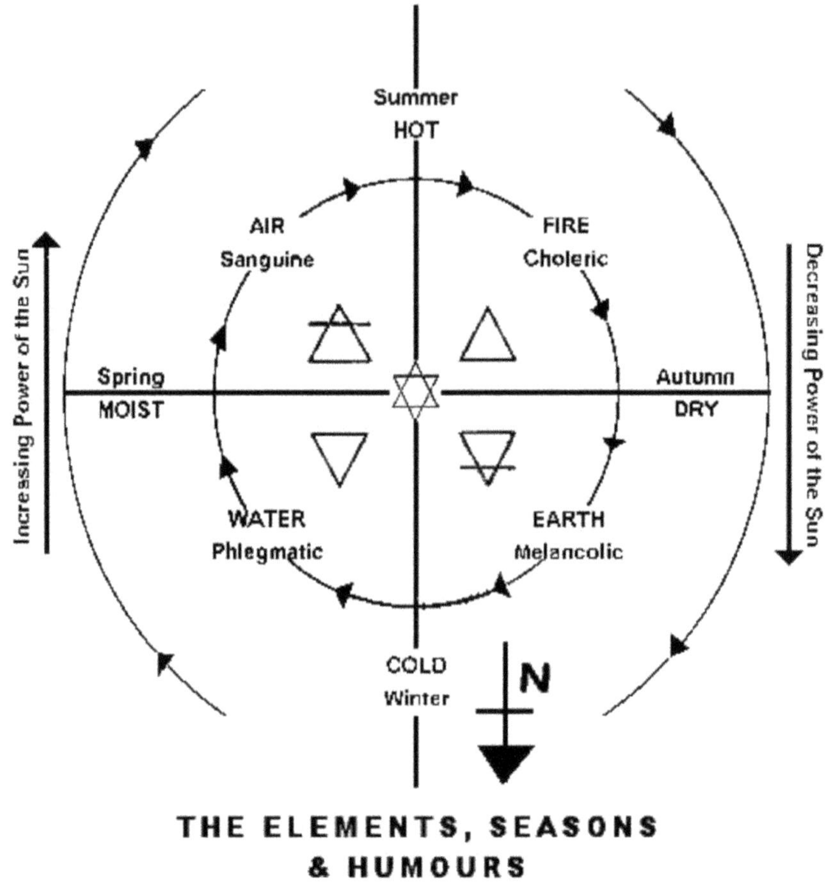

Figure 10.4: The annual cycle of the Elements, Seasons and Humours

Hence, with all the evaporation, the atmosphere feels hot and moist—the very qualities of the Air Element, which rules the Sanguine humour. The first leaves (Air) of sprouting seeds emerge from the soil, while the leaves on woody plants unfurl, to begin their interaction with the Air Element. Thus, the Sanguine humour was visualised as predominating in the Spring.

At the Summer Solstice, the Sun reaches its zenith and its heat dries out any remaining moisture from the Spring. Plants too, generally have reached the zenith of their flowering (Fire) cycle, having attracted pollinators and set seed. After achieving this climax, the flowers fade and the plants start to become desiccated.

Hence, the atmosphere feels hot and dry—the very qualities of the Fire Element, which rules the Choleric humour. Thus, the Choleric humour was visualised as predominating in the Summer.

At the Autumnal Equinox, the Sun starts to lose its heat for the year, the frosts arrive and the Earth cools down. The energy of herbs retreats into its roots (Earth) and tubers within the Earth, while scattered seeds become lodged in crevices in the soil. The atmosphere becomes cold and dry—the very qualities of the Earth Element, which rules the

Melancholic humour. Thus, the Melancholic humour was visualised as predominating in the Autumn.

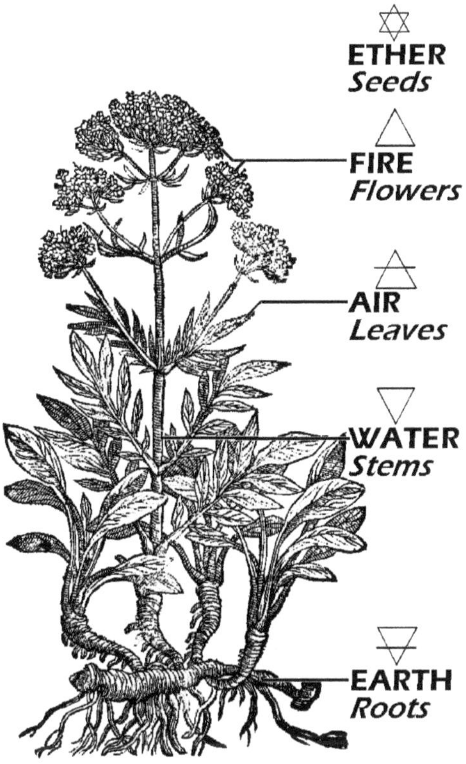

Figure 10.5: The Elemental correspondences to the parts of a plant

At the Winter Solstice the Sun's power is at its lowest ebb. It has insufficient heat to dry out the moisture that accumulates from winter rain and snow. The Water, however, starts the germination of seeds (Ether), and the unfolding of the next cycle of their Elemental stages. Hence, the atmosphere feels cold and moist—the very qualities of the Water Element, which rules the Phlegmatic humour. Hence, the Phlegmatic humour was visualised as predominating in the Winter.

The five circular beds contained in the garden layout would reflect the cosmology of the Five Elements. The central bed would represent Ether, their quintessence, while the circular beds in each quadrant would represent the Four material Elements. Thus, clockwise from the top left quadrant, the circular bed would represent Air, surrounded by its association of herbs with the Sanguine humour. In the top right quadrant, the circular bed would represent Fire, surrounded by its association of herbs with the Choleric humour. In the bottom right quadrant, the circular bed would represent Earth, surrounded by its association of herbs with the Melancholic humour. In the bottom left quadrant, the circular bed would represent Water, surrounded by its association of herbs with the Phlegmatic humour.

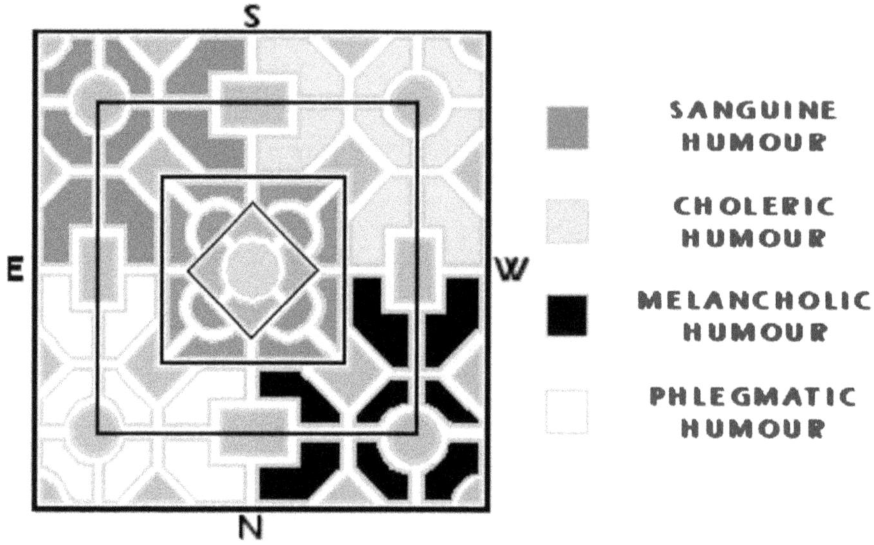

Figure 10.6: Arrangement of the beds according to the seasons

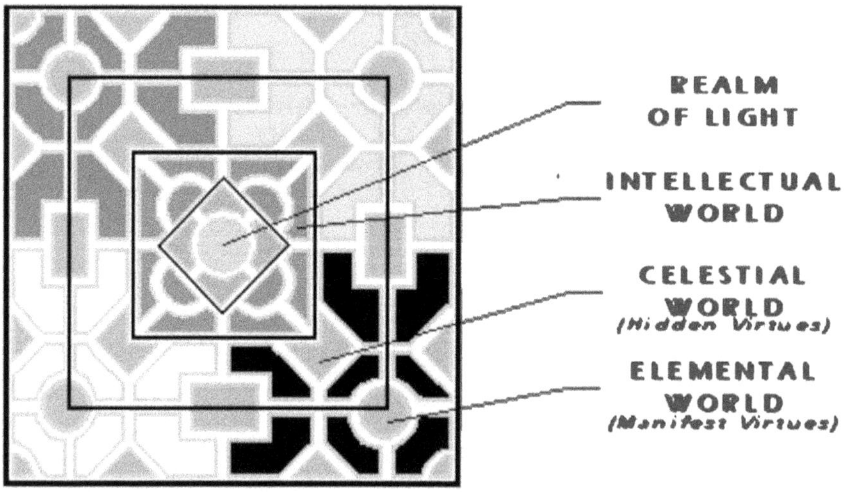

Figure 10.7: Hermetic Three World view in relation to the beds

As has been shown in Chapter 4, the Four material Elements were used to visualise the Hermetic Three World view. The order of these Worlds—the Elemental World, the Celestial World, the Intellectual World and the Realm of Light—is represented by the three concentric squares, with the central diamond shape, respectively. The Celestial World is ruled by the Planets, as used by Galen to describe the Hidden Virtue of the herbs. The Elemental World is ruled by the Elements, whose qualities of hot, cold, dry and moist were used by Galen to describe the Manifest Virtue of the herbs.

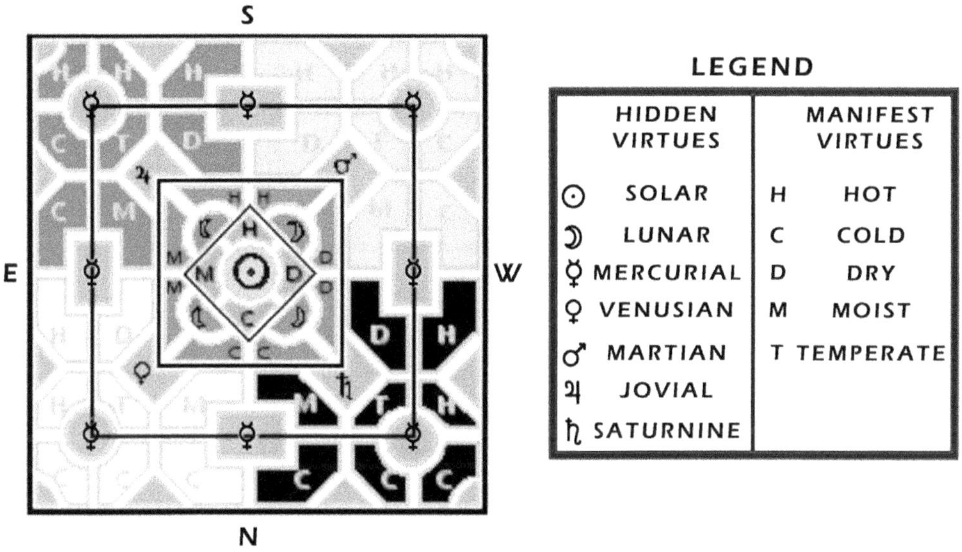

Figure 10.8: The Planetary Virtues and temperatures of the beds

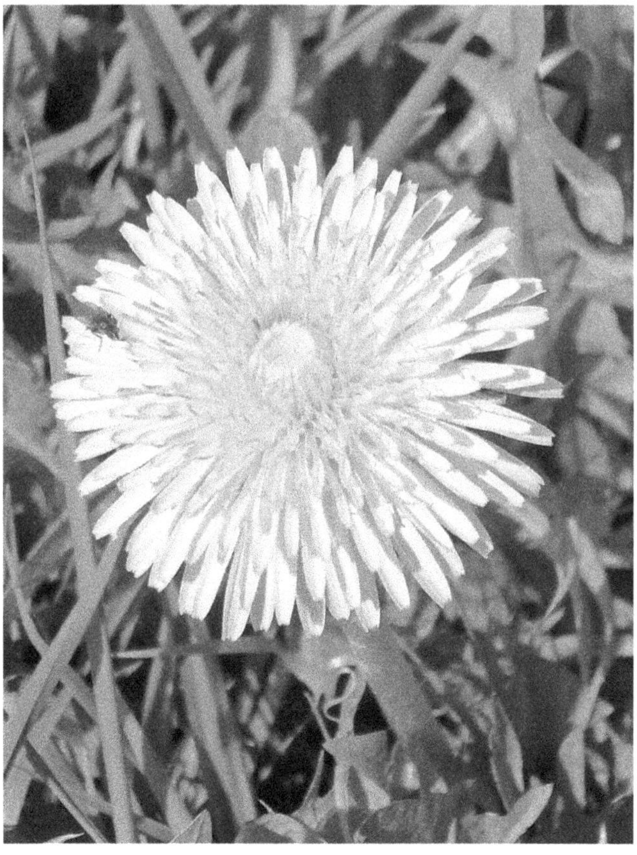

Figure 10.9: Dandelion (*Taraxacum officinale*)

To illustrate the principles of how a physic garden works, a number of herbs can be hypothetically placed within it. If you take the dandelion (*Taraxacum officinale*), it is traditionally ruled by Jupiter and its temperature is identified as temperate and drying to the 1st degree (TD1). The Jovial rulership of the herb (F) connects it to the southeast quadrant of Spring and the Sanguine humour. It is temperate and dry, so it is placed (X) in the temperate bed, next to the bed of drying plants.

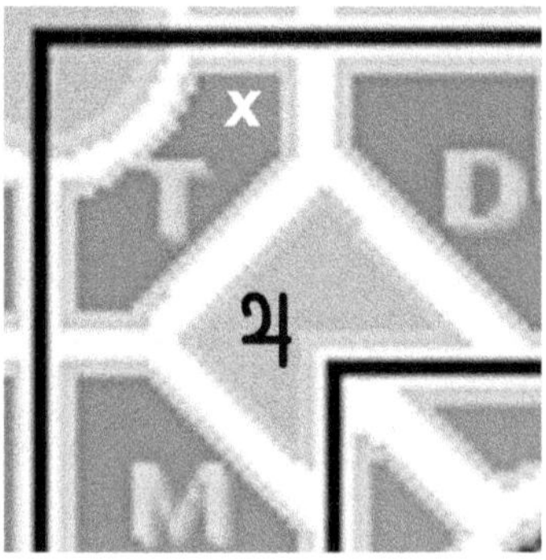

Figure 10.10: Location of dandelion (x)

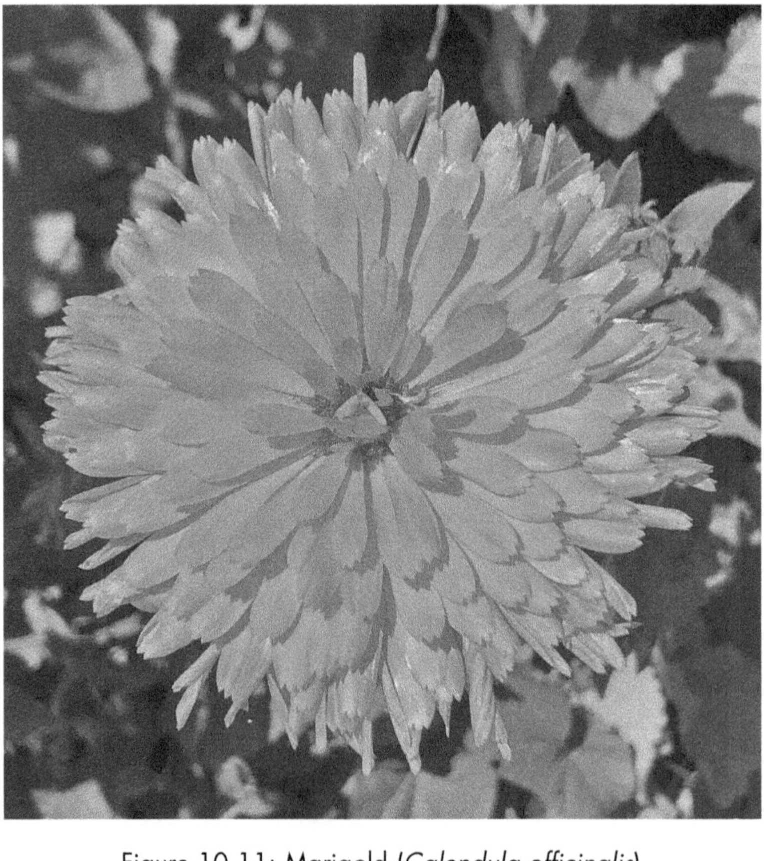

Figure 10.11: Marigold (*Calendula officinalis*)

Another healing herb very likely to have been included would have been marigold (*Calendula officinalis*). Here its Solar virtue would have indicated that it should be planted in one of the central beds. Its temperature is hot and dry to the 1st degree (H1D1), so its placing would be in the hot bed, closest to the adjacent dry bed.

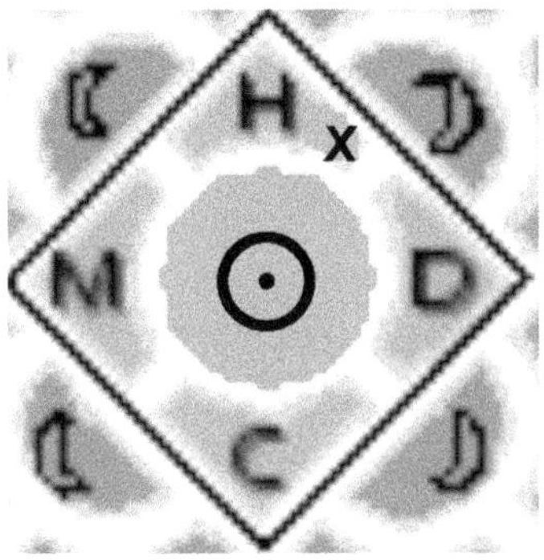

Figure 10.12: Location of marigold (x)

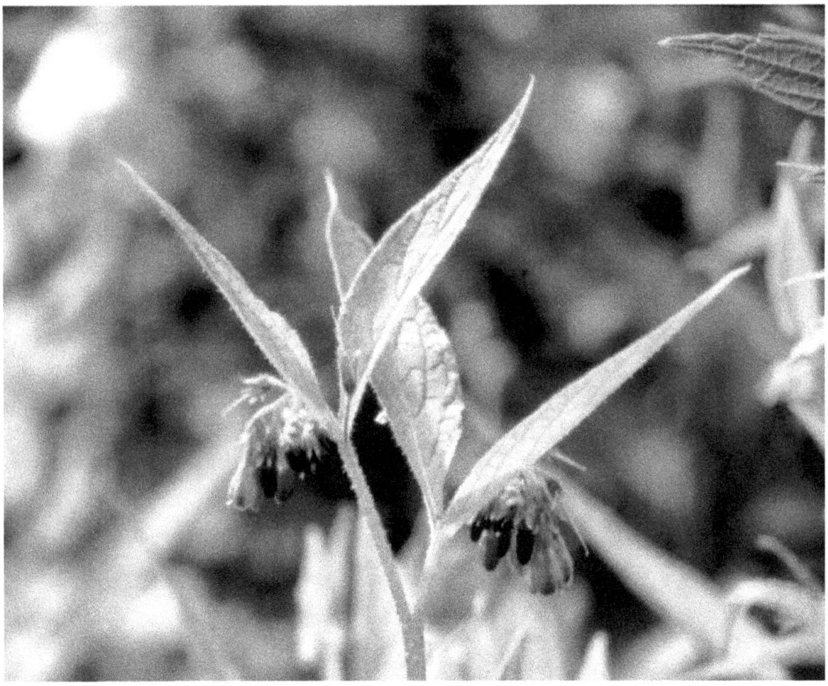

Figure 10.13: Comfrey (*Symphytum officinale*)

No medieval physic garden would have been without comfrey (*Symphytum officinale*). Its Saturnine virtue, along with its temperature being cold and moist to the 3rd degree (C3M3), would have connected it to the northwest quadrant of Autumn and the Melancholic humour. It is cold and moist, so it is placed (X) in the cold bed, closest to the adjacent moist bed.

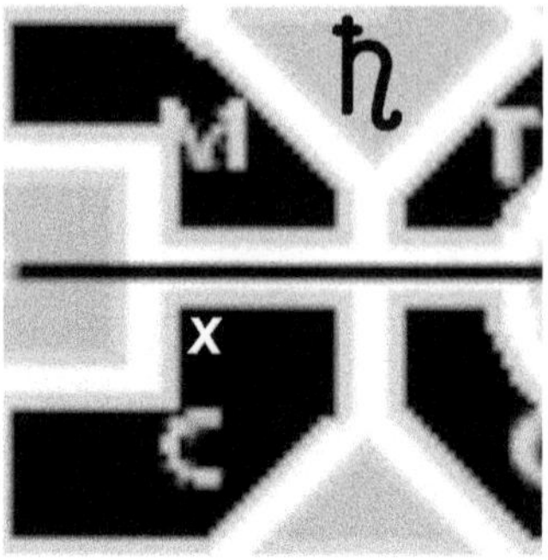

Figure 10.14: Location of comfrey (x)

Using these principles each physic garden would have evolved into a unique arrangement of medicinal herbs. The planting was a combination of herbs found in the location surrounding the monastery with those traded from further afield, in the form of roots and seeds. The design and layout of the beds may have varied between monasteries, but the metaphysical principles on which it was based remained the same.

Tending to the herbs, to maintain their positions in the garden beds, would have served to help aspirants memorise the principles of physic. Even simply walking around the cloisters would have been a meditation on the living herbal mandala.

Having been trained within the monastery, when the monks and nuns left to tend to the sick in the community, as they saw the herbs growing in the hedgerows and gardens, they would have had a visual link to their location in physic garden pf their monastery, reminding them of their herbs' virtues. Alternatively, having made a diagnosis of which humours were out of balance within the visited patient, they could visually refer to the physic garden for herbal options. Thus, if the patient had a fever, displaying an excess of the Choleric humour in the blood, then they could visualise what herbs were growing in the northeast quadrant linked to the Phlegmatic humour. Those that are cooling in temperature would have been especially suited.

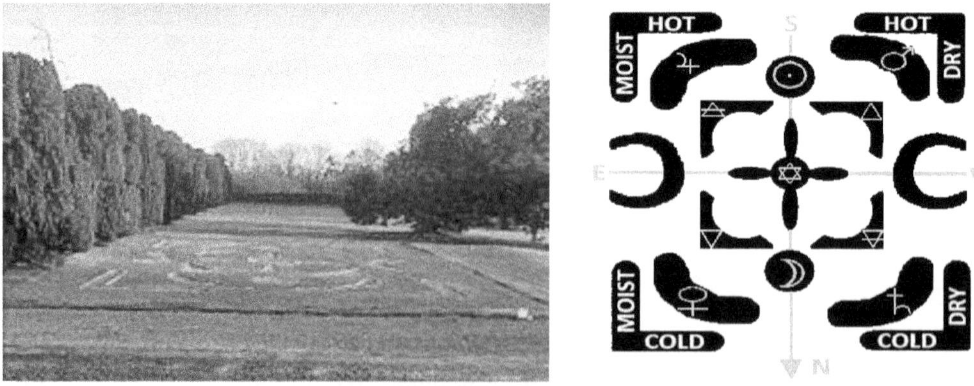

Figure 10.15: Looking down onto the beds of the former physic garden at Knoctopher Abbey, in Ireland. Right: Suggested planting scheme

L'Orto Botanico di Padova

In the 16th century, released from the confines of a cloistered quadrant, the metaphysical principles incorporated into a physic garden reached new heights in the founding of L'Orto Botanico di Padova. This was when Venice was at the height of her trading powers, and plants were brought back from all over the world, including those from the opening up of the New Worlds. Space for a physic garden within the canalled city of Venice was extremely limited, so the walled garden came to be constructed in Padua (Padova), on the mainland.

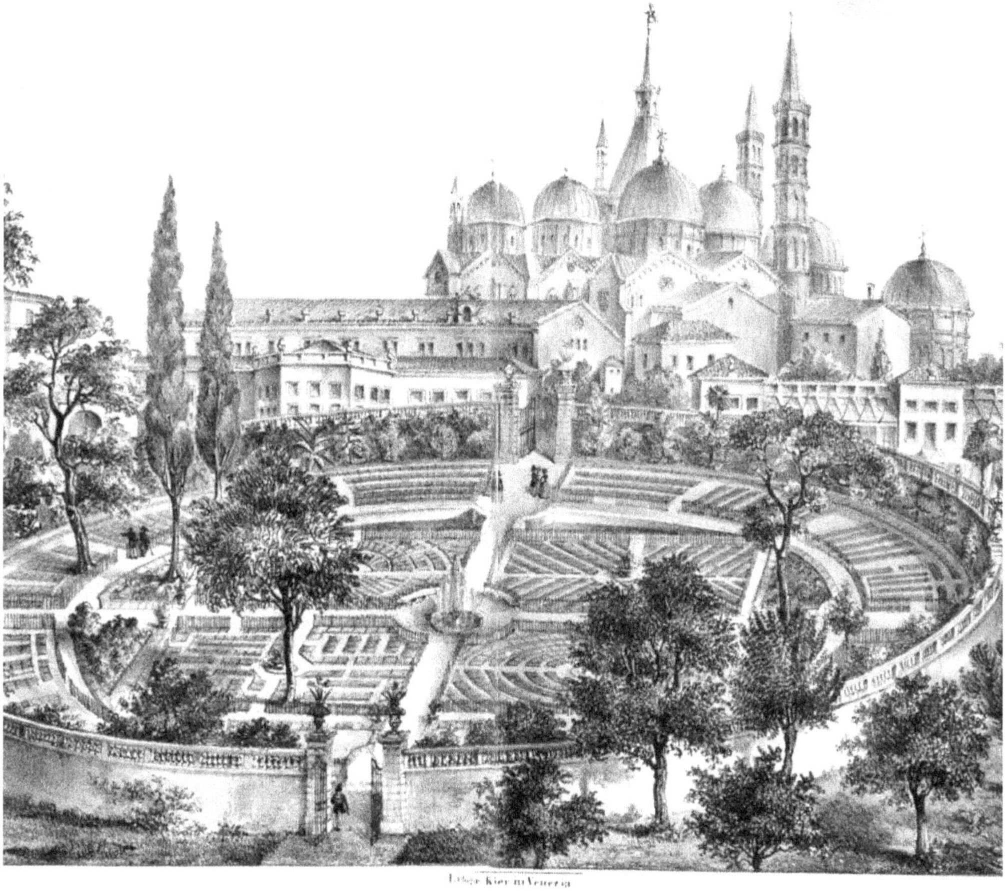

Figure 10.16: L'Orto Botanico di Padova, 1545

In response, the L'Orto Botanico was created, which became the first physic garden in the world outside a monastery. Its design incorporated Galen's principles of physic. The architect was Daniele Barbaro, a Venetian nobleman, a man of vast learning who translated Vitruvius' work *De Architectura*. Consequently, the design of the original botanic garden was based on Vitruvian architectural ideas, which explored the relationship of the Circle and the Square, within the geometry of the Terraces.

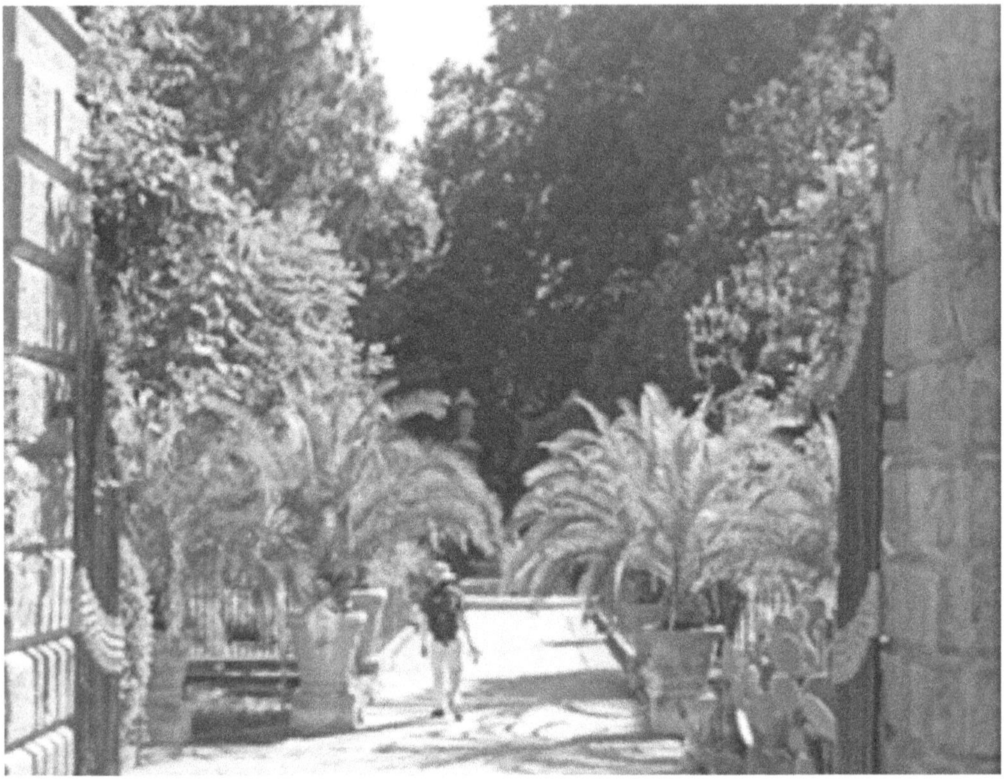

Figure 10.17: View through Main Gate into l'Orto Botanico di Padova

Vitruvius' ideas are perhaps most well-known through Leonardo De Vinci's drawing of "Vitruvian Man". Most commentators think of Leonardo, in this drawing, exploring the proportions of the human body. However, there is symbolic significance in the Man standing betwixt a Square and a Circle, for the Square represents Earth while the Circle represents Heaven. Thus, Mankind is depicted standing between Heaven and Earth.

The original design of the botanic garden also explores the relationship of the Square and the Circle, for in the geometry of the Terraces, in Galen's Hermetic vision, plants too stand between Heaven and Earth.

The astrological symbol for Planet Earth is a Cross within a Circle (M). It can be easily seen how this symbol forms the template upon which the garden, with its four terraces, is based. The four segments within the symbol correspond to the Four Elements on Earth.

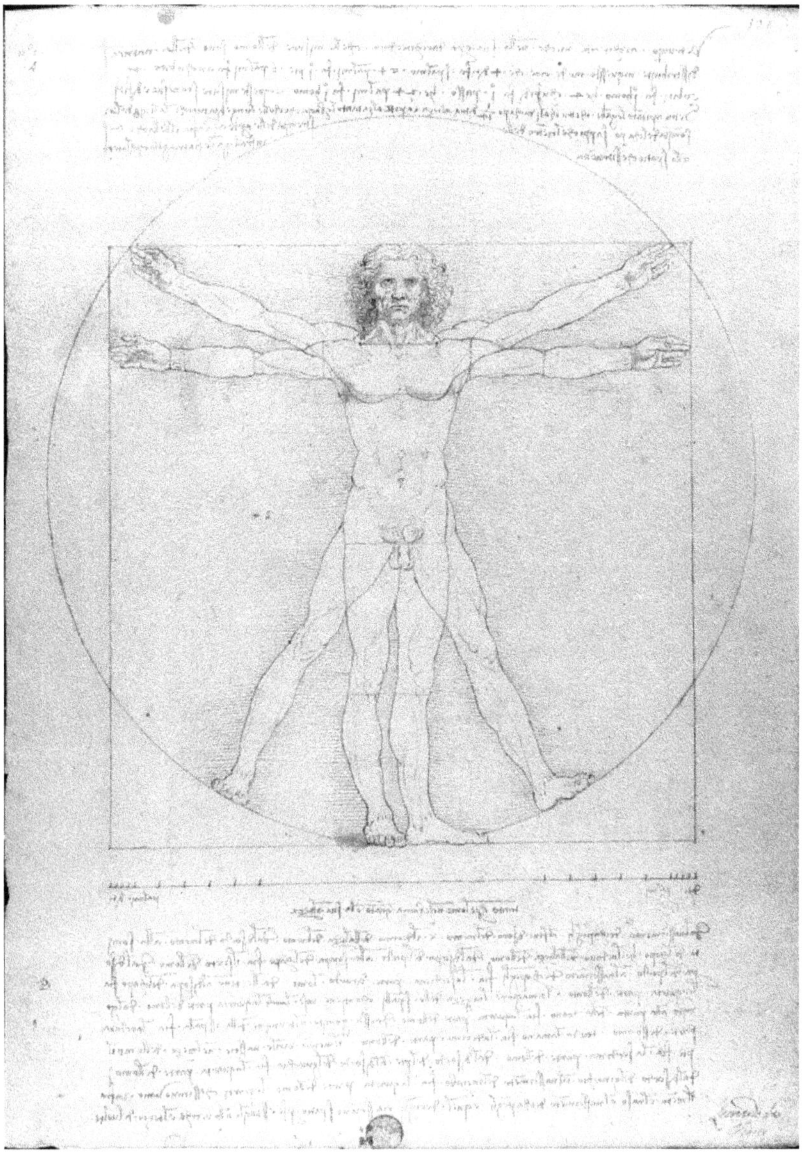

Figure 10.18: Leonardo de Vinci's depiction of Vitruvian Man. Public domain

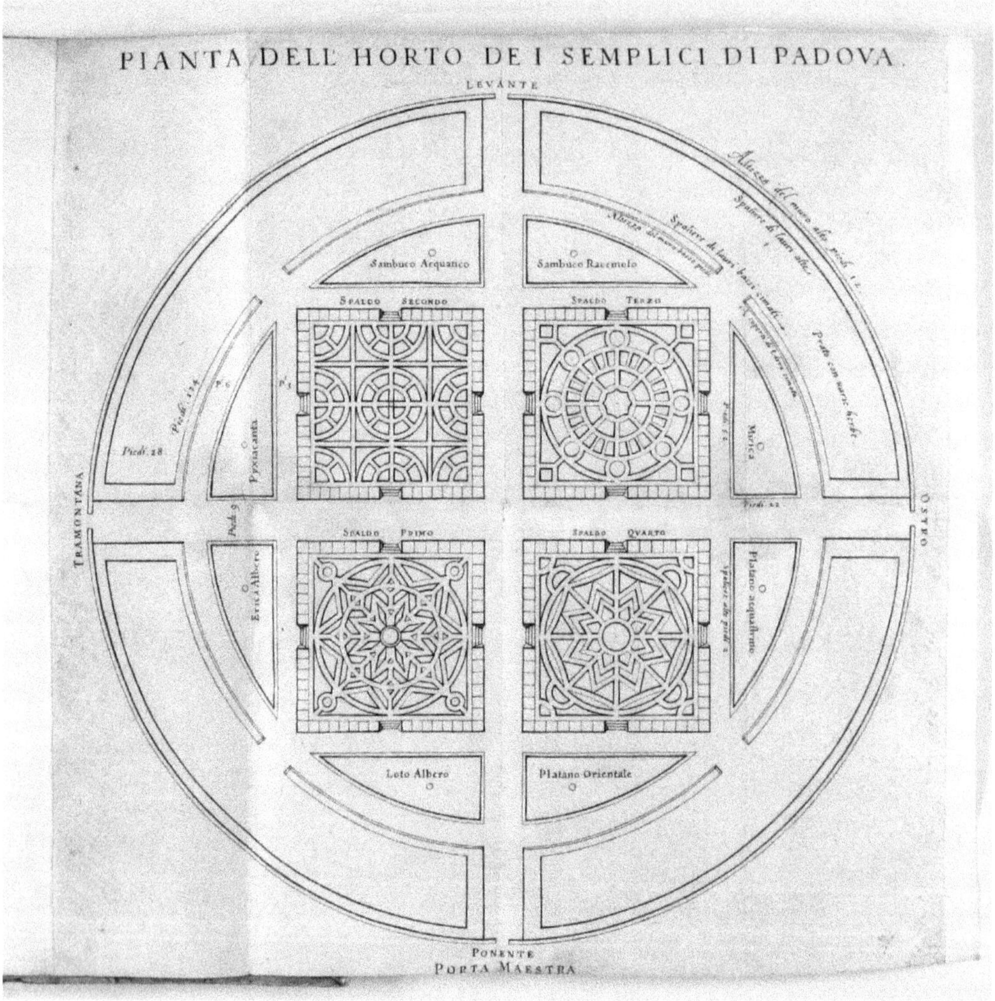

Figure 10.19: The original plans of L'Orto Botanico di Padova, 1545

The extra space in the L'Orto Botanico di Padova allows for the representation of the Four Elements, within each of the four terraces, for each season.

Each terrace is composed of a well-defined perimeter Square, surrounded by beds. These, I would suggest, are trial beds, for when new plants were brought back to Padua, their virtues and the characteristics would have been largely unknown. This enabled plants to be observed, investigated and their temperatures ascertained before being relocated to a more appropriate location in the terrace.

Each terrace has a central point corresponding to the dot of the Sun (☉), so the design of all the terraces explores the dynamic interplay between the Sun and Earth through the seasons. With the Sun generating the Vital Force, the paths can be seen as representing the Vital Force permeating all the constituent beds, like the venation of a leaf.

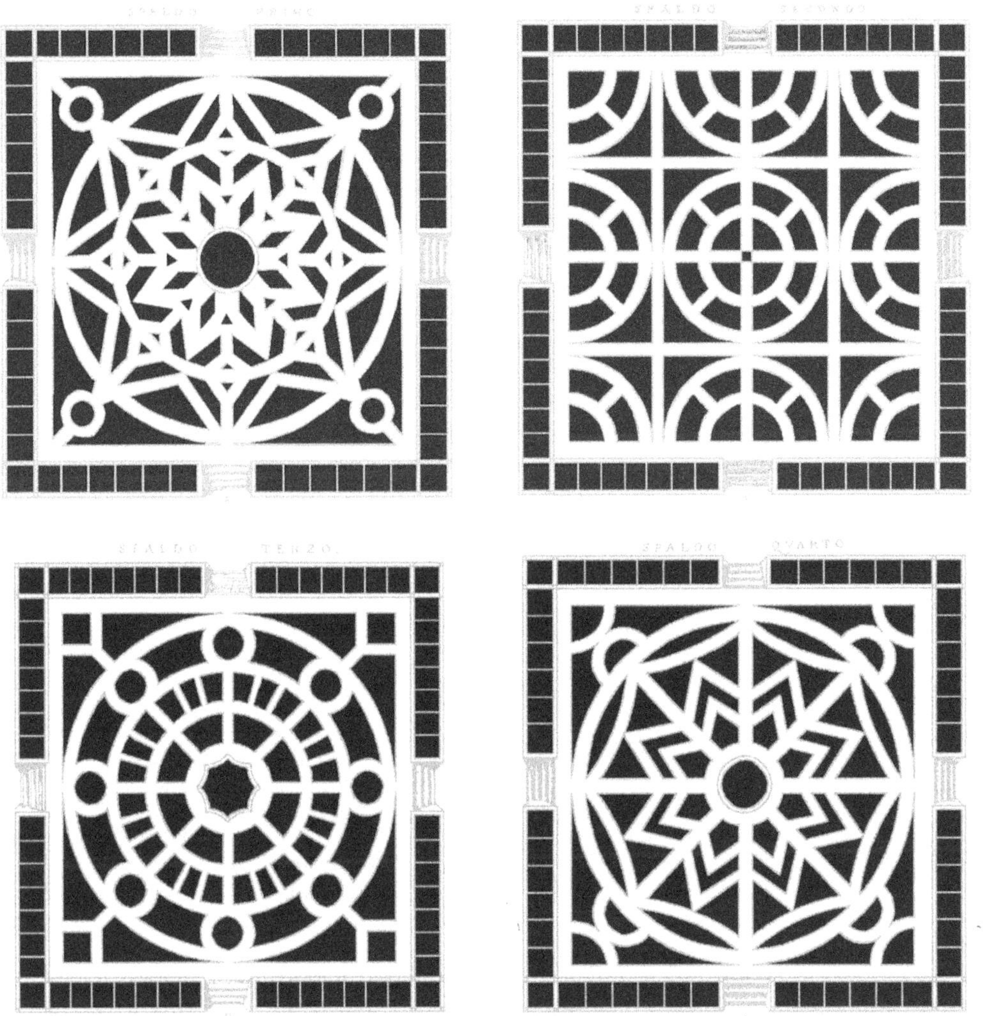

Figure 10.20: Details of the four terraces composing L'Orto Botanico di Padova

The *Spaldo Primo* (1st Terrace) is linked to the Spring season, which is associated with the Sanguine humour. The geometry of the paths, emanating from an eight-pointed star from the central Solar bed, captures the dynamism of the rising energy of the season. Thus, plants that flourish in the Spring would be particularly featured here, such as bugle, periwinkle and ground ivy.

The *Spaldo Secundo* (2nd Terrace) is linked to the Summer season, which is associated with the Choleric humour. Thus, plants that flourish in the Summer would be featured here, such as marigold, St john's wort and wood betony. The Summer Solstice is when the plant kingdom is at its most abundant, hence the complexity of the beds. The Sun is overhead, before declining for the latter half of the year. The Vital Force has achieved its zenith for the year, corresponding to the flowering of the plants.

The *Spaldo Terzo* (3rd Terrace) is linked to the Autumn season, which is associated with the Melancholic humour. Here the eight-pointed star of the Sun has contracted to the central bed, as in the Autumn the Sun's rays weaken. It is the time of harvest, when the Vital Force is concentrated into fruits and seeds. The circular beds that make up the outer Circle can be seen as analogous to seeds.

However, the eight circular beds also correspond to the phases of the waxing and waning Moon, which are important to consider when planting seeds and harvesting herbs for their medicinal uses. Since this is a physic garden, these positions also correspond to the crises and judgmental positions of the Moon used in decumbiture to monitor the course of an illness.

The *Spaldo Quarto* (4th Terrace) is linked to Winter season, which is associated with the Phlegmatic humour. Past the Winter Solstice, the eight-pointed star of the Sun has an ice crystal-like design, giving a sense of contraction before the explosion of Vital Force in the Spring. It captures the potential energy before the germination of seeds and the sprouting of tubers.

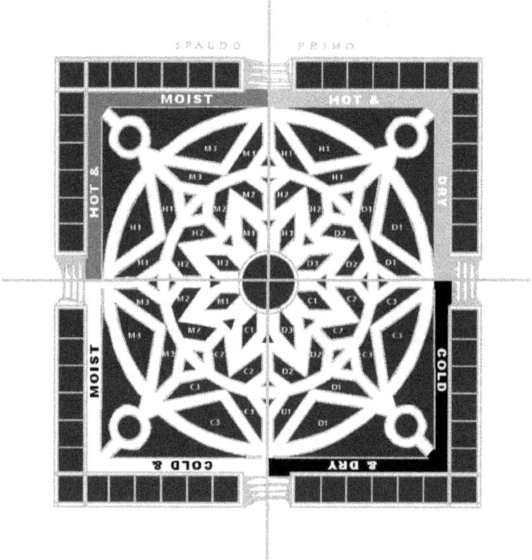

Figure 10.21: Allocation of temperatures to the terraces

With a terrace dedicated to each season, each terrace can be divided by means of the Elemental qualities hot, cold, dry and moist, and used to analyse the herbs within each season.

Additionally, each terrace is generally made up of three concentric circles, which enables the herbs to be placed in order of their degrees of heat or cold. The hottest will be placed in the bed nearest the Sun. Conversely, the furthest away will be the coldest. Similarly, the driest will be closest to the Sun, while the moist most will be furthest away.

For those inspired to visit, sadly, from a metaphysical perspective, the garden today is much more simply laid out in families, using the modern post-Linnaean taxonomy.

Though architectural elements of the garden's original layout can still be seen, the planting now largely ignores its founding principles. However, it has evolved in just under 500 years into a very important collection of plants from all over the world. Despite these enormous changes, the garden still retains a very peaceful, almost reverential, atmosphere. As Monty Don described it in his BBC "Around the World in 80 Gardens" project, *"It is like a temple dedicated to flowers."*

CHAPTER ELEVEN

The Black Death

In the 14th century, Europe was ravaged by the bubonic plague or the "Black Death", as it became more commonly known. The pandemic was first noticed in Eastern Asia, from where it spread to Asia Minor, Arabia, Egypt, North Africa and through Europe, reaching Britain in 1348. As the disease devastated Europe, an estimated 25 million people were thought to have died. Its toll in Britain affected over half the population.

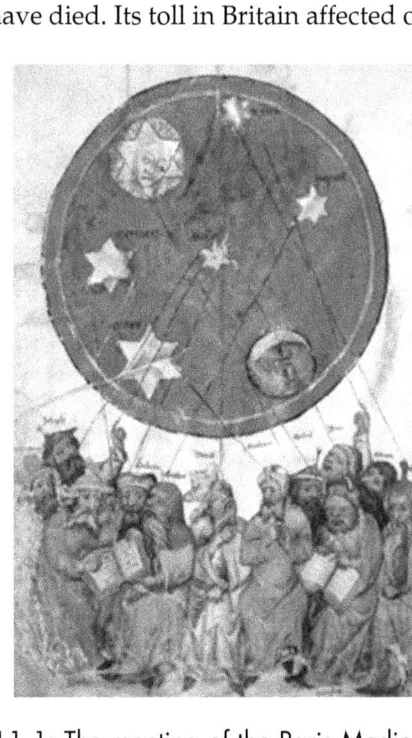

Figure 11.1: The meeting of the Paris Medical Faculty

In 1345 the plague had reached Paris, prompting the Medical Faculty of Paris to make a unique astrological pronouncement:

> *On the 20th March 1345, at 1pm there occurred a conjunction of Saturn, Jupiter and Mars in the house of Aquarius. The conjunction of Saturn notoriously caused death and disaster while the conjunction of Mars and Jupiter spread pestilence in the Air: Jupiter, being warm and humid, was calculated to draw up evil vapours from the Earth and Water, which Mars, hot and dry, kindled into an effective Fire. Obviously, the conjunction of all three planets could only mean an epidemic of cataclysmic scale.*

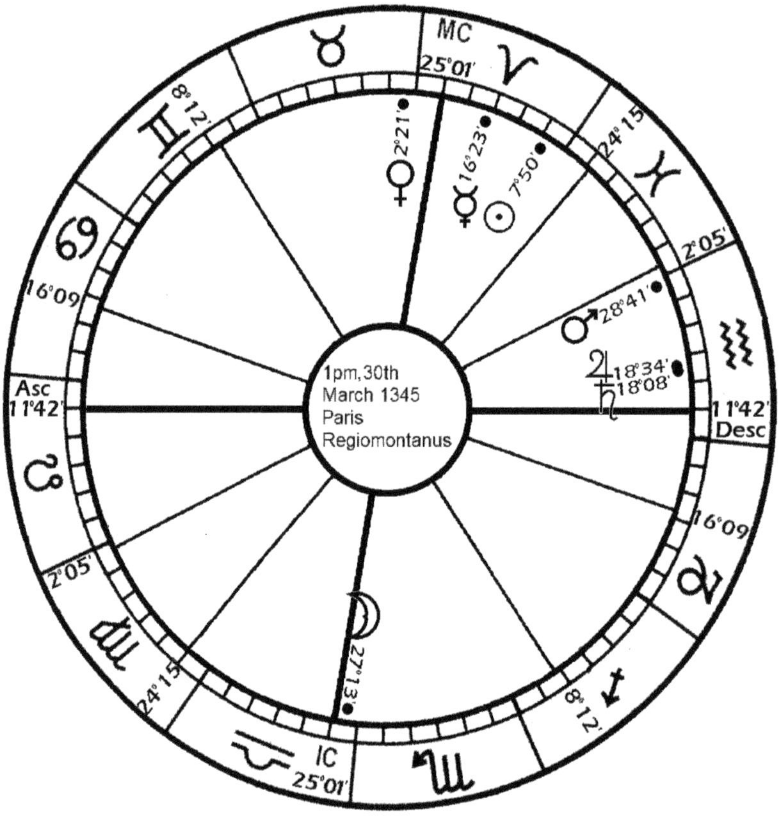

"BLACK DEATH" ANNOUNCEMENT - PARIS MEDICAL FACULTY

Figure 11.2: "Black Death" announcement

This chart has been rectified from the given time of the announcement, compensating for calendrical changes since the 14th century. Grand conjunctions of the slow-moving Planets have always been significant in mundane astrology, their combined lights producing particularly prominent focal points in the sky, which heralded eras of human experience. This rare triple conjunction of Saturn (♄), Jupiter (♃) and Mars (♂), involving the greater and lesser infortunes (♄ and ♂) besieging the greater benefic Planet, Jupiter (♃), must have been viewed with particular foreboding. The combination of

Saturn (♄)—the Lord of Death—with the expansive nature of Jupiter (♃) suggests death on a vast scale. Mars (♂) traditionally rules pestilence—a synonym for the plague—owing to its characteristic high fever.

The conjunction of Mars (♂) with Jupiter (♃), ruling the Air Element, suggests the spreading of the disease through the Air. The line *"Jupiter, being warm and humid, was calculated to draw up evil vapours from the Earth and Water"* sounds a little perplexing, until reflecting that there was no refrigeration at the time. Hot, muggy weather would have been associated with the rotting of food, decaying of dung heaps and stinking stagnant water. Hence the idea of *"evil vapours"*. Symbolically transposed to the blood, this describes the breakdown of the Sanguine humour. Disease connected to Jupiter (♃):

> *... gives all infirmities in the liver, pleurisies and inflammations of the lungs, palpitation and trembling of the heart, cramps, pain in the back bone, quinsies and flatulence; all putrefaction in the blood, or fevers proceeding from too great abundance thereof.*

Mars (♂) rules the Choleric humour, so the description, *"kindled into an effective Fire"* alludes to the fever arising out of this distemper.

The astrological chart of the Paris Medical Faculty announcement focuses on the nature of the disease. Saturn, the Lord of Darkness, ruling the sign of Capricorn, is the ruler of the 6th house of disease. This signification immediately highlights the importance of the Saturn (♄), Jupiter (♃) and Mars (♂) grand conjunction. Jupiter (♃), through rulership of Pisces (♓), is the lord of the 8th house, of Death. It is a fitting signification for the disease, which came to be known as the "Black Death". Mars, separating from the triple conjunction, suggests the rapid spread of the disease. Technically, the 10°orb is too wide to be considered part of the grand conjunction, however the Moon (☽), in Libra (♎) does symbolically reunite them, by translating light from Saturn (♄) and Jupiter (♃) to Mars (♂). Fittingly, the Moon (☽) in medical astrology is *"a general Significatrix in all Diseases"*.

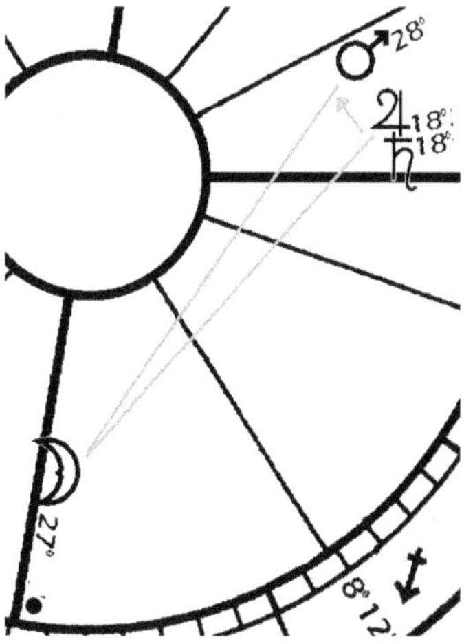

Figure 11.3: The Moon translating the Light from Saturn and Jupiter to Mars

As seen, the chart shows the announcement by the Paris Medical Faculty. The principal of the faculty is reflected by Leo (♌) ascendant, making the Sun (☉) the significator for the head spokesman. It is exalted in Aries (♈), in the 9th house of higher learning. This reflects the Faculty's authority in making this pronouncement.

Jupiter is the lord of the 9th house, conjunct Saturn, significator for the disease. The conjunction reflects the physicians looking into the nature of the disease. Mercury is the ruler of the 3rd house and a natural significator of communication. It is located in the 9th house, sextile to the conjunction of Saturn and Jupiter, and separating from a conjunction with the Sun. This powerfully echoes the principal making the pronouncement about the plague.

With Saturn strongly dignified in Aquarius, where Jupiter by contrast is weak, it conjures up the image of the physicians' helplessness in dealing with the virulence of the disease. Furthermore, Mars' location in the 7th house, moving towards the cusp of the 8th house of death, provides an image of the fever rapidly leading to death.

Modern medical understanding of the pandemic explains the Black Death as caused by a bacterium, *Yersinia pestis*. This bacillus is transmitted by two vectors, the rat and the flea. Primarily the bacterium infests the blood of rats and, consequently, is predominantly spread via fleas, which feed upon their blood. The blood of an infected rat dying of the plague will contain many bacilli. The flea feeding on its host takes in the bacteria while ingesting the blood. The bacteria multiply rapidly in its stomach, causing it to become obstructed. The flea becomes hungry from not being able to ingest any more blood. When the rat host finally dies, the hungry flea desperately searches for sources of fresh blood, usually other rats, but this is the point where humans are bitten instead.

When the flea bites another host the obstruction still prevents it from feeding. In desperation the flea regurgitates some of the infected blood, enabling the bacteria to gain entry to the host's blood via the bite hole. Once the flea's stomach is empty, the flea is free to feed again. The bacteria may also pass through the flea in its faecal material, so the infection can be spread in dust contaminating cuts or abrasions in the skin.

This understanding would clearly have been denied to the physicians in the 14th century, but the chart from this announcement does contain fascinating symbolic details that concord with a contemporary understanding of the disease.

Yersinia pestis is known to be carried by both black and brown rats. Though historically the plague was said to be carried by the "black rat", in the context of the fear associated with the pandemic, the "black rat" has a more mythical role. In the announcement chart, the 6th house also represents small animals. Saturn, its ruler, is a particularly fitting significator for the "black rat". The list of animals traditionally ruled by Saturn includes the following:

> *... Mouse ... [and] all manner of creeping creature breeding of putrefaction, either in the Earth, Water or ruins of houses.*

Notably, the rat is not found in this list, but with Jupiter conjunct Saturn, then symbolically a "mouse", particularly one "breeding of putrefaction", would surely qualify as a description of a rat!

The second vector, the flea, living on the black rat, must be identified by the ruler of the 6th house from the 6th house of the chart, that is, the 11th house. Gemini is found at the 11th house cusp, signifying the flea. Mercury, with its volatile, ethereal nature symbolises the elusive agility of a flea. Furthermore, its placing in the Fire sign of Aries reflects the burning irritation caused by its bite. Here too, its placing in the 9th house (with its Sagittarian associations) reflects the insect's powerful rear legs. enabling it to jump more than 200 times its own body height. The sextile aspect between Mercury and the Saturn/Jupiter conjunction reflects the relationship between the flea and the disease/rat.

Mars, the natural significator of the pestilence, disposes Mercury (which also rules the 4th house from the 11th house, that is, the flea's stomach) from Aries, which suggests the insect regurgitating the blood, allowing the infection to get through the bite hole into the victim's blood. The separating conjunction with the Sun (which now signifies the patient, as the Sun rules the Ascendant), suggests the patient has been bitten and the flea has hopped off.

The plague has a high fever, which starts a few days after the infection and is associated with headaches and great lassitude. The body temperature rises to 39.5°C and more. This Choleric response (hot and dry) is further shown by the lips and tongue becoming covered with dried saliva crusts from the excessive dehydration. The patient becomes rapidly prostrated.

After about the third day, as the organism spreads through the blood, small black spots or petechiae appear on the skin. As a harbinger of worse symptoms to come, it is likely these contributed to the name "Black Death". The spots are caused by areas of haemorrhage and gangrene under the skin. They even swelled up into blisters that burst forming an ulcer, the so-called "carbuncle".

The motion of the Moon in a decumbiture chart describes the developmental sequence of the disease. The Moon is separating from an opposition to Mercury and translating the light of the Saturn/Jupiter conjunction to Mars. This suggests the time taken for the infection to develop into a fever. According to "The Generally Accepted Measure of Time", since the Moon is in a cardinal sign and in an angular house, the 12°'s from the opposition to Mercury to trine with Mars, it indicates the fever would start about 10 days after the infection, reaching a peak at about 12 days.

The physicians at the Paris Medical Faculty would have been familiar with Hermes Trismegistus' "Upon the First Decumbiture of the Sick". According to this text:

> *The Moon in Libra, oppressed of Mars, by Conjunction, Quartile, or Opposition—Much blood offends the sick, causing intense Feavers, with high pulses, much waking, and the whole body in flames; … without the help of the fortunes* [Jupiter and Venus], *the sick will be in a great danger when the Moon comes to the body of Mars.*

Though the Moon here is applying to a trine aspect to Mars, the combined maleficity of the triple conjunction would far outweigh any benevolence of the trine.

The Moon is also present in the Via Combusta, which runs from 15°'s Libra to 15°'s Scorpio. The luminaries are said to be weak when placed here, because the Sun and Moon have their falls in Libra and Scorpio, respectively. The two malefics, Saturn and

Mars, are exalted and dignified in these two signs respectively, and hence able to dispose the luminaries. 25–30°'s Libra and 1–6°'s Scorpio are under the terms of Mars, which makes this zone even more inhospitable to the luminaries. Saturn and Mars in this chart strongly indicates the nature of the disease, further suggesting the gravity of the illness.

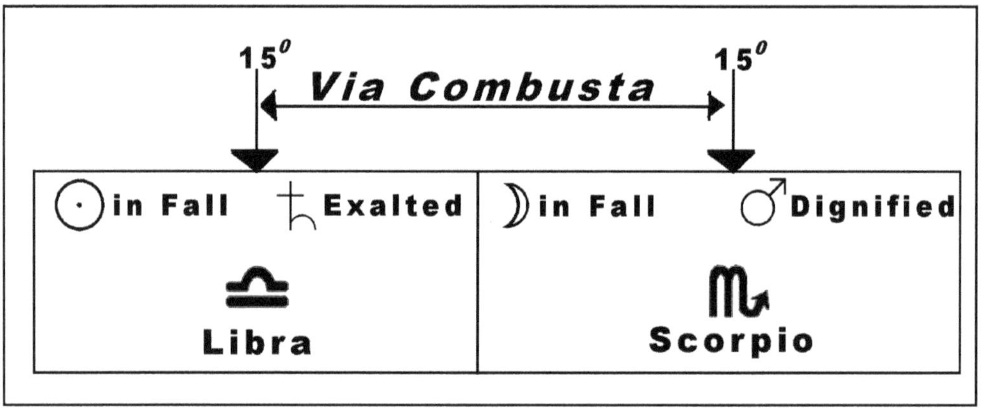

Figure 11.4: The Via Combusta

The name "bubonic plague" comes from the characteristic development of the buboes. The lymphatic glands, which drain the part of the body proximally to where the flea bite occurred, became rapidly and prominently swollen. This caused considerable pain as the lymphoid tissue responds to the invading bacterium. Later the lymph nodes often became haemorrhagic, leading to necrosis (death) of its tissues. The swollen buboes often burst, discharging their purulent contents through the skin.

The lymphatic system was not recognised in medieval medicine, with its physiology only becoming clearly understood in the last fifty years. Very simply, the lymphatic system is a series of channels and ducts that drain fluid from the tissues and return it once more to the blood in the venous circulation. In medieval physiology, the Sun in the sign of Leo ruled the heart and circulation, respectively. The blood was visualised as radiating from the heart to the rest of the body, like the light radiating from the Sun and illuminating all things. Aquarius the "Water carrier" is the opposite sign of the Zodiac to Leo and thus the most appropriate to rule the complimentary lymphatic system, which carries the "water" of the lymph back to the main circulation.

The Moon rules the Phlegmatic humour, which includes such secretions as sweat, tears and urine. Lymph is formed from the fluid that seeps out of the capillaries as the blood perfuses the tissues, and it too can thus be included in the Phlegmatic humour. This is confirmed by the Moon being traditionally used to indicate oedematous swelling, such as dropsy.

The triple conjunction placed in the sign of Aquarius would reflect this extensive involvement of the lymphatic system. Mars and Jupiter would thus indicate the inflammation and swelling of the buboes, while Saturn represents their necrosis.

The infection also affected the nervous system, causing intensely painful muscular spasms. Mercury rules the nervous system, and in the announcement chart Mercury is sextile the Saturn/Jupiter part of the grand conjunction, while located in Aries, the sign that rules. The muscles too are ruled by Mars, so Mercury's placing here would symbolically capture the intense muscular spasms. After four or five days of the fever starting, patients normally died an extremely agonising death.

The 10th house of the chart rules the medicine; in the announcement chart, Aries is at the mid-heaven or 10th house cusp, which indicates Mars is the nature of the medicine. This must have been alarming to the physicians since Mars, with its connection to the fever, was perceived to be highly descriptive of the malevolence of the disease. Surely Martian medicines would amplify and accelerate the disease. This paradox was resolved in the physicians' choice of herbs. Butterbur (*Petasites hybridus*) stands out as one of the herbs chosen.

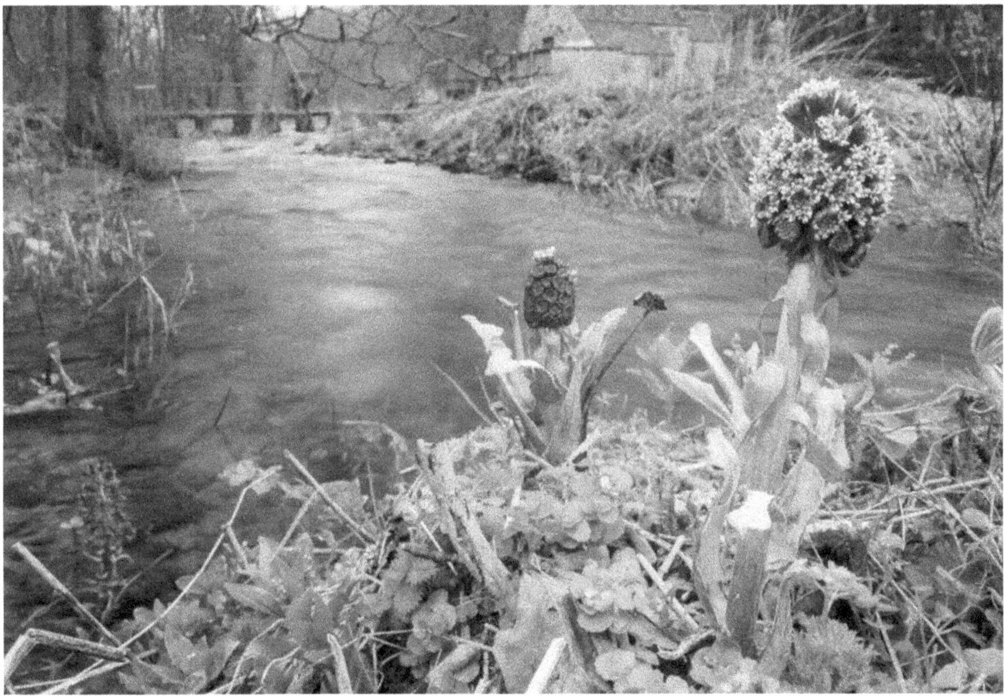

Figure 11.5: Butterbur growing beside the River Lathkill. Photo credit *Stephen Middleton*

The morphology of butterbur exhibits a powerful Martian signature, with the reddish-pink, phallus-like, flower spike growing from a bulbous base, being analogous to the Mars glyph. Thus, the Martian herb was thereby seen to have an affinity with the ravaging fever. However, butterbur is always found growing next to rivers and streams, a habitat associated with the Water sign of Cancer. Therefore, the growth of herb in its preferred habitat exhibits a fuller signature of Mars in Cancer. Astrologically the Fiery Planet Mars was seen to have its fall in the Water sign of Cancer—thereby its energy becomes extinguished. Thus, the medieval physicians visualised the virtue of this herb as having an affinity with the fever and then being able to weaken or attenuate it.

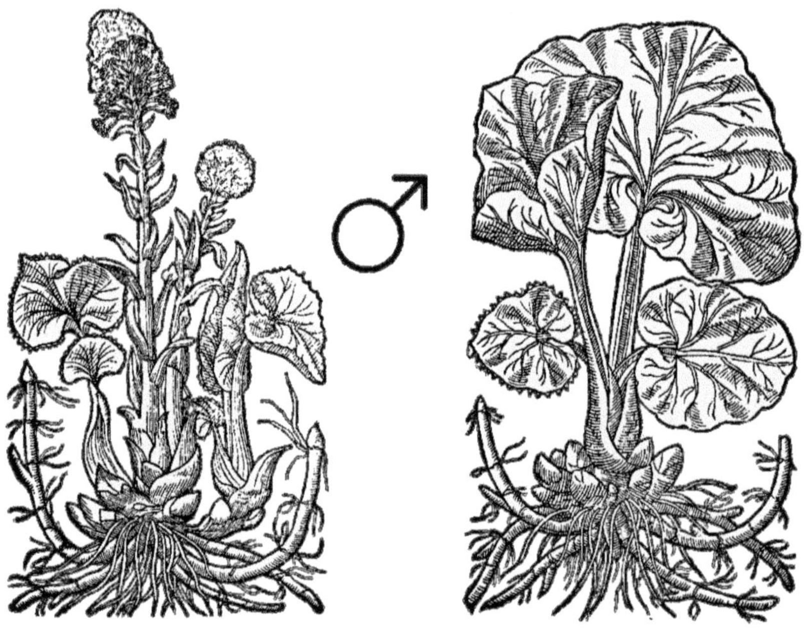

Figure 11.6: Woodcut of butterbur from *The Herball* by John Gerard, 1633 Edition

To quote from Gerard's *Herball*:

> *The roots of Butter-Burre stamped with ale, and given to drinke in pestilent and burning fevers, mightily cooleth and abateth the heat thereof ... is a soveraigne medicine against the plague and pestilential fevers, because it prouvoketh sweat, and driveth from the heart all venome...*

Butterbur is a dioecious herb, that is, having separate male and female plants. Appropriately, it is the male butterbur plants that most powerfully exhibit this Martian signature. The flowering spike of the female plants by contrast has a much more feathery, expansive structure and consequently fails to fulfil the signature. It is notable that in the woodcut print from Gerard's *Herball* only the male plant is shown, as if the author were unaware of the existence of the female plant.

When the Black Death reached England in 1348, via the port of Weymouth, three years after the Paris Medical Faculty made their announcement, butterbur roots and rhizomes, following the successful use on the continent, would have been hastily introduced to Britain to counter the spread of the pandemic. In this haste, the male plants were specifically chosen, leaving the female plants behind. The imported herb would have been passed along the trade routes that supplied the monasteries, whose infirmaries functioned as local hospitals for the surrounding community. Monks and nuns would have planted the roots in waterways in the vicinity of the infirmaries, to generate an immediate supply for their patients.

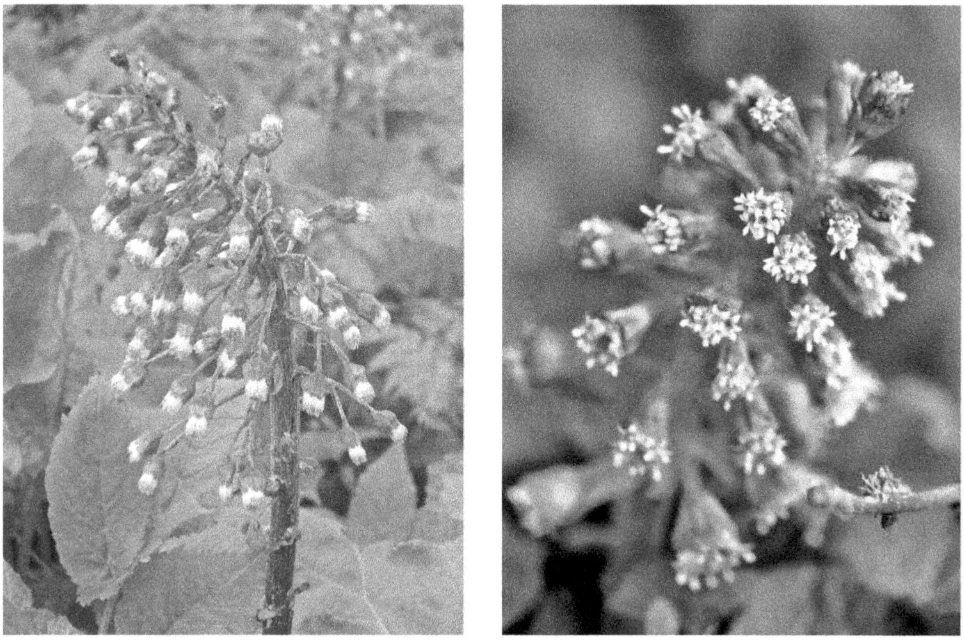

Figure 11.7: The flowers of butterbur: female (left) and male (right)

The most extraordinary legacy of the butterbur lies in the fact it has only been able to grow vegetatively, so where it is found today is largely a continuation of where it was planted 800 years ago. Thus, finding the plant in the wild provides a rough and ready indicator of where the scourge of the Black Death once struck the population of Britain.

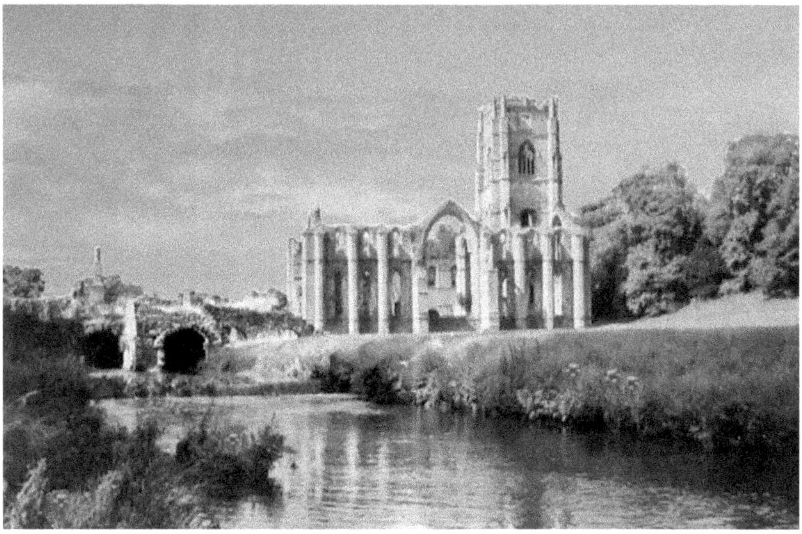

Figure 11.8: Fountains Abbey, Yorkshire. The infirmary foundations are located on the left-hand side

Fountains Abbey was one of the Cistercian monasteries that acted as a hospital for the local populace. Among the ruins patches of butterbur can still be seen growing in the water and on the banks of the River Skell, as it weaves its way through the monastery grounds. In this picture postcard view, the bridge-like structure is all that remains of the foundations to one of the two infirmaries at Fountains there. Just a stone's throw away, the large distinctive leaves of butterbur can be seen in the wear. So, where it is found today is largely a continuation of where it was planted 800 years ago. Clearly these plants are descendants of the herbs used by the monks to treat the plague. Genetically, they may even be all parts of the same plant!

The plague spread across the rest of Britain, reaching Wales in 1349. The horror of the time was captured by the Welsh poet Jean Geuthin, who would himself perish in the pandemic that same year. He wrote:

> *We see death coming into our midst like black smoke, a plague which cuts off the young, a rootless phantom which has no mercy or fair countenance. Woe is me of the shilling in the arm-pit; it is seething, terrible, wherever it may come, a head that gives pain and causes a loud cry, a burden carried under the arms, a painful angry knob, a white lump. It is of the form of an apple, like the head of an onion, a small boil that spares no-one. Great is its seething, like a burning cinder, a grievous thing of an ashy colour. It is an ugly eruption that comes with unseemly haste. It is a grievous ornament that breaks out in a rash. The early ornaments of black death.*

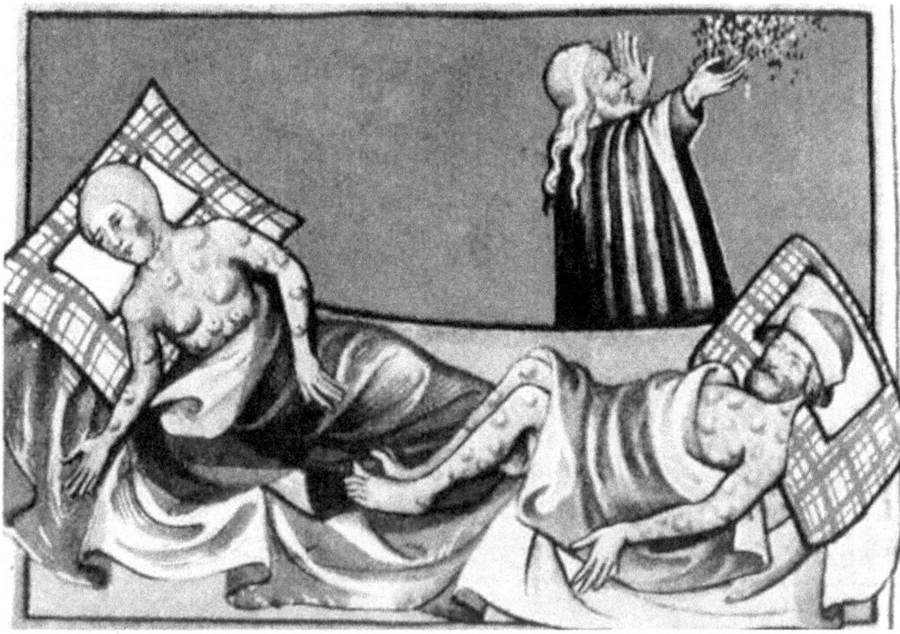

Figure 11.9: An image of the Black Death, showing distended buboes, from the Toggenburg Bible, 1411

Another important plant in the story was the lesser spearwort (*Ranunculus flammula*). From Jean Geuthin's description, among the prominent symptoms of the plague were the swollen and painfully distended lymph nodes called buboes. As we have seen, the lymphatic system is a series of vessels, as distinct from the blood vessels, which carry the fluid from around the tissue cells and return it to the blood. At the confluence of two lymph vessels there is a lymph node, which is essentially a concentrated area of immune cells that filters the lymphatic fluid and swallows (phagocytoses) bacteria and other micro-organisms. When an infection is present the immune cells rapidly multiply to fight it, causing the node to increase in size.

In the case of the bubonic plague, the rapidly proliferating organism evoked a particularly strong immune response in the lymph nodes. The combination of the immune cells fighting large numbers of bacteria caused congestion of the nodes, which swelled up from all the cells and lymph being blocked there. These huge glands or buboes occasionally burst, discharging a black, putrid-smelling liquid. It was then that physicians noticed that those patients whose buboes burst were the ones that recovered from the Black Death. It dawned on them that if they could burst the buboes, they could help the patients recover.

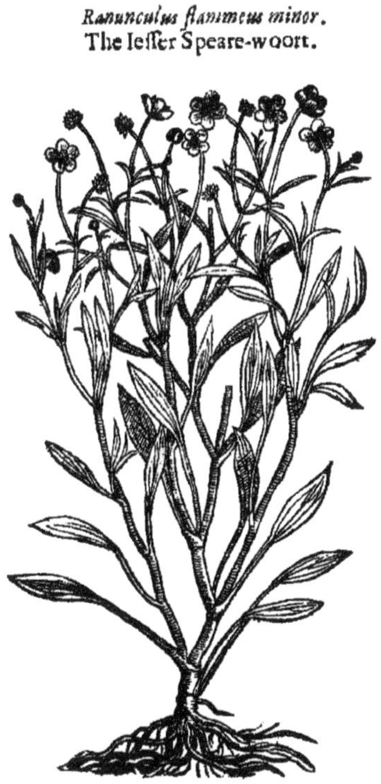

Figure 11.10: Woodcut of Lesser Spearewort from *The Herball* by John Gerard, 1633 Edition

One herb they chose for this purpose was the lesser spearwort, which is found at the boggy edges of ponds or lakes. Like the butterbur, it too was also seen to have a Mars in Cancer (♂ in ♋) rulership. The Martian signature here derives from the reddish hue to the stem and the slender, sharp-pointed leaves, hence the name spearwort.

For such a small plant the tips are remarkably sharp to touch, making it an ideal instrument to lance the buboes. The juice of the spearwort too is a strong rubefacient, causing redness and blistering of the skin on contact. This property gives the herb the specific name *flammula*, for it literally inflames the skin. This action is described in Gerard's *Herball:*

> *The leaves ... stamped and applied to any part of the body, causeth the skin to swell and blister.*

He goes on to specifically refer to the buboes or carbuncles:

> *The leaves stamped and applied unto any pestilentiall or plague sore, or carbuncle, staieth the spreading nature of the same, and causeth the venomous or pestilential matter to breath forth, by opening the parts and passages in the skin.*

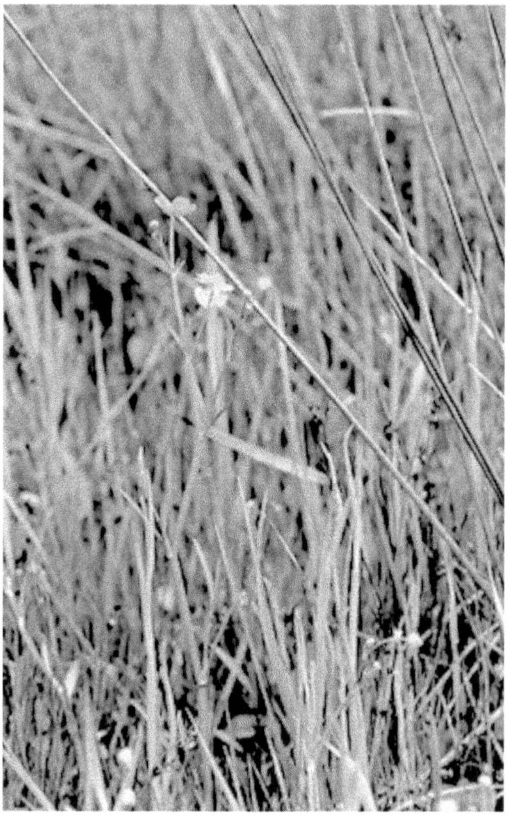

Figure 11.11: Lesser spearwort (*Ranunculus flammula*)

The third herb that was chosen was angelica, known to Gerard as great angelica (*Angelica archangelica*). When the Church authorities saw the distinctive black buboes and black petechiae, they took the attitude that it was sign of the Devil, so the reason people were succumbing to the disease, was because they were doing the work of the Devil and now getting their reward!

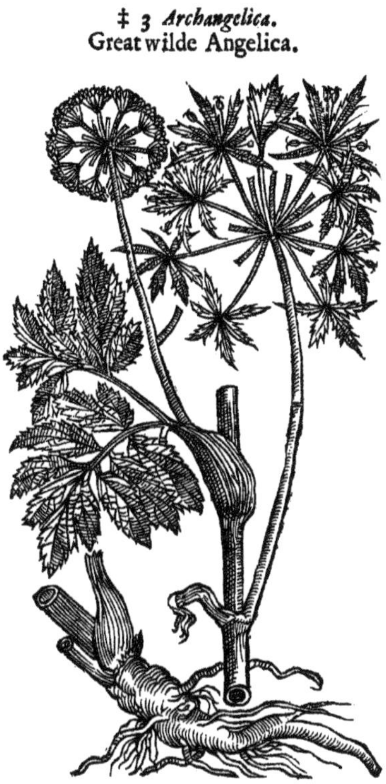

Figure 11.12: Woodcut of Great Wild Angelica from *The Herball* by John Gerard, 1633 Edition

The great angelica is one of the most revered ancient herbs. As a Solar herb, it was used in ancient ceremonies for protection and to banish any evil spirits. In the Gothic era the spherical orb of the seedhead was thought to be analogous to the halo, used in Christian art to depict the inner illumination of saints and angelic beings. Its large leaves too can be seen to be analogous to the wings of an archangel.

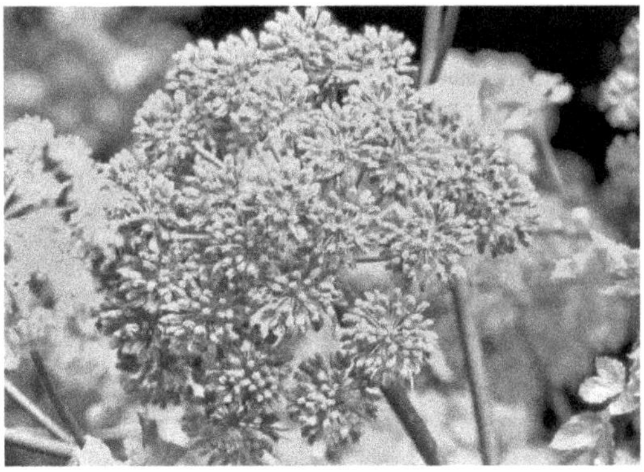

Figure 11.13: The seedhead of *Angelica archangelica*; in Catholic theology thought to be analogous to the halo of saints

Consequently, angelica was also known as "the root of the Holy Ghost" and thereby conferring protection against sorcery and witchcraft. The dried stems with the seedheads were lit and carried as a ferrule in the celebration of St Michael—the archangel associated with the Sun—during the medieval service of Michaelmas, which was then held on 16 October. The archangel Michael was known to be the slayer of dragons and demons, so his presence was invoked to slay the demons that inflicted so much suffering on the people.

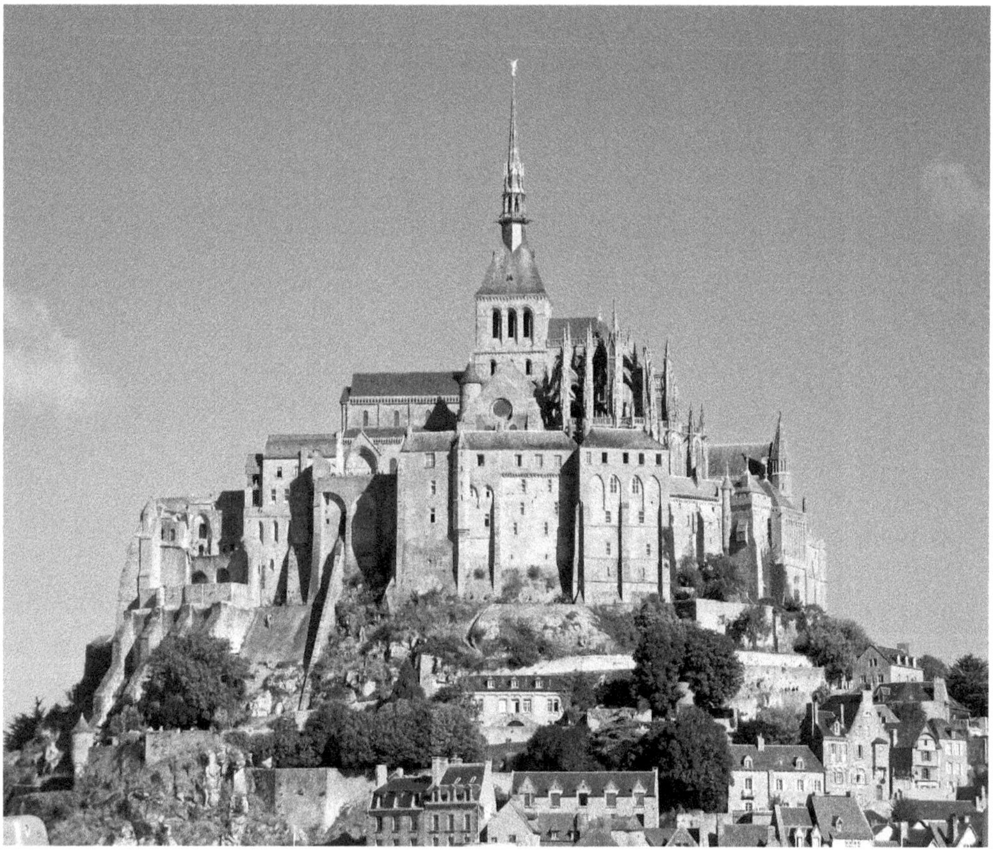

Figure 11.14: Mont-Saint-Michel, Normandy with a gold statue of St Michael atop its spire

St Michael is associated with churches built atop hills, symbolically surrounded by water. Mont-Saint-Michel, near St Malo in Normandy, is arguably the most spectacular, with its magnificent golden statue of St Michael at the top of the spire, situated in the tidal estuary of the Couesnon River. In medieval times Mont-Saint-Michel was an especially important centre for pilgrimage and healing. Similar associations can be found in Britain with St Michael's Mount off the Cornish coast and St Michael's Church at the top of Glastonbury Tor.

Such powerful associations to Catholic theology meant that angelica came to be highly regarded as a herb and used as a preventative, and for protection against contagions such as the plague, for purifying the blood and curing many infectious diseases. As Gerard's *Herball* describes the uses of Angelica:

> *The roots of garden Angelica is a singular remedy against poison, and against the plague, and all infections taken by evil and corrupt aire; if you do but take a peece of the root and hold it in your mouth, or chew the same between your teeth, it doth most certainly drive away the pestilential aire ...*

But when the clergy were seen to be covered in black spots and dying from the disease, the Catholic Church experienced a huge loss of confidence among its followers. The sight of the clergy exhibiting the signs of the Devil and, furthermore, being powerless to do anything about it, challenged the faith of many Christians.

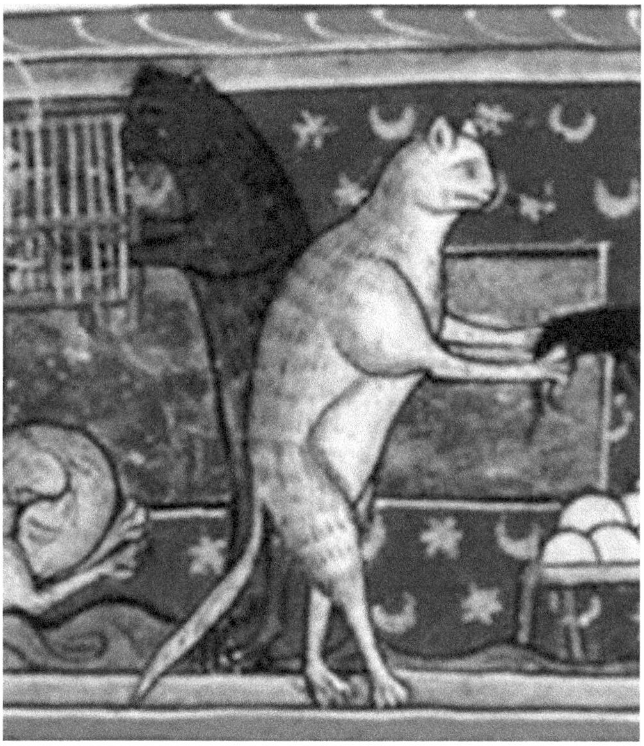

Figure 11.15: Cats from a medieval manuscript

Ironically, the Catholic Church might well have played a part in bringing this cataclysm onto themselves and the population of Western Europe, for in 1232 Pope Gregory IX declared that cats, especially black ones, were evil and consequently were associated with witchcraft and the Devil. Even owners of black cats could be killed under this Papal decree. Over the next century this led to the mass extermination of cats in an attempt to rid the world of the perceived evil. Consequently, with their major predator gone, the rat population exploded, unwittingly creating the ideal conditions for the proliferation of the bubonic plague in 1345.

The Black Death had a momentous impact on all aspects of society. The loss of so many lives tore gaping holes in its fabric, so that much of the feudal order fell apart. There was a shortage of labour to do the basic tasks of farming the land and providing food. Whole villages died out. The cultural momentum of the Gothic era effectively came to a grinding halt. The extravagant building work of the cathedrals stopped. Monasteries and universities would have lost the knowledge of key people. Without their expertise education became stunted.

In the fight against the pandemic, many who administered herbs must have perished, thereby being no longer able to pass their knowledge on. Much herbal knowledge as a living art would have been lost, while the training of physicians, too, would have been suspended.

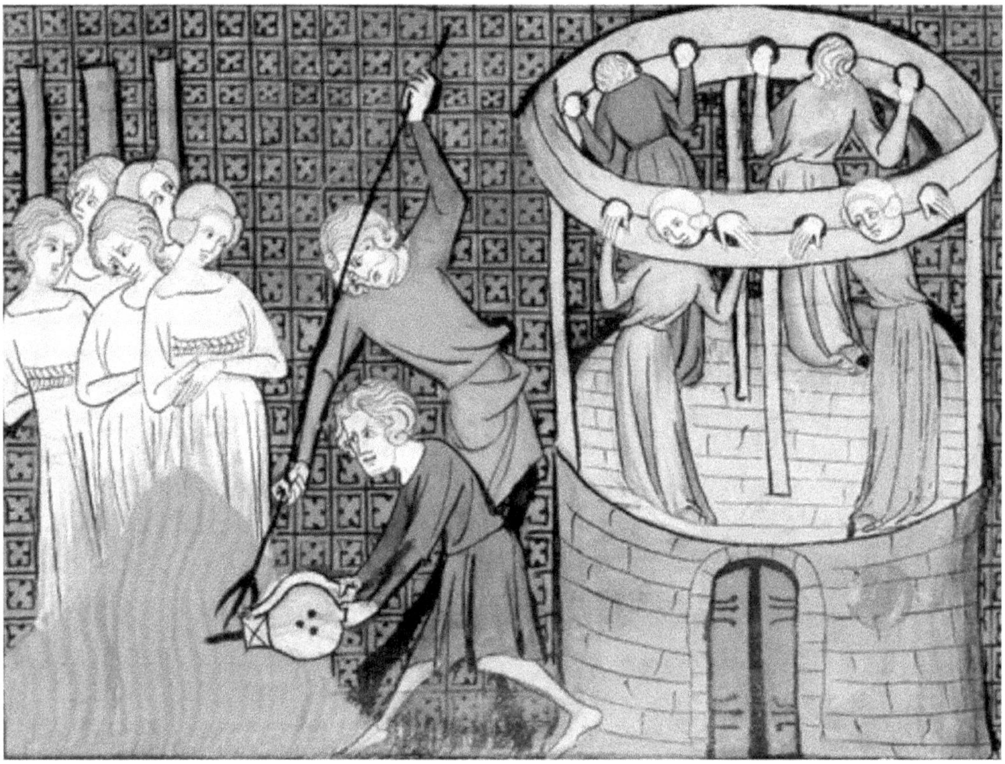

Figure 12.1: Torturing and execution of witches from a medieval miniature. Public domain http://molcat1.bl.uk/IllImages/Ekta%5Cmid/E124/E124110.jpg

CHAPTER TWELVE

The witch hunts

The witch hunts are perhaps the ugliest phase of our herbal history, whose impact has had a huge lasting impact on women's social and political status to the present day. The aftermath of the Black Death left a massive crisis of confidence in the Church's authority. indeed so much that had been previously organised by the Church, as the ordained world under the feudal system, fell apart. People lost faith in their teachings. Essentially the Church had to eat humble pie—or maybe spotted dick! To regain their authority the Church sought a scapegoat, and chose the witches, who were blamed for practising black magic, which, it was said, had brought so much devastation and suffering into the civilised world.

The Catholic Church was formed in the 4th century in Roman Empire when the Emperor Constantine converted to being a Christian. Prior to his conversion, the emperor boasted of the number of Christians he had killed during his rule. Then he had an epiphany moment, and, piqued by guilt from his former actions, he sought to make amends.

Under Constantine's rule Christianity supplanted Mithraism to become the official religion of Rome, and consequently started to spread with the zeal and conquering ambition of the former Roman Empire.

Constantine instructed St Jerome to collect and compile Jesus' teachings from about two dozen gospels that had been written down from the teachings of his disciples and their followers. Of these only four were selected to be included in the Bible. The teachings became strongly patriarchal in nature, as evidenced by the missing second verse of the Lord's Prayer, which is dedicated to Our Mother:

> *Our Mother which are upon earth, hallowed by thy name. Thy kingdom come, and thy will be done in us, as it is in thee. And lead us not into sickness, but deliver us from all evil, for thine is the earth, the body and the health. Amen.*

The new Catholic faith was seen as a powerful civilising influence on the common man and sought intellectual control over society instead of the military one that characterised the Roman Empire. The founding fathers of the Catholic Church wanted to convert everyone to the new faith.

In 595, Pope Gregory the Great chose Augustine, a Christian monk, for a mission to Britain in order to Christianise King Æthelbert, ruler of the Kingdom of Kent, from Anglo-Saxon paganism. Augustine became the first archbishop of Canterbury in the year 597.

The word "pagan", from the Latin *paganus*, simply means a heathen, literally "someone who lives on the heath". Such people were generally more attuned to the seasons and the rhythms of nature since the success of their survival depended on understanding them. Therefore, they had a spiritual connection to the land involving the veneration of Nature and the Elements that sustained them through the seasons.

The women who were the herbal healers in the community embodied these qualities and consequently were well-respected. As Christians sought to convert the pagans, they naturally encountered the authority of the wise women.

The patriarchal authority of the Catholic Church would have been powerfully challenged by the strength of the Elders' matriarchal authority. In the ensuing power struggle, the Church deliberately discredited the matriarchs' authority by calling them witches and their work demonic.

Where the Church had the support of the State, then soldiers would arrest witches on behalf of the Church. In the zeal of the Church to assert its authority, witches were typically tortured into confessing their "sins", then sentenced to death.

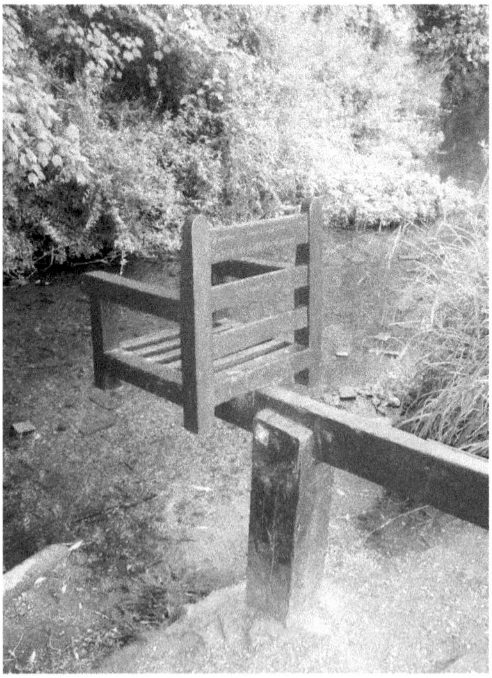

Figure 12.2: The ducking stool on the River Avon, Christchurch, Dorset

Though the burning of the witches had been occurring in Britain since the 10th century on a minor scale, this scapegoating after the Black Death gave the witch hunts extra focus and intensity. Their perceived evil had to be purged from society if it was to be brought back under control of the Church's authority.

So, under the full authority of the Church, an offensive was launched against the women in the villages and communities throughout Britain and Europe. Any woman suspected of the slightest magical powers or sorcery was investigated by the magistrates and cruelly subjected to interrogation and torture, administered with "heads we win, tails you lose" justice.

The ducking stool was a typical example: a priest would bless the water, be it a pond, lake or a river, and the suspected woman was tied to the chair, then lowered into the water. If she drowned, it was because she was innocent and was taken to heaven. If she survived, it was because she was rejected by the water and therefore found guilty and consequently burnt at the stake. Once again, the priest would bless the flames as the fire took hold, so that it was God's will that the woman should perish in the fire.

The reality was that the "wise woman" in villages, with their traditional herbal knowledge and skills in childbirth serving their community, were held in higher respect than the priests and monks, with all their learning, that had been seen to be so ineffectual in the plague. The women held a power and respect that the Church had lost. By burning so many witches, the hunts led to the deliberate removal of herbal knowledge from the community, back into the monasteries, under the control and authority of the Church.

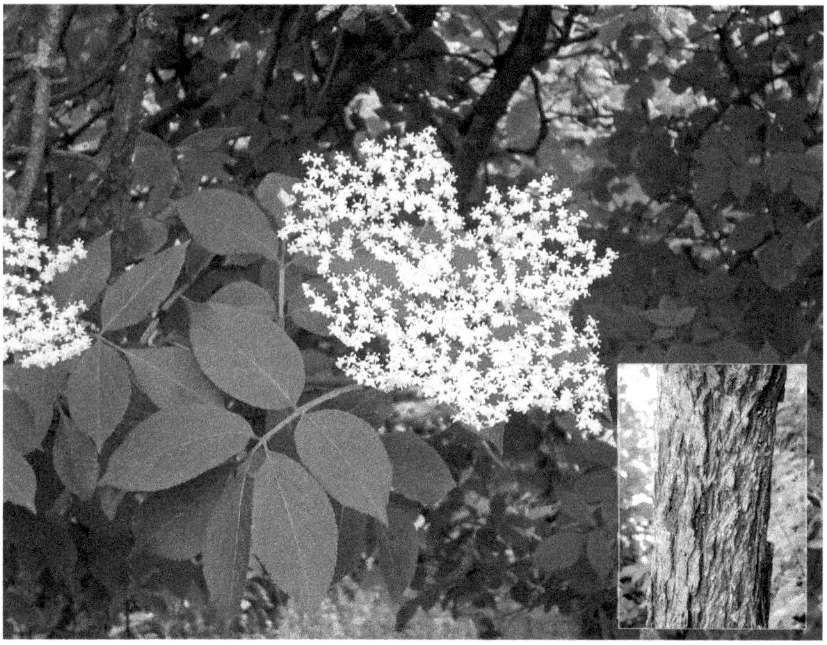

Figure 12.3: The common elder or crone's tree (*Sambucus nigra*) with bark: see inset

The elder or crone's tree has a long tradition as a healing tree. When the soldiers and magistrates came in search of the wise women suspected of being witches, the villagers often sought to hide and protect them. Having secreted them away, they then told the pursuers that the witches had used their powers to transform into an elder bush. Its gnarled bark even resembling the withered skin of an aged body, added to the deception. Without anything to be gained by arresting an elder bush the pursuers left empty-handed. Furthermore, the wood from the elder tree is so full of sap that burning it is almost impossible!

Thus, the crone's tree came to be associated with the healing powers of wise women. Perhaps it should be seen as a living memorial to all those women who were brutally murdered by the witch hunts. Consequently, this association led to the folk belief that cutting down an elder bush would bring bad luck, for the act would be symbolic of killing the wise woman—not to mention destroying a valuable healing tree in the village.

CHAPTER THIRTEEN

The Dissolution of the Monasteries

In the 16th century King Henry VIII was to have an enormous impact on the practice of physic in Britain, which has affected herbal medicine to the present day. In particular, it was through the Dissolution of the Monasteries, which, as has been shown, were important cultural centres of education and caring for the sick.

Events that led to the Dissolution of the Monasteries started with issues surrounding the divorce of Henry VIII from his first wife, Catherine of Aragon. They had been married in accordance with Catholic law, which expressly forbade divorce. Henry needed a son and heir to his throne. Sadly, Catherine was unable to provide him with a son, so he sought a divorce from her.

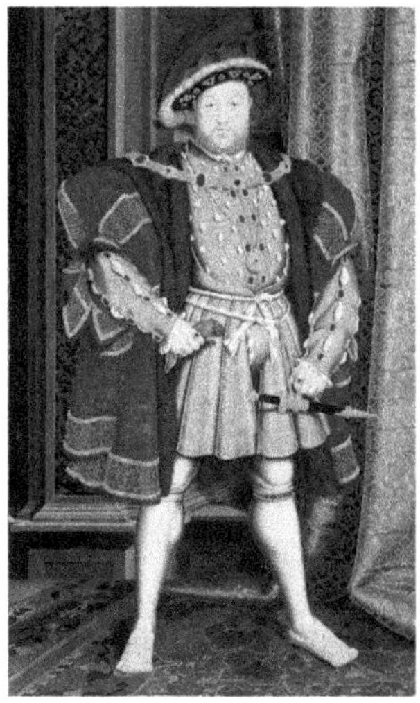

Figure 13.1: After Hans Holbein's portrait of Henry VIII. Public domain

Cardinal Thomas Wolsey, who was then also the Archbishop of York, was unable to secure a divorce to Henry, so fell out of favour. Prior to this moment, Wolsey had had an illustrious career. He had been appointed by Henry VIII as Archbishop of York in 1514. He was then chosen by Pope Leo X To become a cardinal, representing the Catholic Church in Britain. Henry's trust in him was further rewarded by making him his Lord Chancellor, in 1515. He retained this post till 1529 when he fell from grace.

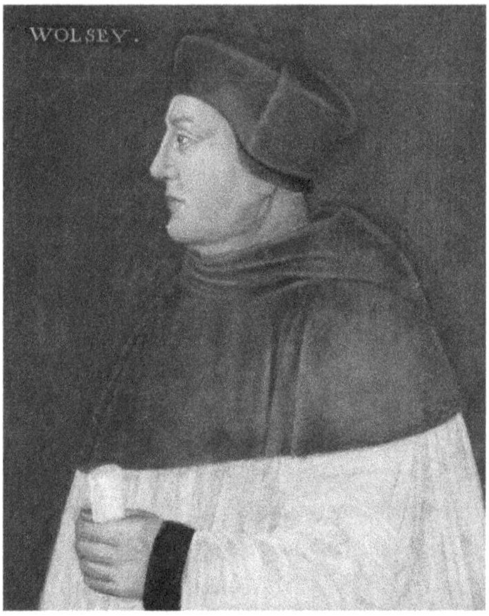

Figure 13.2: Cardinal Thomas Wolsey (1475–1530), royal minister, Archbishop of York. Public domain

In his capacity as a cardinal, Wolsey would have had to travel to visit the Pope at the Vatican in Rome. While he was in Italy, he became inspired by seeing the universities of Padua—with its reputation for medicine, Bologna—with its reputation for law, and Milan—with its reputation for theology, and wanted to found a similar institution in Britain. On his return, he shared his ambitions with Henry, who was interested in the project but refused to supply any funding for it.

Wolsey had a plan. He knew of the convent of St Frideswide, in Oxford. She was an Anglo-Saxon saint and healer whose holy well in medieval times had become an important place of pilgrimage and healing. By the time of Henry's reign, the convent barely functioned but had amassed considerable wealth from its former importance. Wolsey suggested that the convent could be sold, and the money used to build his new college. Henry granted Thomas his wish.

Originally called Cardinal College and today Christ Church College, this was Thomas Wolsey's brainchild. By exploring the symbolism within its structure, most clearly seen from the aerial view, you can appreciate Thomas' vision for the college. The paths of the quadrangle define the symbol for Earth (⊕). Each quadrant is linked to each of the four material Elements, Earth, Water, Air and Fire, in a similar way to the orientation already described in the chapter on physic gardens.

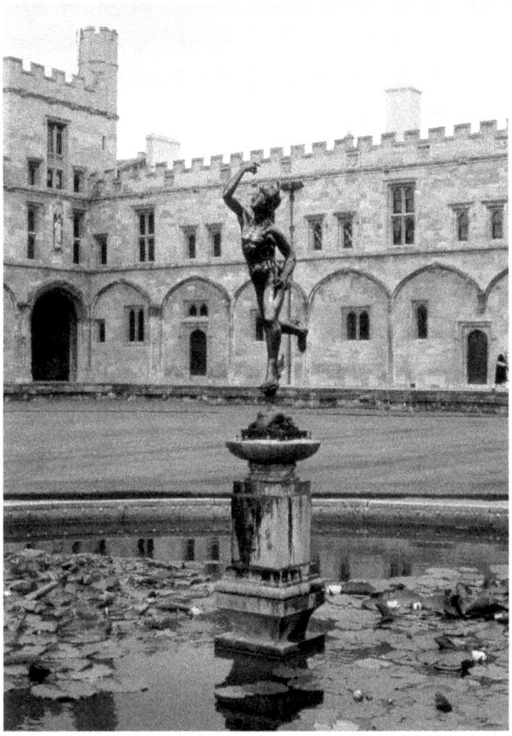

Figure 13.3: Christ Church College, Oxford University

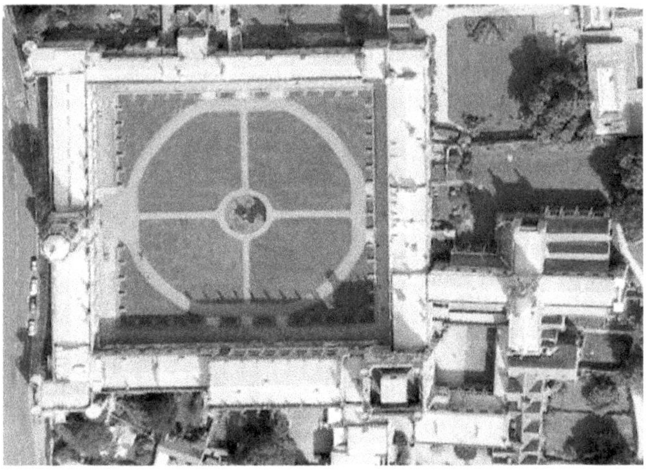

Figure 13.4: Aerial view of Christ Church College

This means the pond at the centre of the quadrants represents Ether, the Fifth Element, also known as Aqua Vitae or Water of Life. The symbolism has been perfected by the placing of a stature of Mercury at its centre. It is in fact a fountain, so when it is working, the statue shows Mercury, the winged messenger of the gods, flying through the Waters of Life or Aqua Vitae.

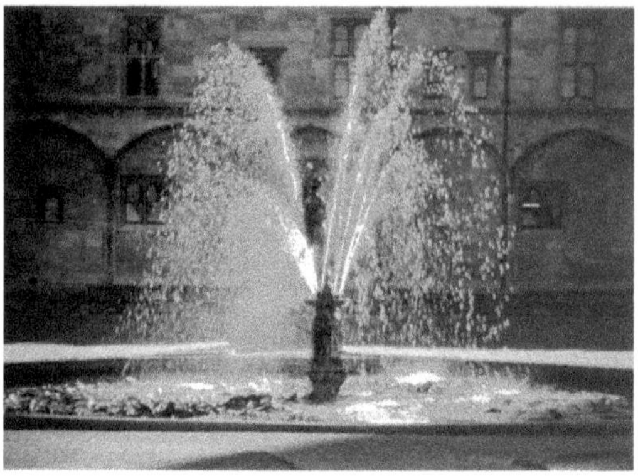

Figure 13.5: The Fountain

Each flank of the college buildings surrounding the quadrants represents a different Element of the material world, as well as, the four levels of learning—the literal, tropological, allegorical and anagogical.

The Hermetic Three World view can also be seen. Hence the Intellectual World above is mediated down through the Mercury/Ether (Celestial World) to the Elements (Elemental World) below. To the bottom right in the aerial view, Christ Church Cathedral can be seen adjoining the college quadrant. Thus, the fountain is symbolically fulfilling the connection between heaven and earth.

The gateway into the quadrant resembles a Vesica Piscis, a symbol of the Universal Mother. The words "matter" and "material" are derived from the Latin *mater*, meaning "mother". Entry into the university, through this gate, is called matriculation, while the campus was called the *alma mater*, meaning "bounteous mother".

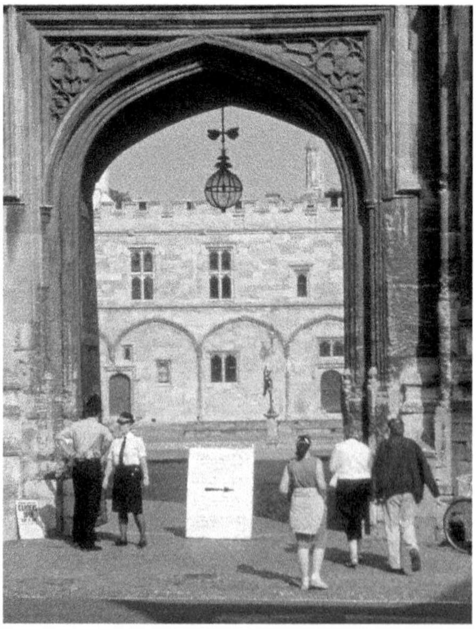

Figure 13.6: Looking through the main gate into Christ Church College

Looking through the gateway, you can see the statue of Mercury—the spirit of education was to symbolically look through the material world and see the spiritual within it. After achieving their Mastery of the Arts, the student graduated and was reborn out into the world.

Wolsey was never able to complete the college before he fell from favour, owing to his failure to get the Pope to grant a divorce for Henry's marriage to Catherine of Aragon. Wolsey had intended the quadrangle to have a cloistered walkway around it. In the distance only the traced outline of arches in the stonework on the college walls can be seen, essentially capturing the moment of his fall. His name, however, has been affectionately preserved by students as Tom's Quad. When you see the similarities of design between L'orto Botanico di Padova and Christ Church College, it is tantalising to ponder whether Wolsey saw the garden at Padua in his travels.

Ironically, with the high educational ideals Wolsey had for the college, in selling off the convent of St Frideswide, he had sown the seeds for the massive destruction of the Catholic faith in Britain, for in the Dissolution of the Monasteries, Christ Church College became its template. The building of Christ Church College made Henry aware of just how much wealth was locked away in the monasteries.

When the Pope excommunicated Henry VIII in 1538, Henry assumed control of the Church in Britain by appointing himself as head of the new Anglican Church. Thomas Cromwell, his new chancellor, was dispatched to make a full inventory of all the monastic institutions throughout the kingdom. He noted the wealth of their treasuries and their annual income, whether from indulgences, rents or tithes, and how many monks or nuns were resident, as well as the quality of their discipline.

Following the two Acts of Dissolution, Cromwell and his officers started the process of dissolution. First in their sights were the monasteries that only had a few monks or nuns using them. After the impact of the Black Death, a number of monasteries never fully regained the power they formerly had, leaving only had a handful of monks or nuns occupying them. A similar fate happened when its resident monks or nuns had become apostate—in other words, had become negligent in their religious practices, often instead living up the high life on the monastery's wealth.

After the lesser monasteries had received their fate in 1535, the larger and more wealthy monasteries in turn were dissolved in 1539. The purpose of the Acts was to deliberately strip the monasteries of their assets for the Crown, and to make their priests, abbots and priors renounce their allegiance to the Pope in Rome and instead become beholden to the Anglican Church.

To this end, senior clergy were given the choice to accept the changes and receive a pension or be executed. The monastic buildings were destroyed, most commonly by setting fire to the wooden rafters in the roofs, and letting them collapse, so allowing in the wind, rain and frost to dissolve the rest of the fabric of walls. Local villagers were encouraged to freely use the abbey walls as quarries for building their houses and barns—a symbolic act of allowing the laity to take back their portion of the Church's former wealth. It is still possible today to see older buildings within villages that were constructed from the stone taken from the local monastery.

This wilful vandalism on the monasteries had a huge cultural effect. The monasteries were no longer able to maintain their infirmaries or provide their medical services to the community, such as educating and caring for the sick. Physicians were lost, and the training of others disrupted. Manuscripts, including medical texts, were burnt. Physic gardens were abandoned, while the knowledge preserved within them vanished and the schools they formerly encouraged were dispersed. Though manuscripts and works of art have survived, a vast amount of artwork was later destroyed or covered up with the cultural purge of the Reformation. Little remaining stonework that contained esoteric symbolism that smacked of "Popery" escaped the hammer of the iconoclasts.

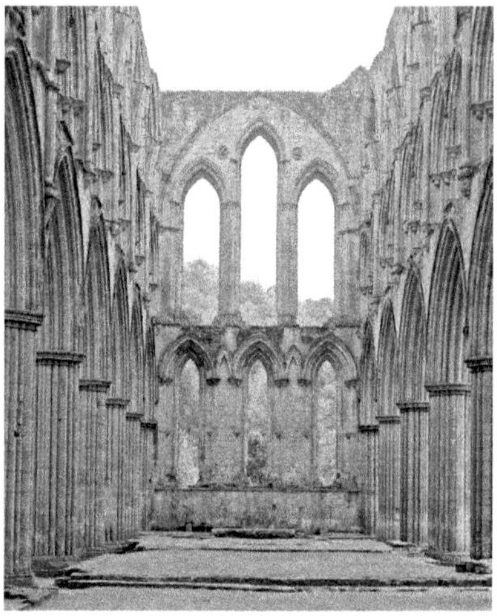

Figure 13.7: Looking East along the main nave of Rievaulx Abbey, Yorkshire

The teaching and practice of physic was a major casualty of this upheaval. Realising the impact on the suffering of the sick that the Dissolution had caused, Henry passed the Herbalists Act in 1542. Basically, this gave anyone who had the faintest knowledge of herbs the common law right to practise physic, thereby encouraging anyone to help heal the sick—so desperate this situation had become.

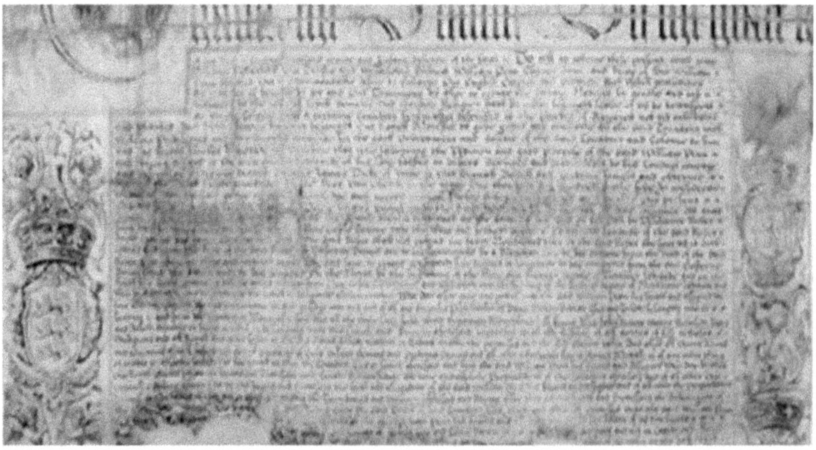

Figure 13.8: The Herbalist's Charter of Henry VIII of 1542: "An Act that Persons, Being No Common Surgeons, May Administer Outward Medicines"

The Act states:

> *In consideration whereof, and for the Ease, Comfort, Succour, Help, Relief and Health of the King's poor Subjects, Inhabitants of this Realm, now pained or diseased:*
>
> *Be it ordained, established, and enacted, by Authority of this present Parliament, That at all Time from henceforth it shall be lawful to every Person being the King's subject, having Knowledge and Experience of the Nature of Herbs, Roots, and Waters, or of the Operation of the same, by Speculation or Practice, within any part of the Realm of England, or within any other the King's Dominions, to practice, use and minister in and to any outward Sore, Uncome Wound, Apostemations, outward Swelling or Disease, any Herb or Herbs, Ointments, Baths, Pultess, and Emplaisters, according to their Cunning, Experience, and Knowledge in any of the Diseases, Sores, and Maladies beforesaid, and all other like to the same, or Drinks for the Stone, Strangury or Agues, without suit, vexation, trouble, penalty or loss of their goods; ...*

Though the standard was not particularly high, it nevertheless gave herbalists the common law right to practise herbal medicine, enabling it to survive to the present day, unlike other countries of continental Europe where herbalism is banned.

CHAPTER FOURTEEN

Continental Hermetic developments

While Britain was experiencing the turmoil of the reign of Henry VIII, Hermetic teachings were quietly flourishing in continental Europe. The medieval city of Nuremberg in Germany was a clear focal point of these developments.

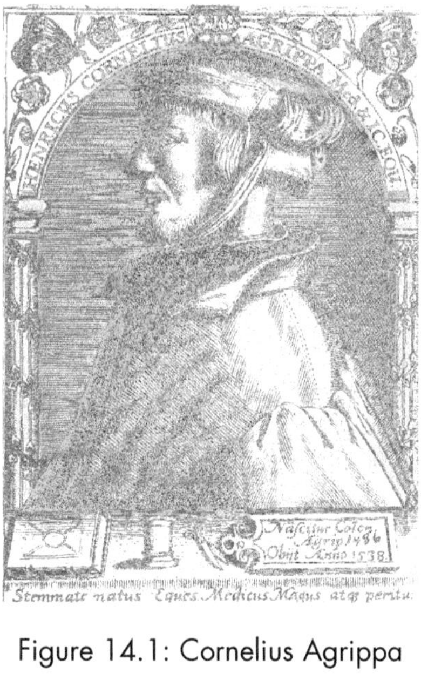

Figure 14.1: Cornelius Agrippa

The connection stems from the controversial figure of Cornelius Agrippa (1486–1535), a Hermetic philosopher whose teachings were written down in his *De Occulta Philosophia* (Of the Hidden Philosophy). Among his followers was Albrecht Dürer, who lived in Nuremberg. Dürer was a prolific artist who explored religious and metaphysical themes, and was also keen to explore the new medium of copperplate engraving that followed on the development of the printing press. These engravings enabled detailed graphic illustration of texts.

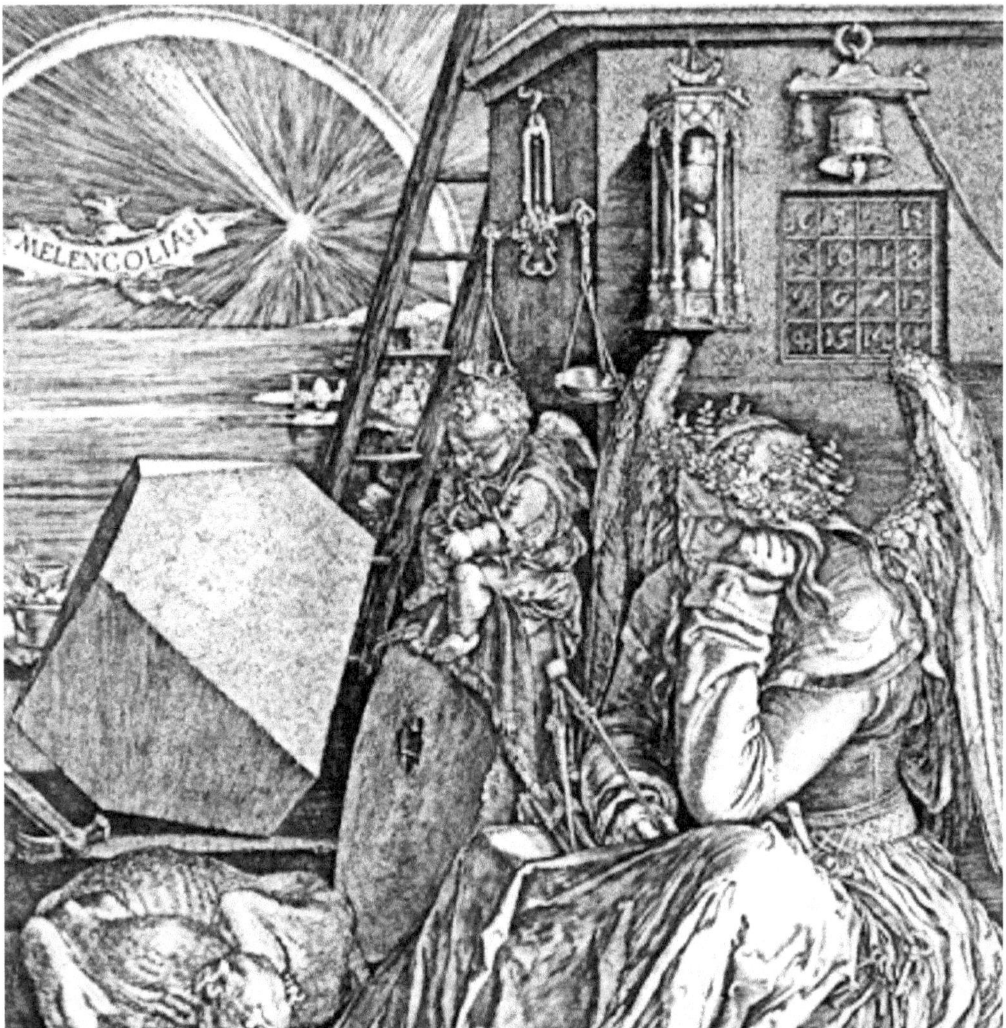

Figure 14.2: Albrecht Dürer's "Melancholia I", 1514

Arguably, one of his most important and powerful illustrations is Dürer's engraving "Melancholia I", completed in 1514. The artist was no stranger to experiencing melancholia himself, and the title "Melancholia I" alludes to the particular form of melancholia experienced by artists, according to Cornelius Agrippa.

The engraving is Dürer's attempt to express the complexity of the emotion, within the context of Hermetic teachings. It is an extraordinary study too of the symbolism of Saturn, which rules the Melancholic humour. It serves to reveal just how sophisticated Hermetic teachings had become in the 16th century.

The central figure is a melancholic angel, weighed down by pondering the gravity of issues in life. In the Hermetic vision, angels are beings that live in the Intellectual World, illuminated by the Light of Creation. When a Soul incarnates it leaves the Intellectual World and descends through the Planetary Spheres of the Celestial World and acquires a physical body in the Elemental World.

The highest of the Planetary Spheres linked to Saturn was known as the "The Gate of the Soul". By contrast, the lowest of Planetary Spheres linked to the Moon and was known as "The Gate of the Body".

When the influence of Saturn is very strong, it creates fears, doubts, obstructions and blockages, such that the Gate of the Soul becomes sealed, shutting people off from contacting their inner light and their spiritual inspiration. Hence the melancholic angel represents someone whose Soul is trapped in the physical world and is no longer free to fly in the Intellectual World and receive inspiration from the Light of Creation.

This descent into a physical body is echoed by a ladder leaning against a plinth in the background. Its seven visible rungs correspond to the descent of the Soul through the seven Planetary Spheres into mortal form, and also serve as a reminder of the need of the Soul to ascend through the Planetary Spheres once more.

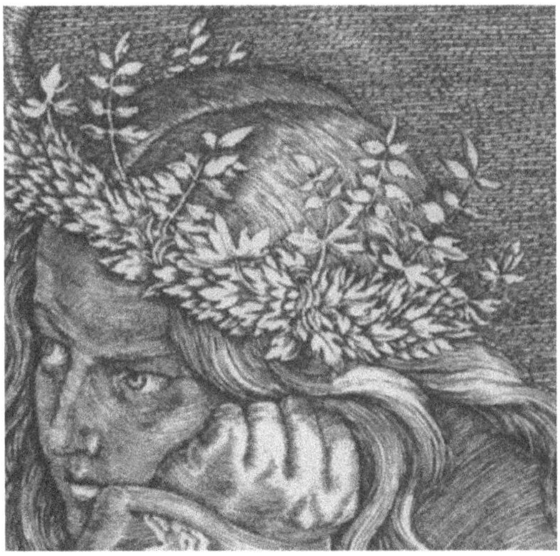

Figure 14.3: Detail of Garland

The melancholic angel wears a garland of flowers, which has been identified by botanists as a species of anemone. The common wood anemone (*Anemone nemorosa*), with its dull red stems, is associated with the Planet Mars (♂).

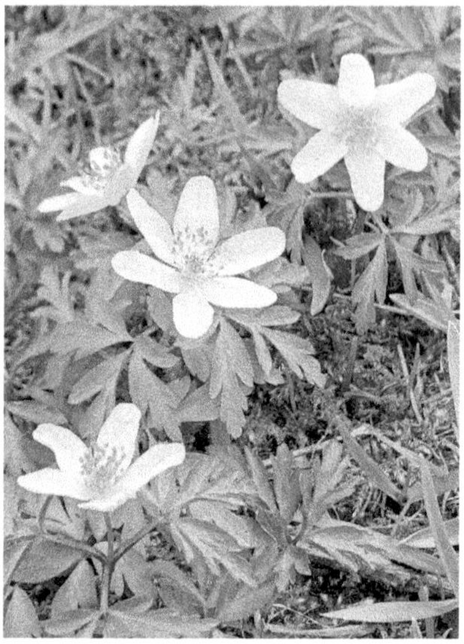

Figure 14.4: Wood anemone (*Anemone nemorosa*)

Analogous to a halo depicting the inner virtue of saints, the garland instead captures the mental anxiety and frustration from the angel's inability to break out of his inertia. The stagnation of his energy in melancholia manifests as a lack of will power and motivation to do anything.

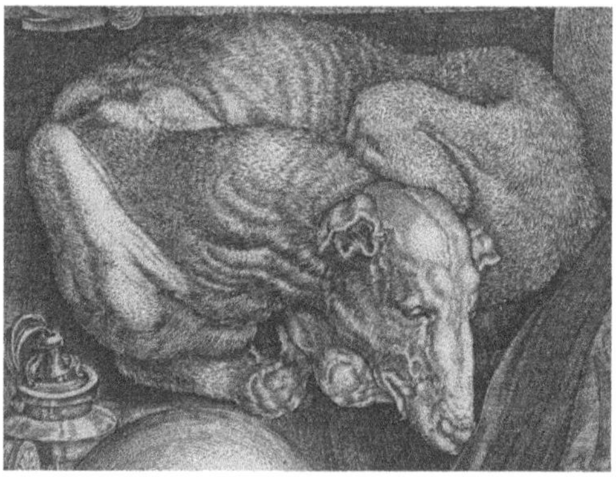

Figure 14.5: Detail of the galgo

This lack of motivation is echoed by the sleeping dog. Dogs generally are ruled by Mars. Here Dürer has depicted a *galgo*, a Spanish hunting dog, which when they are not hunting are known for sleeping excessively. Dürer portrays this dog as though it has been asleep and has not eaten for a long time, and its bones, ruled by Saturn, stand out of its flesh as if it was dead.

Such is the loyalty of the dog, however, that as soon as its master stirs it is ready for the chase. But with its owner crippled by melancholia, and lacking drive and motivation as a consequence of the melancholia, the dog just remains fast asleep.

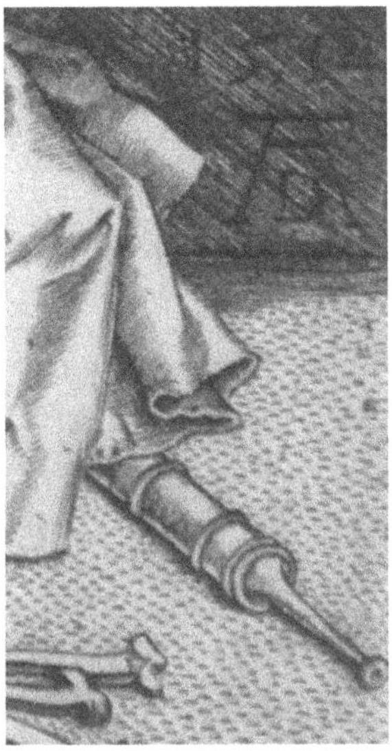

Figure 14.6: Detail of clyster

At the bottom right, hiding under the angel's robe, a clyster can be seen. This syringe-like device was inserted anally to pump laxative herbs into the colon as an enema to relieve constipation. Constipation had long been recognised as a symptom of an excess of the Melancholic humour, since it rules the retentive virtue. Evacuation of the bowel markedly elevates the mood of people. In medieval medicine the excess of the Melancholic humour was considered a major cause of mental illness; therefore, its remedy was to purge it from the body.

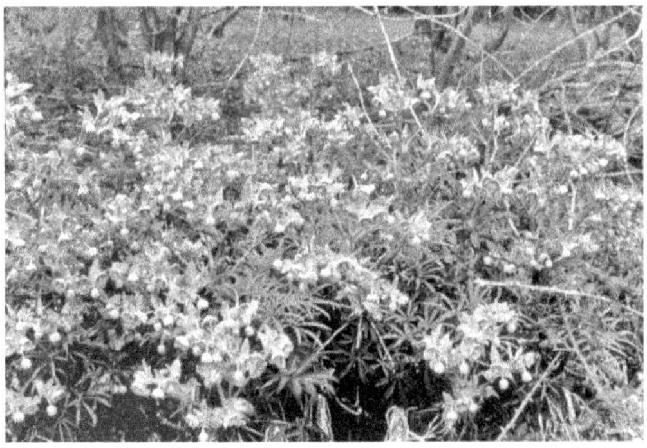

Figure 14.7: Stinking hellebore (*Helleborus foetidus*)

Though now considered too poisonous a herb for medicinal use, the Saturnine stinking hellebore (*Helleborus foetidus*), with its black, smelly leaves, was administered to mental patients, right up until the Second World War.

The present author learnt from an old man who grew up by the Wychwood Forest in Oxfordshire that as a boy in the 1930s he remembered this herb being collected there every year and sent to St Thomas' Hospital in London.

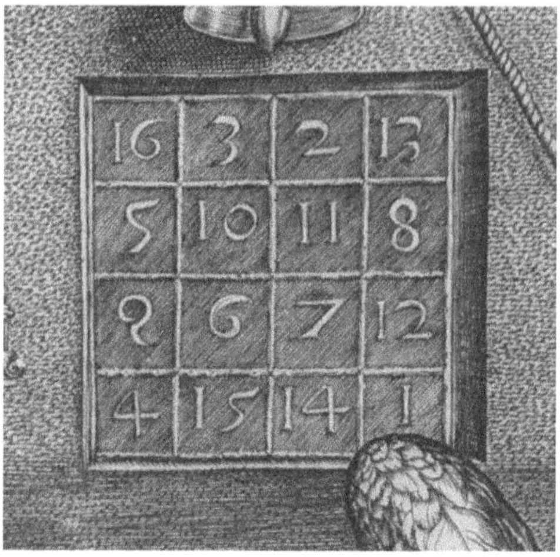

Figure 14.8: Detail of the magic square of Jupiter

A fascinating detail in the engraving is the inclusion of the magical square for Jupiter above the angel's head. Each of the seven traditional Planets has a corresponding magical square, based on its planetary number.

The number corresponding to Jupiter is 4, and the numerals within the square consist of 4 rows and 4 columns, containing numbers that all add up 34, whether added vertically or horizontally. Magical squares were a key part of Agrippa's teachings, but what is Jupiter's square doing, among the Saturnine theme of melancholia?

Art historians have observed that Dürer rearranged the numbers of the square, so they reflect the date of 1514 at its base, the year of the engraving's completion as evidenced by his AD monogram, located in the shadow just above the clyster.

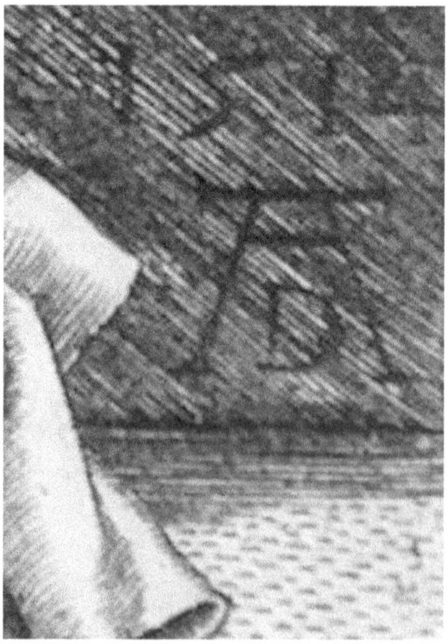

Figure 14.9: Detail of monogram

In the monogram, the A has been stylised as a doorway, which is a visual pun on the artist's surname Dürer, for in German it means "a door". Thus, Dürer saw his artwork as opening up doors of perception, enabling the beholder to grasp its deeper teaching.

When you compare Dürer's square to the traditional square of Jupiter, you can see he has inverted the order of the rows and swopped the positions of 2nd and 3rd columns, in order to place 1514 at the bottom. What is the significance of this inversion?

4	14	15	1
9	7	6	12
5	11	10	8
16	2	3	13

Figure 14.10: Magical square of Jupiter, after Agrippa

Jupiter (♃) is the symbolic opposite to Saturn (♄), which is shown by their respective glyphs. In Jupiter's the Crescent of the Spirit is exalted over the Cross of Matter, while in Saturn's the Cross of Matter is exalted is exalted over the Crescent of the Spirit.

This inversion of the square of Jupiter instantly makes the square become more Saturnine. If the Jupiter square placed above the angel's head symbolises hope and inspiration, then this inverted square means a denial of hope and lack of inspiration.

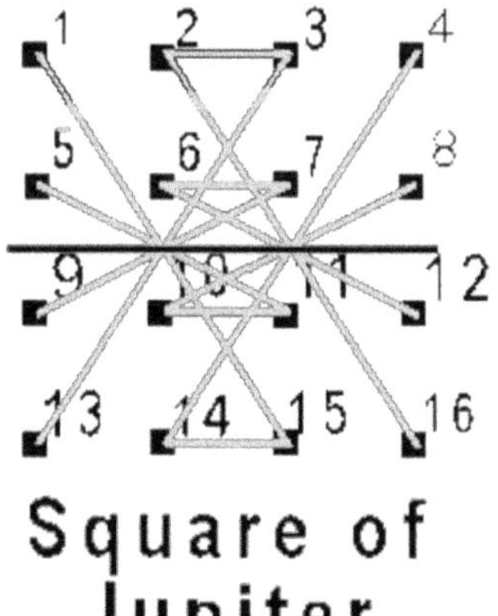

Figure 14.11: Graphic expression of Jupiter's Square

The magical squares contain intricate geometries, which have inspired architectural masterpieces of the Gothic era. When the numbers of the square of Jupiter are joined in sequence to the numbers in each row of the square, it generates the symmetric pattern shown. Jupiter represents the drawing down of the spirit into the physical world.

When a horizontal midline is drawn through the pattern, between the central columns the viewer can now see a pentacle with a triangle at its apex above, which is then mirrored by its counterpart below—"As above, so below."

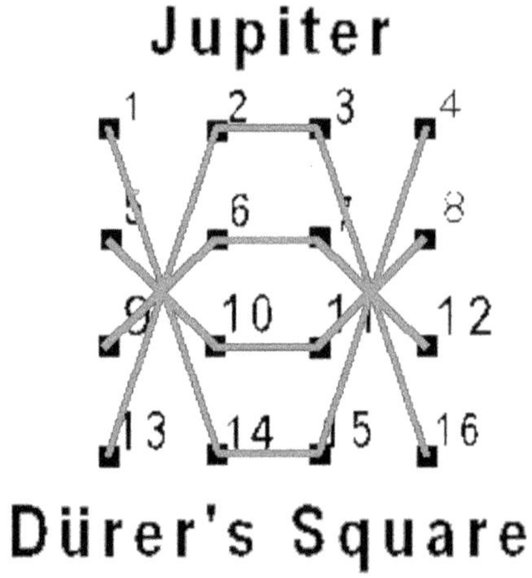

Figure 14.12: Graphic expression of Dürer's Square

Contrast this pattern of the Square of Jupiter with the pattern generated by the numbers in Dürer's Square. The symmetrical dynamism of the pentacle and triangle reflected above and below has been replaced by horizontal lines that just delineate separation. In summary, Dürer's Square is showing the loss of the symbolic perspective—"As above, so below." Thus, in a symbolic sense, it is showing a dark night of the soul, where all things lose their inner meaning.

To the left of the hourglass a set of scales hangs unused from a hook. The scales refer to the Zodiacal sign of Libra, where Saturn is exalted.

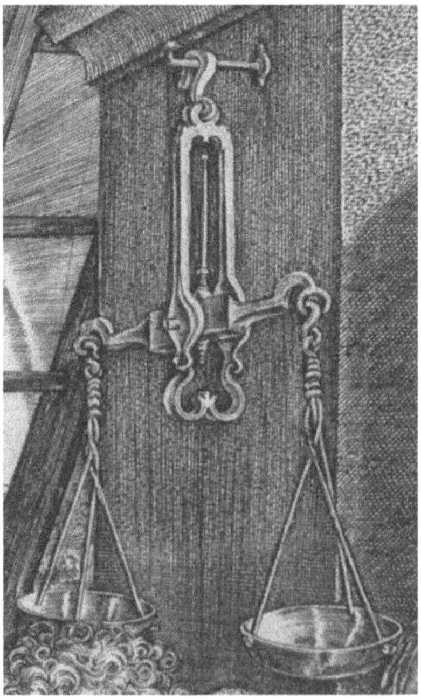

Figure 14.13: Detail of scales

Libra (♎), the 7th Zodiacal sign, is also linked to the Seven Liberal Arts—grammar, didactic, rhetoric, music, mathematics, geometry and astronomy—which were the foundation of the medieval education syllabus. The Liberal Arts were deliberately arranged to facilitate the Soul's return through the Planetary Spheres.

Normally, Saturn (♄) here would provide the discipline and concentration needed to facilitate their study. Here the scales are idle, suggesting the melancholic angel is unable to pursue any studying.

Between the magic square and the set of scales hangs an hourglass with a small sundial on top. Saturn (♄) is traditionally linked to time, giving rise to the word "chronology" (Gk *Khronos*). Saturn is very much a part of these instruments of time, for in the day as the Earth moves around the Sun, the needle of the sundial casts a shadow across its face, pointing to the hour of the day.

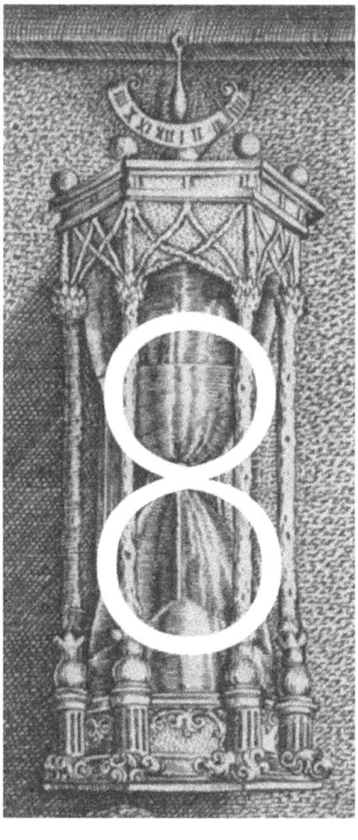

Figure 14.14: Detail of the hourglass

The shape of the glass vessel is analogous to the figure of 8, the number for Mercury. The vessel too is housed in an octagonal wooden structure. Its four visible wooden spindles are analogous to the four Elements.

Gravity (♄) pulls the grains of sand through the aperture of the hourglass, down from the chamber "above" to the chamber "below", defining the hour. Thus, the instrument is also a metaphor for one's time upon the Earth, in which to learn the lessons of the Planetary Spheres.

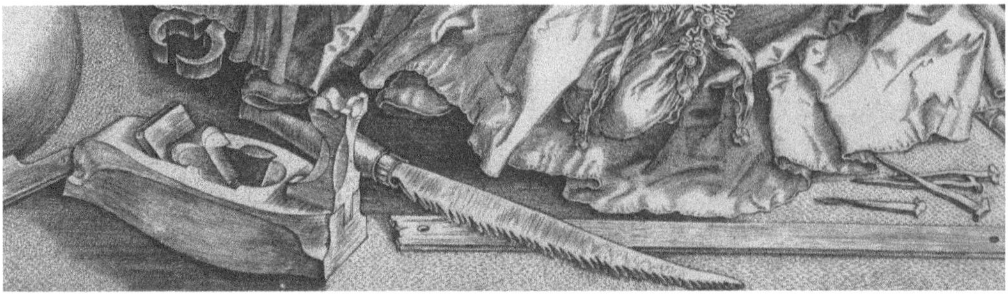

Figure 14.15: Details of carpentry tools

Below the melancholic angel's feet there is a scattered assortment of carpentry tools such as nails, a ruler, a saw, a hammer, a pair of pincers, a plane and a device to ensure the uniformity of moulding contours. A heavy sphere too has rolled away from the angel's control and come to rest out of reach.

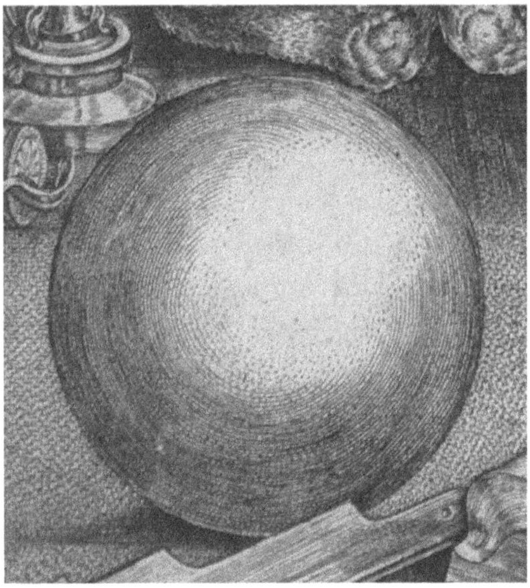

Figure 14.16: Detail of sphere

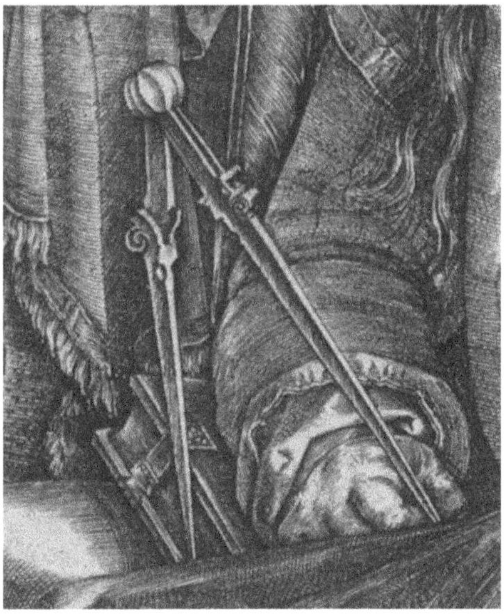

Figure 14.17: Detail of compass

The angel is clearly bored and distracted while fiddling with a compass. This shows he is unable to meaningfully engage in understanding the creative process of the universe. His lack of philosophical interest is echoed by the dishevelled array of carpentry tools, revealing his lack of motivation to do any carpentry. Carpentry here is a metaphor for the building of the physical world, and the compass is a symbol representing the beginning of creation, where duality arises out of the oneness. The frontispiece from the Gothic *Bible Moralisée*, illustrated here, depicts God, with a compass in hand, creating the world.

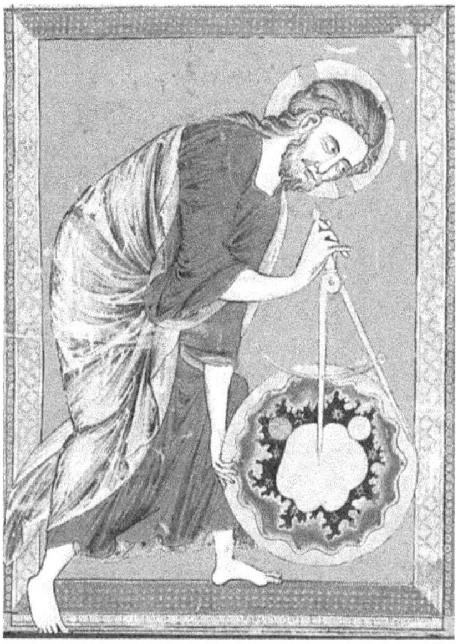

Figure 14.18: Frontispiece from the Gothic *Bible Moralisée* (13th century)

Within the radius of the compass, the Planet Earth, surrounded by representations of the Water, Air and Fire Elements, along with the Sun and Moon, can all be seen. So how does God with the compass create the Elements and life upon Earth?

In drawing a circle from a central point, the central dot and the circumference define the glyph for the Sun (☉) as the source of light and creation.

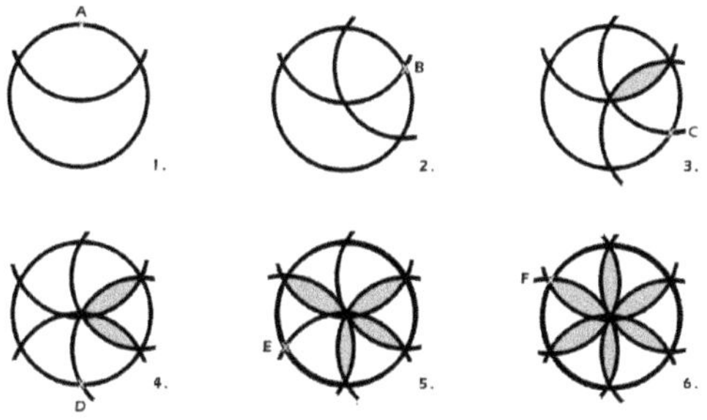

Figure 14.19: The geometric creation of the Flower of Life with a compass

When from any point, as in (A) on the circumference of the Solar glyph (B), an arc is drawn with the compass using the same radius of the circle, it creates an elliptical shape of a Vesica Piscis. Taking one end of this intersection (B), another arc is drawn. This is then repeated four more times at intersections (C), (D), (E) and (F), creating the petals of a six-pointed flower.

From each petal tip, six more circles can then be drawn. These in turn can generate six more petals, forming a geometric pattern known as the Flower of Life.

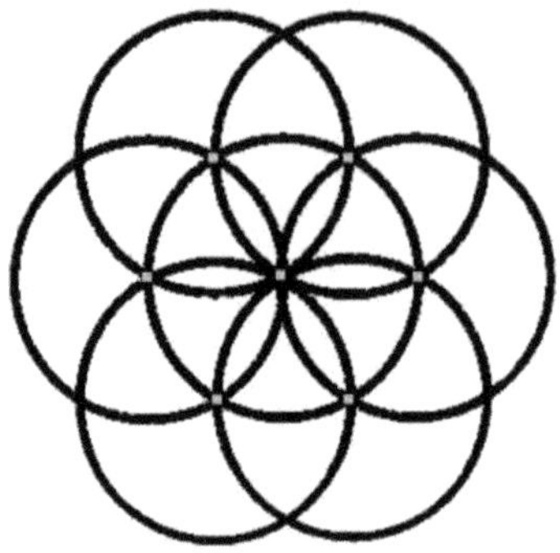

Figure 14.20: The Flower of Life

If each Solar glyph (B) represents one day, then with the six more glyphs surrounding it in total, this symbolically represents the Seven Days of Creation, named after the seven Planets.

- Monday = Moon's day
- Tuesday = Mars' day
- Wednesday = Mercury's day
- Thursday = Jupiter's day
- Friday = Venus' day
- Saturday = Saturn's day
- The middle glyph represents Sunday, the 7th day of rest.

As already explained in Chapter 1 on the Westminster Palace Rose Window, from all the Vesica Pisces, within the Flower of Life, the triangular shapes of the Elements are born.

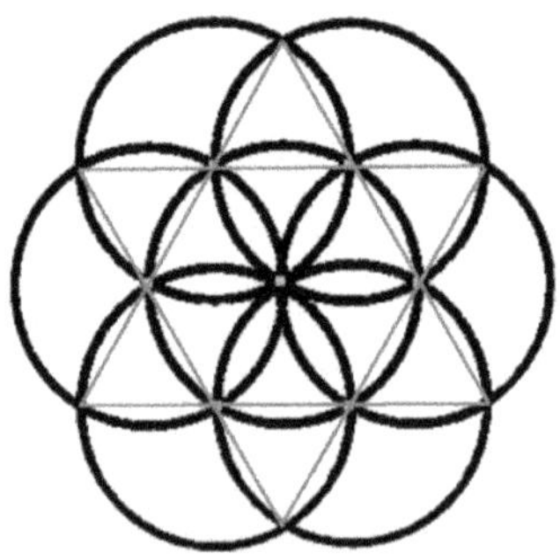

Figure 14.21: Creation of the Elements

Note too, this reflects the shape of the flower of the wood anemone, thus the garland and the angel's fiddling with a compass illustrate the frustration of not being able to resolve his existential conflicts.

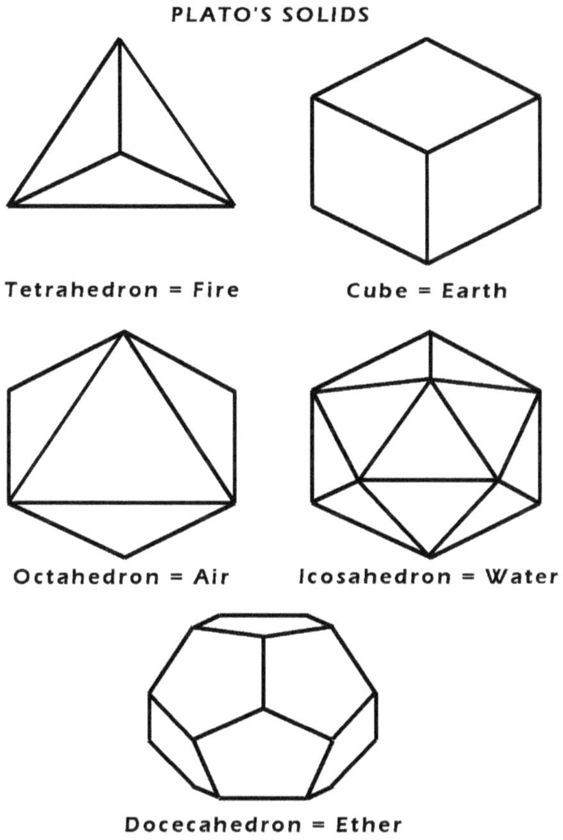

Figure 14.22: Plato's Solids

Of all Plato's Solids that evolve out of the Flower of Life, the dodecahedron is the most relevant here, for it represents the Fifth Element of Ether, symbolising the Vital Force. Additionally, owing to its 12 faces, it is linked with the 12 signs of the Zodiac, and thus the universe in general.

Considering the metaphysical progression of Plato's geometric solids, Dürer's inclusion here, at the base of the ladder, of an irregular eight-sided solid is significant. Its irregular structure, which has come to be known as the "Dürerhedron", is composed of six interlocking, elongated pentagons united by two equilateral triangles at the top and bottom.

The pentagonal faces clearly refer to the harmonious structure of the dodecahedron, although what Dürer wished to convey was that the gravity of melancholia had elongated and distorted it out its regular, concordant symmetric shape. Thus, it symbolically showed how much melancholia depressed the Vital Force, literally making it solid. The metaphor for fear is to be petrified, which literally means "to turn to stone". As a powerful symbol it conveys how much out of tune with the universe a person feels with the intensity of melancholia.

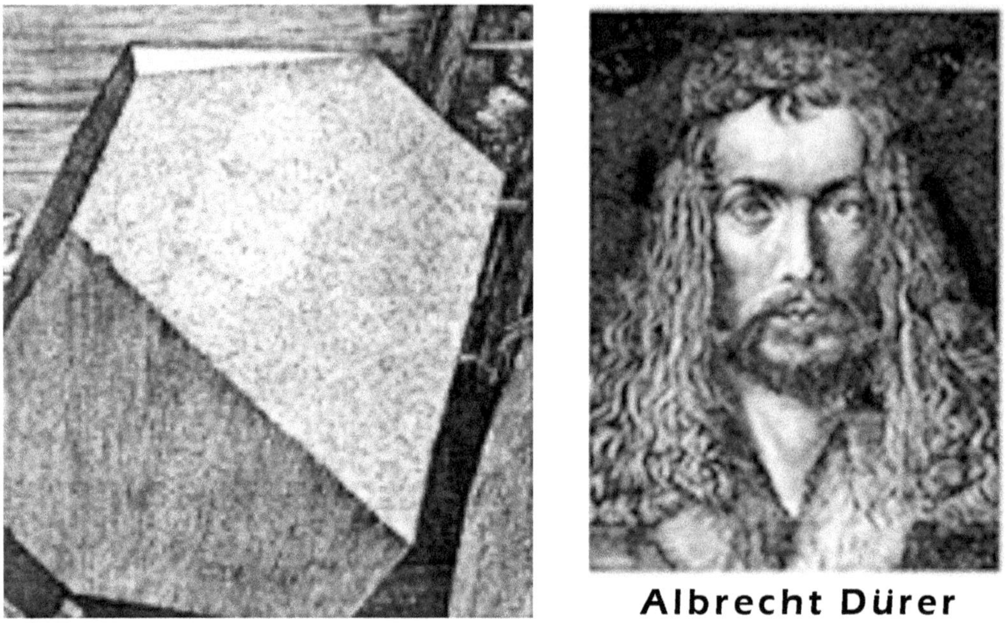

Figure 14.23: The "watermark" of Dürer reflected in the "Dürerhedron" compared to his self-portrait

The angel gazes at the upper pentagon of the "Dürerhedron"—facing the observer—which has the faint, oblique "watermark" impression of the face of Dürer himself. This cannot mean anything other than the artist is clearly identifying with this crushing weight of melancholia, depressing his vitality and making him feel "out of synch" with the universe.

The sheer weight of the emotion is preventing him from climbing back up the ladder of the Planetary Spheres. It is important to note that not all reproductions of this image have this subtle detail clearly visible. Considering how many copies were run off the printing press in his day, it was only when the surplus ink was used up that this detail became visible.

The little angel or cherub sitting on a millstone would thus describe the artist as a solitary, solemn child. Clearly, the artist suffered from melancholia since childhood, though probably largely unaware of the extent of his suffering then.

The engraving does, however, contain a powerful image of hope and resolution. Hanging from the angel's waist is a collection of six keys. Dürer was particularly fascinated by keys in his artwork, as symbols for unlocking hidden knowledge in his images. The largest, sixth key is suspended separately from a ribbon containing the name "IBIS", an allusion to Thoth, implying that Hermetic teachings contain the key. In other words, the sixth key is the one for unlocking the enigma of the Planetary Spheres and escaping the hold of melancholia.

Six is the number of the Sun. In the background the Sun is found shining with an arc of a rainbow above it, from across the sea. It is an allusion to the myth of finding gold at the end of the rainbow. Most people interpret this myth as the futile search for a crock

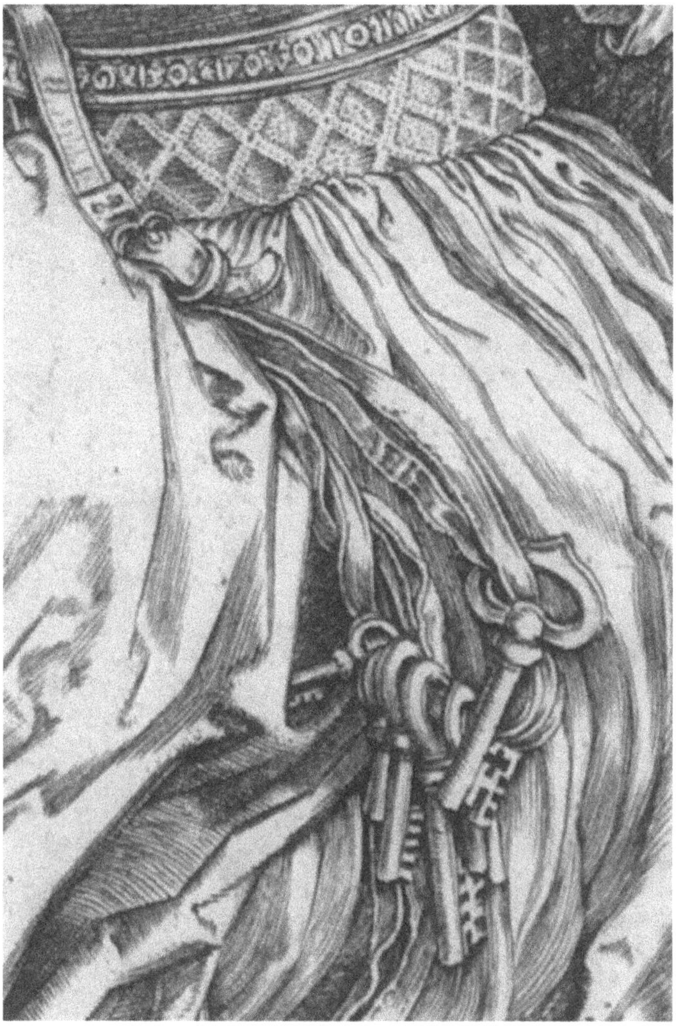

Figure 14.24: Detail of keys

of physical gold—as is well known as fast as you rush towards a rainbow in the attempt to reach the ends of its arc, so it recedes. You can never reach the end, yet alone find gold there! Hence chasing rainbows is considered a foolish activity. But Dürer knew that symbolically there *is* gold at the end of every rainbow.

If you look at the rainbow and then turn around 180°, you will be confronted by the gold of the Sun shining at you. You will no longer see the rainbow, which as a consequence has "ended". Instead of pursuing ephemeral goals, the myth is actually about turning within towards the light of the inner Sun of the Soul.

The Sun rules the Zodiacal sign of Leo, which is the opposite sign to Aquarius, ruled by Saturn. It shows that the heat and light of the Sun can disperse the cold and darkness of Saturn's influence, thereby elevating a person from the paralysing gloom and despondency of melancholia, to be free to ascend through the Planetary Spheres.

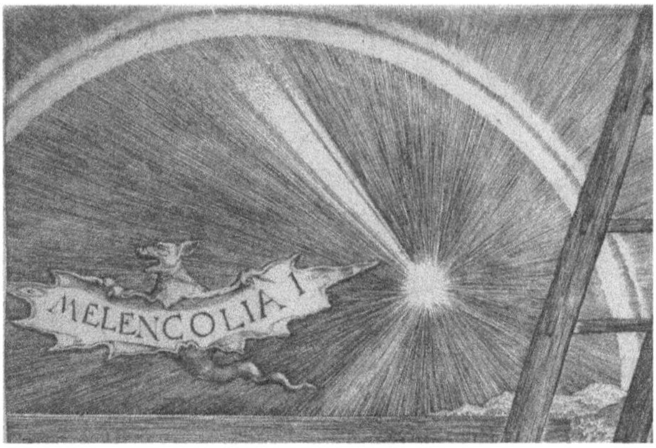

Figure 14.25: Detail of rainbow

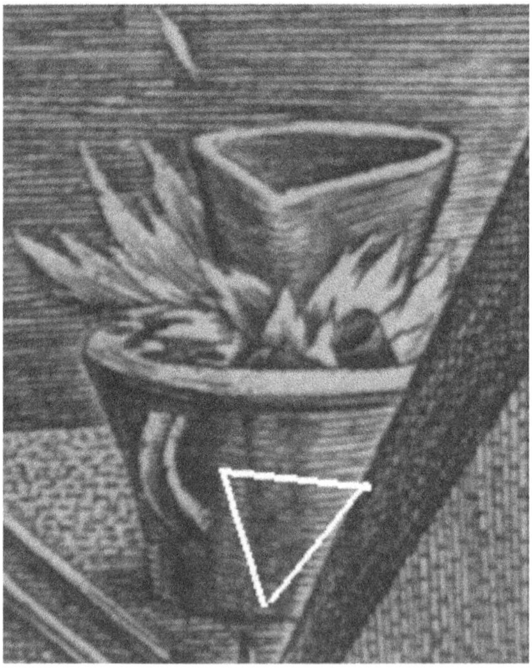

Figure 14.26: Detail of crucible

Furthermore, a detail that eludes the attention of most observers is located to the left, behind the "Dürerhedron". It consists of a crucible amid the glowing coals of a brazier. The crucible is deliberately depicted as being triangular in shape, forming the inverted triangle of the Water Element.

Water is the Element of cleansing and connection. Under the Saturnine influence of fear, the Vital Force becomes dense and leaden. Cold water flowing over the body washes the dross out of the Vital Force, whereby it releases the psyche from fear, making a person more receptive to inspiration from the Intellectual World. As the Water warms, so it releases tension from the muscles of the body, where the fear has become locked.

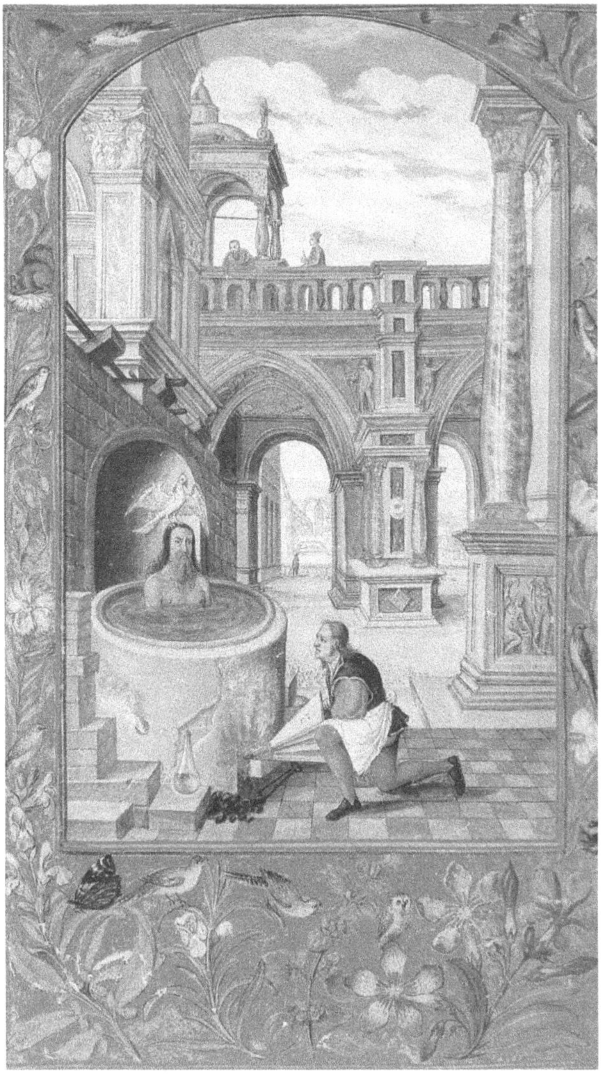

Figure 14.27: "Decoction", from the *Splendor Solis*. Public domain

This theme is shown in a plate, called "Decoction", from the sixteenth-century illuminated alchemical work, the *Splendor Solis*. Though its artist is unknown, the original work was also composed in Nuremburg, at the same time as Dürer lived there.

The central motif is a man sitting in a bath with a fire underneath, and an alchemist pumping a pair of bellows, driving up the flames. A white dove—a symbol of the Holy Spirit—has settled on the bather's head. This suggests that with his aura cleansed from the dross, he is able to connect with his higher self. Thus, this transmuting of lead (♄) into gold (☉) facilitates the inner journey of his Soul through the Planetary Spheres.

CHAPTER FIFTEEN

The Elizabethan Era

When Elizabeth I came to the English throne in 1558, she inherited religious conflict and uncertainty in the aftermath of her father's excommunication by the Pope and subsequent Dissolution of the Monasteries, followed by the short and bloody reign of her half-sister Mary (1553–58), who attempted to undo these changes and restore Catholicism to Britain.

Public display of the Catholic faith became very dangerous, yet despite this many noble families privately maintained their Catholic beliefs. They covertly celebrated the Catholic mass in their homes, often conducted by priests who had not completely renounced their faith, and who had to be quickly secreted away in priest holes if enforcement officers arrived at their door.

With all the religious uncertainty, there became a need to conceal metaphysical knowledge to all but the initiated. The language and imagery of alchemy, prevalent on the European continent, became a popular medium for both concealing and communicating this knowledge.

We will examine the work of two prominent and influential intellectual men from this era, and see how they adapted the metaphysical knowledge in their writings to the political climate. The first of these is the astrologer, John Dee and the second is the bard, William Shakespeare.

John Dee

John Dee (1527–1608), who was the royal astrologer and close confidant of Elizabeth I, was deeply inspired by the teachings of Hermeticism. He would have witnessed the conflict, suffering and deaths occasioned by religious conflict in England. His way ahead came to him, as he reflected on this conflict, through a powerful symbol that would, he believed, enable those who studied it to transcend the limitations of formal religious structures.

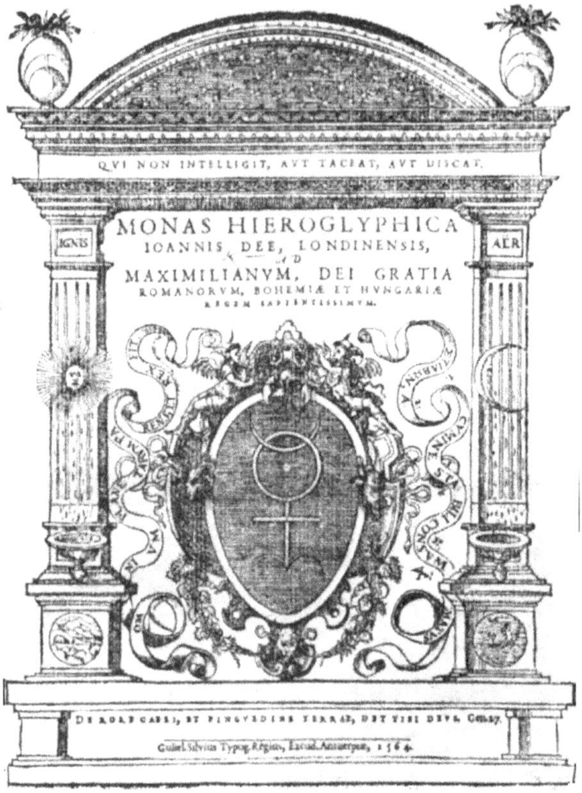

Figure 15.1: John Dee's *Monas Hieroglyphica*

For Dee the Hermetic teachings were revealed inwardly as a composite symbol, his *Monas Hieroglyphica*. He was particularly excited by this revelation, for it embodied many aspects of esoteric knowledge into a single unity (*Monas*).

His hope was by unifying all these ideas into a single symbol, when meditated upon it would generate peace and harmony, thereby connecting people to the source of the Hermetic teachings and enabling them to overcome their religious differences. He saw the symbol, which he named "The London Seal of Hermes", as capable of revealing the secrets of the entire creation. Within its intricate structure a dazzling array of astrological, alchemical and mathematical ideas can be found. This symbol deserves close attention, for it encapsulates both the cosmology and symbolism of Hermeticism, knowledge that would have previously required the study of the Seven Liberal Arts to have obtained.

The genesis of the hieroglyph is reflected in its central motif of an egg, which contains the Planetary glyph for Mercury (☿), located above a flattened form of the Zodiacal glyph for Aries (♈). When Mercury is equated with the god Hermes, and Aries to the head—the part of the body traditionally ruled by Aries—one can visualise an image of the wisdom and knowledge of Hermes coming down and entering Dee's head.

This same image is descriptive of the nature of Hermetic revelation. Since Aries (♈) is a Fire sign it indicates that energy needs to be focused onto the symbol in order to derive knowledge from it. Hermetic philosophy visualises the universe as having three distinct Worlds manifested out of a realm of Light. When transposed into man the Intellectual World corresponds to the spirit, the Celestial World to the soul and the Elemental World to the body.

This tripartite cosmology is reflected within the glyph of Mercury (☿), as the three component shapes respectively: the Crescent of the spirit, the Circle of the soul and the Cross of matter. The Crescent corresponds to the Intellectual World, the Circle to the Celestial World and the Cross to the Elemental World.

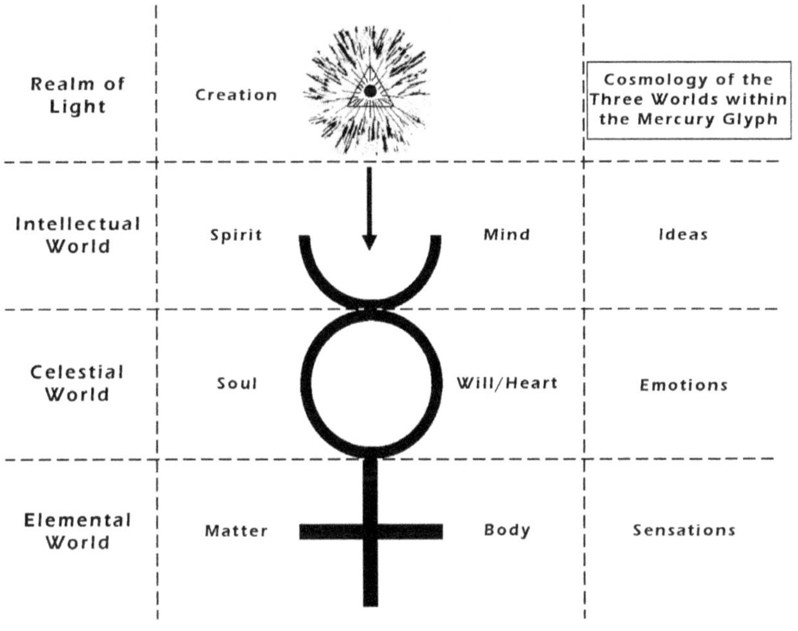

Figure 15.2: The cosmology of the Mercury glyph

The location of the central glyph within an egg is important, for this is an ancient Egyptian symbol that alludes to the source of Hermetic knowledge. In the Egyptian pantheon, Hermes is associated with Thoth, the scribe of the gods, who is depicted with the head of a sacred ibis. Its egg has as its sequel the hatching out of a baby chick, which ultimately learns how to fly. The flying of the bird through the Air, or the Intellectual World of spirit, is symbolic of Man's spiritual unfoldment. Thus, the reception of Hermetic knowledge leads to spiritual insight and development.

The archway of the *Monas Hieroglyphica* symbolises Creation as perceived within Hermetic philosophy. Despite the substantial appearance of the pillars that compose the arch, the stars located in its dome suggest that Creation should be interpreted on a universal cosmic scale. The crescent-shaped dome is separated from a much larger circle.

If this circle was completely present its circumference would encompass both the bottom corners of the pillars. Taking the complete circle to symbolise the unity of life, then the two pillars splitting away off the crescent dome symbolically show the generation of duality out of unity.

Embodied in the shape of the pillared archway can be found the Roman numeral II—the glyph for the Gemini (♊). Gemini traditionally rules London, hence Dee's appellation for his symbol—"The London Seal of Hermes". Being an Air sign Gemini relates to the mind. Furthermore, Mercury, its ruler, is synonymous with the god Hermes. Thus, the Latin inscription at the top the pillars, *Qui non intelligit, aut taceat, aut discat*, meaning, "He who does not understand should be silent or learn," indicates the necessary attitude for receiving the Hermetic teachings.

On the left-hand pillar there is an image of the Sun, and on the right-hand pillar an image of the Moon. Thus, between these two pillars the whole range of duality is symbolised, including day and night, light and darkness, masculine and feminine, positive and negative, Sulphur and Salt, manifest and hidden, hot and cold, and dry and moist.

At each of the four corners, at the top and bottom of the pillars, are found representations of the Four Elements: top left, *Ignis* (Fire); top right, *Aer* (Air); bottom left, a rural vista (Earth); and bottom right, the Lunar goddess Diana swimming in the waves (Water).

The Four Elements have a quintessential relationship to the Fifth Element Ether, whereby they evolve out of the Fifth. Ether was known to the alchemists as the Aqua Vitae, meaning "the Water of Life".

On the pillars of the hieroglyph, the Aqua Vitae can be seen in the "droplets" present between the Luminaries (Sun and Moon) and the basins below. A subtle circulation of the Aqua Vitae is also symbolically described, for on the left pillar the Sun (hot and dry) evaporates it from the Earth, while on the right pillar the Moon (cold and moist) condenses it back to the Water.

The Hermetic Three Worlds are also reflected vertically in the pillars. At the top, above the Luminaries (Sun and Moon), is located the Intellectual World. In the middle between the Luminaries and the basins is located the Celestial World. At the bottom, below the basins where the pillars are substantially larger, is located the Elemental World. Subtle details on the pillars highlight these three realms.

The Elements present in the Intellectual World (the realm of ideas) are shown as words—"ideas"—whereas the Elements present in the Elemental World (the realm of matter) are expressions of their physical forms. The "droplets" of the Aqua Vitae are only found in the Celestial World, since Ether forms the medium of this realm.

An idea central to Hermetic philosophy is that Man is made in the image of the heavens, summed up by the oft-quoted phrase, "As above, so below." The *Monas Hieroglyphica* reflects this correspondence in a variety of ways. In the macrocosm, the Four Elements located at the corners of the pillars correspond to the Four Elements reflected by the four angles of the Cross within the microcosm of the central Mercury glyph. Ether is readily seen in the macrocosm as the "droplets", but its microcosmic counterpart is more abstruse. The Aqua Vitae is also alluded to by alchemists as the Philosophical Mercury. Hence the glyph of Mercury represents Ether in the microcosm within the egg.

The Sun and Moon located on the pillars also have their counterpart in the central glyph, since their symbols (☉ and ☽) are found composing their upper two sections of the glyph. Again, the Three Worlds reflected vertically in the pillars correspond to the three sections of the Mercury glyph.

The three Alchemical Principles—Sulphur, Salt and Mercury—are covertly reflected in the *Monas Hieroglyphica*. The Sun connects with the masculine, dynamic, fiery, Sulphur Principle (🜍) and the Moon with the feminine, passive, watery, Salt Principle (🜔). Their synthesis, the Mercury Principle (☿), is once again reflected by the central glyph. The egg is a common alchemical symbol, for its three main components also reflect the alchemical principles, the yellow yolk with the Sulphur Principle (🜍), the shell with the Salt Principle (🜔) and the white with the Mercury Principle (☿).

The Dot, forming the Solar glyph found inside the Monas Mercury glyph, forms the central point of the pillars. In Hermetic philosophy the "opening of the heart" is central to understanding the nature of the universe. When the Sun is seen to symbolise the heart—the seat of the soul—and the pillars to symbolise the Hermetic vision of the Creation of the Three Worlds, then the concordance between the Dot within the Solar glyph and the centre of the pillars symbolically reveals how the opening of the heart leads to the understanding of Creation. This is a particularly powerful confirmation of Man being made in the image of the heavens.

These ideas concord with Christian teachings in which Jesus says, *"The kingdom of heaven lies within."* The Sun is a symbol of a kingship, as well as of the Soul's residence in the heart: *"Blessed are the pure in heart for they shall see God."* A Christian cross is visible within the shaft of the central glyph. A further Christian connection is made by the Latin inscription found at the base the pillars. This extract, from Genesis 27 means *"May God give thee the dew of heaven and of the fatness of the earth."* Jesus in growing up in Egypt would have been exposed to Hermetic teachings, which, in turn, is reflected in his teachings. Therefore, in Dee's mind, in presenting Hermetic principles afresh, he saw its teachings as offering the potential for harmonising the Anglican and Catholic branches of Christianity, a division that was causing so much suffering and conflict.

At the top of the Monas Mercury glyph, the Crescent of the Moon lies over the Sun, with its concave aspect receptive to the impressions from above. Since the Moon symbolises the visual imagination, this illustrates the importance of the imagination in the development of intuition. Once a person's intuition is developed, they can receive the necessary inspiration for their own spiritual development.

By purifying the heart (☉) and developing the imagination (☽), the inspiration of Hermes (☿) can flow. This point is highlighted by certain Zodiacal signs located around the egg. At the top are the head and claws of Cancer; at the bottom is the head of Leo (♌); on the right is the head of Aries (♈); on the left is the head of Taurus (♉). The two twins of Gemini (♊) are found, one on either side of Cancer, each bearing a caduceus (a further Hermetic symbol).

To see the significance of this we must refer again to the three main Planetary glyphs found within the central glyph. Traditionally the Sun is dignified in the sign of Leo and exalted in the sign of Aries. The Moon is dignified in Cancer and exalted in Taurus. Mercury is dignified in Gemini. Thus, symbolically these are the conditions that enhance the hatching out of the egg—in other words, a person's spiritual unfoldment.

The Intellectual World embraces the mind, where ideas are formed out of spirit. The Celestial World of the soul is the source of will. It is also connected with the flow of emotions through the heart. The Elemental World of matter corresponds to the physical body and its sensations.

The Cross of matter situated below the Circle in the glyph for Mercury describes the manifestation of the Four Elements from the Ether. The Crescent of spirit, with its concave surface uppermost, shows the receptiveness of the Ether to the inspiration descending from the Intellectual World. This symbolically describes how ideas are formed within consciousness.

The alchemists saw the shining liquid mercury or quicksilver as symbolising the Fifth Element, Ether. They called the metal *Hydrargyre,* which literally means "the water that joins together", coming from the Greek *hydor,* meaning "water" and *ageiro,* "to gather, bind or join". The name *Hydrargyre* alludes to their perception of Ether as permeating all Three Worlds, joining everything together. So strong are these symbolic connections that the name mercury for the metal is derived from the Roman deity Mercurius, the "Messenger of the Gods". In modern chemical textbooks Hg, short for *Hydrargyre,* is still found as shorthand for the metal.

Surrounding the egg and the Zodiacal symbols in Dee's *Monas Hieroglyphica* is a scroll that twists around the central Monas motif. Its Latin inscription means *"Mercury* [Stilbon] *becomes the parent and the King of all planets when made perfect by a stable pointed hook."* This enigmatic phrase alludes to the alchemical perception of Mercury as symbolically embodying all the other Planets. Just as Ether is seen as the Quintessence of the Four Elements, so too, Mercury embodies all the qualities of the other six traditional Planets.

This idea is likely to have arisen from alchemy, where the corresponding metals for each planet were all perceived as dissolving into the quicksilver. This is not strictly chemically true, for while it is known that gold and silver readily dissolve into quicksilver at room temperature, copper, iron, tin and lead do not do so easily. However, with heat inside a furnace it is likely they observed the metals melting and thereby able to fuse with the liquid metal.

The *"stable pointed hook"* refers to the Dot in the central glyph forming the Solar glyph. Once this Dot is in place all other Planetary glyphs can be found within the glyph for Mercury, hence the idea of it becoming a parent. The Sun is symbolically connected with kings, so the presence of a Solar glyph at the centre of the Mercury glyph makes it *"King of all planets"*. The name *Stilbon* is Greek, meaning the "Glistener", another allusion to the Fifth Element, Ether.

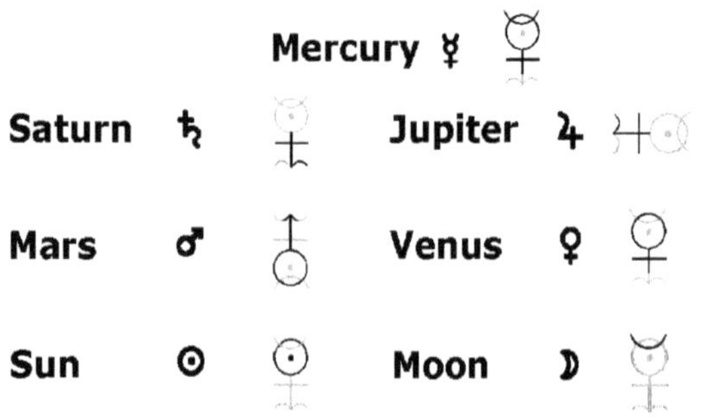

Figure 15.3: The Planetary glyphs concealed in the *Monas Hieroglyphica*

The inclusion of the Dot in the *Monas Hieroglyphica* is significant, for it represents the source of Light or God (Fire), which in each incarnation leaves the Intellectual World of the Air Element and descends through the Planetary Spheres of the Celestial World, where it acquires an emotional body and resides within the heart as the soul. Here the soul remains with the potential for mankind's inner illumination.

Understanding these Planetary qualities facilitates the return journey of the Soul back through the Planetary Sphere to reconnect with the light. In other words, this glyph captures the essence of the Seven Liberal Arts formerly taught within the monasteries but no longer available since their Dissolution.

Among the complex interaction of astrological and alchemical symbols, Dee described the symbol as embodying the "octonary" in a "most secret manner". The octonary is significant because the number 8 was traditionally attributed to the Planet Mercury in the Ptolemaic order of the Planets.

In Agrippa's teachings mathematical "magic" squares have been worked out for the numbers between 3 and 9. These have been utilised in various ways to express or engender the energy of the corresponding Planet into diverse things, ranging from the architectural design of Gothic cathedrals to the shape of the violin. Exploring the mathematical correspondence for Mercury launches the *Monas Hieroglyphica* into quite a different dimension.

Magical Square of Mercury

8	58	59	5	4	62	63	1	260
49	15	14	52	53	11	10	56	260
41	23	22	44	45	19	18	48	260
32	34	35	29	28	38	39	25	260
40	26	27	37	36	30	31	33	260
17	47	46	20	21	43	42	24	260
9	55	54	12	13	51	50	16	260
64	2	3	61	60	6	7	57	260
260	260	260	260	260	260	260	260	

Figure 15.4: The Magical Square of Mercury, after Agrippa

Mathematically, the square of 8 (8^2) is 64. As can be seen from the Magical Square for Mercury, the numerical configuration consists of 8 rows and 8 columns, whereby all the numerals between 1 and 64 are arranged in such a way that they all add up to 260. Numerologically, this number can be reduced to eight once more, as in the following progression, $2 + 6 + 0 = 8$.

The full significance of the mathematical symmetry embodied in these squares cannot be appreciated until these numbers are expressed graphically. If a grid of 64 dots is drawn on graph paper, laid out in a square of 8 rows and 8 columns and then numbered, then the numerical sequence of the magical square can be expressed by drawing a straight line between the appropriate dots. For example, the top row of the square reads; 8, 58, 59, 5, 4, 62, 63, 1, which can be drawn as shown.

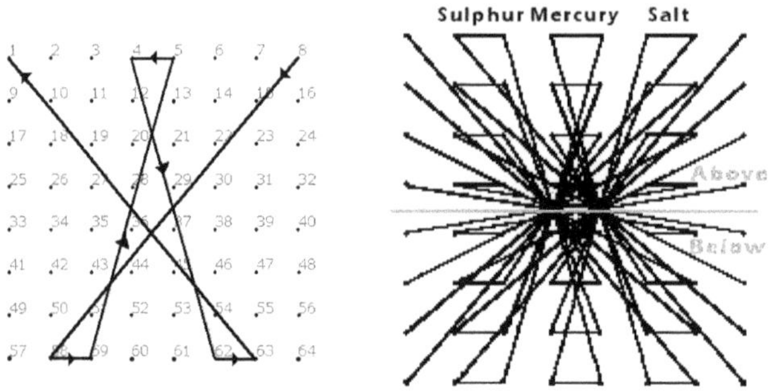

Figure 15.5: Graphical expression of the Magical Square of Mercury

After repeating the technique through all the rows, the resultant completed geometric pattern reveals a remarkable symmetry along its equatorial axis. The pattern above the line reflects through two foci the pattern below, which in turn reflects the ancient Hermetic maxim, "As Above in the Heavens, So Below on Earth." The pattern reveals three distinct columns, which once again corresponds to the Three Alchemical Principles of Salt, Sulphur and Mercury.

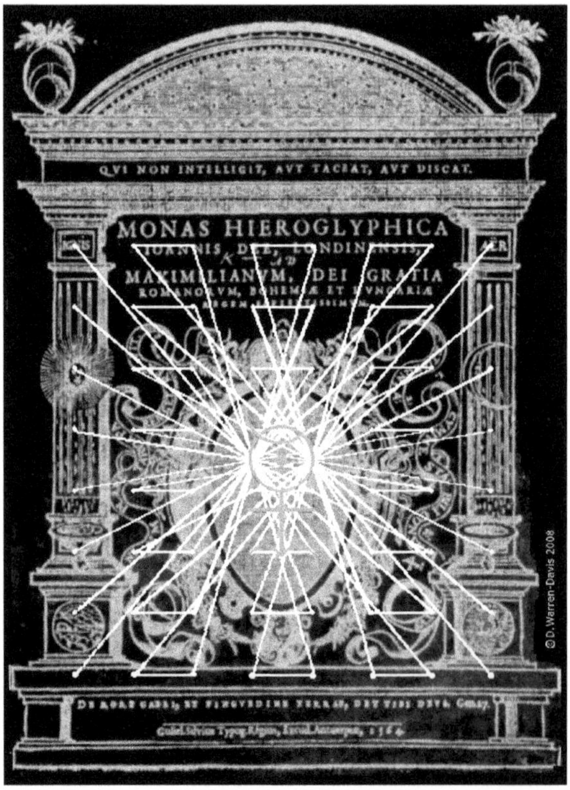

Figure 15.6: Projection of the geometric expression of the Magical Square for Mercury onto the *Monas Hieroglyphica*

The enigma of the symbol revealing the "octonary" in a most secret manner becomes apparent when this graphical pattern is projected onto the *Monas Hieroglyphica*, so that the two foci fit onto the sides of the Circle of the Soul within the central motif. The lines of the pattern connect key components of the design, confirming that the Mathematic Magical Square of Mercury was used as the foundation for Dee's design. The image has been intentionally inverted, as in an X-ray, which enables the subtle details to be seen more clearly.

William Shakespeare

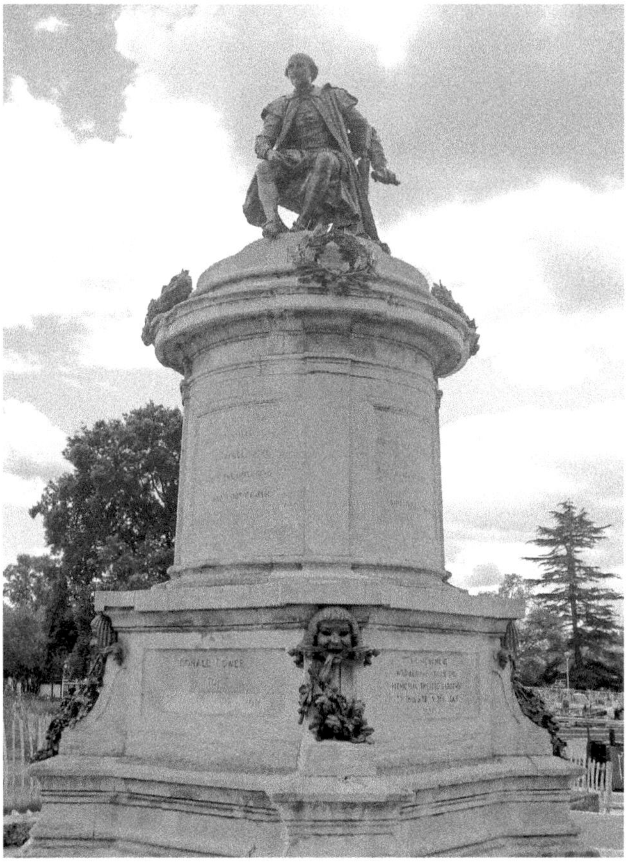

Figure 15.7: Statue of William Shakespeare in Stratford-upon-Avon

William Shakespeare was born into a Catholic family, so he too had to be very careful not to reveal his birth Catholic beliefs. Despite this stricture, his plays contain many examples of metaphysical ideas and imagery, revealing his profound wisdom.

A simple example is his description of the Seven Ages of Man woven into the dialogue of *As You Like It* spoken by the melancholy Jaques in Act II Scene VII. The monologue alludes to the return journey of the Soul, after it has learnt its lessons within each Planetary Sphere.

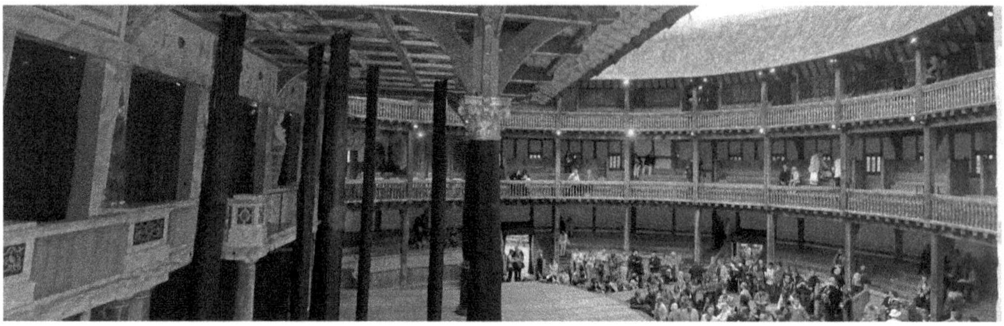

Figure 15.8: Reconstruction of Shakespeare's Globe Theatre on the South Bank, London. Note the Three World view in levels of the auditorium

All the world's a stage,
And all the men and women merely players:
They have their exits and their entrances;
And one man in his time plays many parts,
His acts being seven ages. At first the infant,
Mewling and puking in the nurse's arms.
And then the whining school-boy, with his satchel
And shining morning face, creeping like snail
Unwillingly to school. And then the lover,
Sighing like furnace, with a woeful ballad
Made to his mistress' eyebrow. Then a soldier,
Full of strange oaths, and bearded like the pard,
Jealous in honour sudden and quick in quarrel,
Seeking the bubble reputation
Even in the cannon's mouth. And then the justice,
In fair round belly with good capon lin'd,
With eyes severe, and beard of formal cut,
Full of wise saws and modern instances;
And so he plays his part. The sixth age shifts
Into the lean and slipper'd pantaloon,
With spectacles on nose and pouch on side,
His youthful hose, well sav'd, a world too wide
For his shrunk shank; and his big manly voice,
Turning again toward childish treble, pipes
And whistles in his sound. Last scene of all,
That ends this strange eventful history,
Is second childishness and mere oblivion;
Sans teeth, sans eyes, sans taste, sans everything.

The idea of the world being like a stage is a clear reference to the Hermetic incarnation of the Soul, down through the Planetary Spheres. A lifetime can be divided into seven stages of experience and learning, represented by the Planets, through which the

Soul evolves, in order to prepare for its return back to the light. Thus, the Lunar age is reflected in the "mewling and puking" infant; the Mercurial age in the "whining schoolboy"; the Venusian age in the "lover sighing like furnace"; the Martian age by the soldier; the Jovial age by "justice in fair round belly"; and finally, the Saturnine age is represented by the "lean and slipper'd pantaloon".

To those familiar with the "Seven Ages" will have noticed the absence of any reference to the Solar age in this monologue, which contrasts with the large number of lines devoted to the Saturnine age. Thus, Shakespeare wished to convey to his audience that Jaques had failed to find his calling, listen to his heart and express his creativity within. Instead, he had sought fame—"the bubble reputation"—leaving him in his melancholic old age, as he loses his strength and vitality, to regret that all he achieved came to nothing.

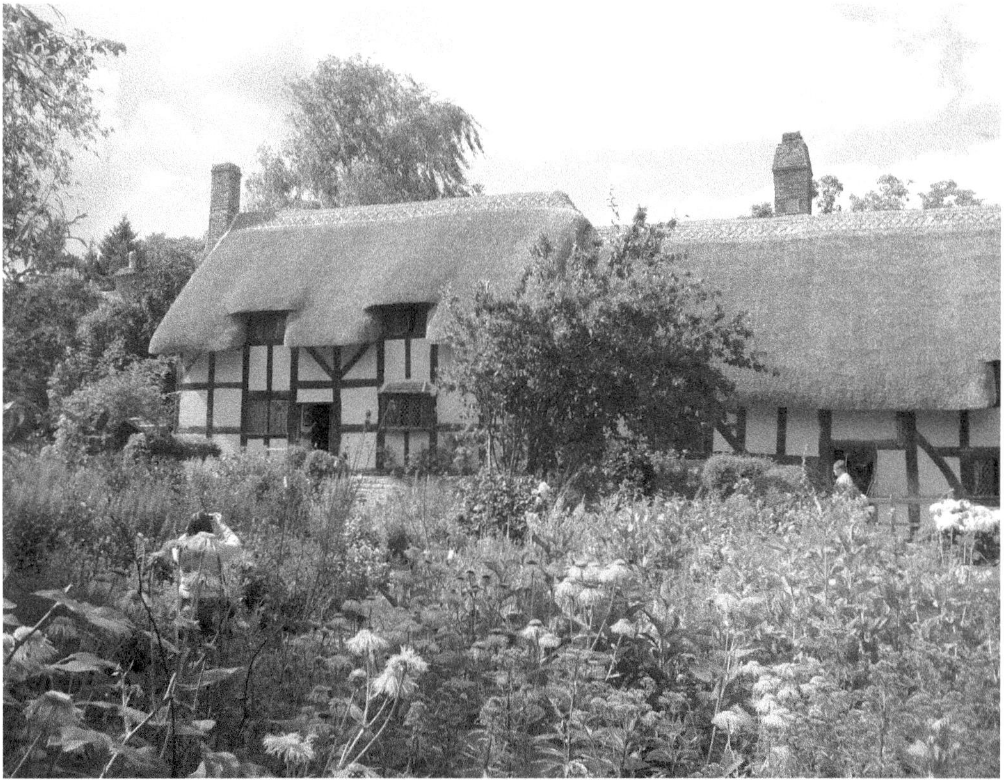

Figure 15.9: The garden at Anne Hathaway's Cottage, where William wrote a number of his plays

His plays also show how familiar William was with the myths and uses of herbs. An outstanding example, from a herbal perspective, is Friar Laurence's soliloquy in *Romeo and Juliet*, Act II Scene III:

The grey-eyed morn smiles on the frowning night,
Chequering the eastern clouds with streaks of light,
And flecked darkness like a drunkard reels

From forth day's path and Titan's fiery wheels:
Now, ere the sun advance his burning eye,
The day to cheer and night's dank dew to dry,
I must up-fill this osier cage of ours
With baleful weeds and precious-juiced flowers.
The earth that's nature's mother is her tomb;
What is her burying grave, that is her womb,
And from her womb children of divers kind
We sucking on her natural bosom find,
Many for many virtues excellent,
None but for some, and yet all different.
O, mickle is the powerful grace that lies
In herbs, plants, stones, and their true qualities:
For naught so vile that on earth doth live,
But to the earth some special good doth give,
Nor aught so good, but, strain'd from that fair use,
Revolts from true birth, stumbling on abuse:
Virtue itself turns vice, being misapplied,
And vice sometimes by action dignified.
Within the infant rind of this small flower
Poison hath residence, and medicine power:
For this, being smelt, with that part cheers each part;
Being tasted, slays all senses with the heart.
Two such opposed kings encamp them still
In man as well as herbs, grace and rude will;
And where the worser is predominant,
Full soon canker death eats up that plant.

Shakespeare chose the names of his characters deliberately to communicate a deeper dimension to his plays. Here he has chosen Friar Laurence as his herbalist and not using the more usual spelling of Lawrence. This spelling links his character to the laurel or bay tree, the emblem of the god Apollo. This alludes to the Hippocratic Oath, which opens with the line, "*I swear by almighty Apollo,*" thereby linking the friar to the Asclepiad medical tradition.

Fittingly, the opening lines of the friar's soliloquy poetically describe a sunrise.

Now, ere the sun advance his burning eye,
The day to cheer and night's dank dew to dry,

This encapsulates a snippet of Galen's temperatures in action for the hot and dry temperature of the Sun in the heavens is described as drying out the cold and moist dew of the Moon below on Earth.

The sunrise too is used metaphorically as illuminating the principles of herbal medicine, since the metaphysical principles underlying physic had become suppressed.

The dawn is the time when the Vital Force is strongest and its energies start to rise for the day, consequently it is a beneficial time generally for gathering herbs, hence the description.

I must up-fill this osier cage of ours
With baleful weeds and precious-juiced flowers

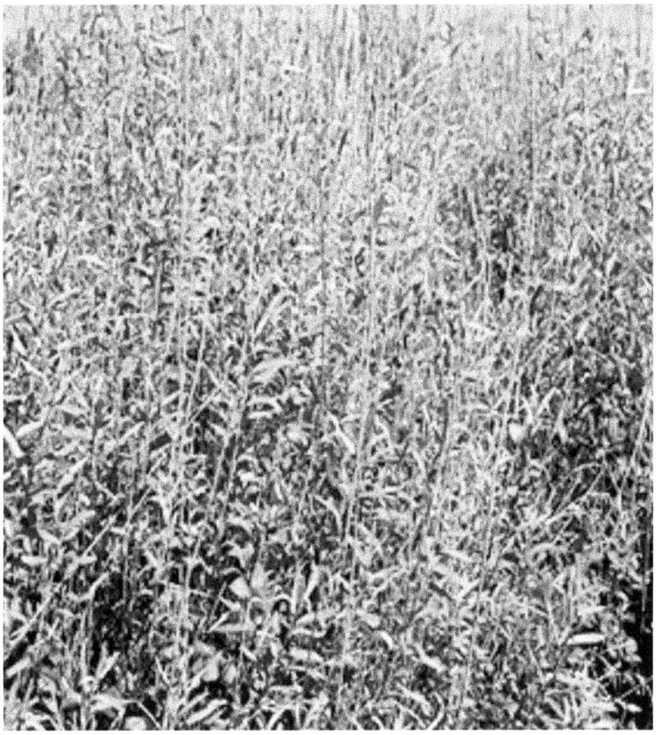

Figure 15.10: Common osier (*Salix viminalis*)

Osiers are the species of willow whose withies are chosen for weaving wicker baskets, hence make the ideal receptacle to collect herbs in. However, since willows are linked to the Moon, which symbolises the imagination, Shakespeare is subtly suggesting the importance of the receptivity of the imagination in understanding the virtues of herbs, whereby a physician can distinguish between poisonous weeds and valuable healing herbs. The juice or sap is where the virtue of the herb resides.

The earth that's nature's mother is her tomb;
What is her burying grave, that is her womb:
And from her womb children of divers kind
We sucking on her natural bosom find,
Many for many virtues excellent,
None but for some, and yet all different.

Profound respect is given to Mother Nature, and how she provides the floral diversity, in her annual cycle of life and death. "Sucking" refers to the Galenic tasting of herbs, identifying their temperatures—hot, cold, wet and dry—whereby their virtues can be worked out.

> *O, mickle is the powerful grace that lies*
> *In herbs, plants, stones, and their true qualities:*

In other words, fickle and elusive, while abundant, is the Vital Force that lies within plants, herbs and stones, which is linked to their therapeutic properties.

> *For naught so vile that on earth doth live,*
> *But to the earth some special good doth give;*
> *Nor aught so good, but, strain'd from that fair use,*
> *Revolts from true birth, stumbling on abuse:*

There is a no herb that is so poisonous that it kills itself. Shakespeare highlights that there is a balance to the virtues of herbs, and even the noxious ones do have purpose while valuable ones never give up on their qualities despite being over-used.

> *Virtue itself turns vice, being misapplied,*
> *And vice sometimes by action dignified.*

Because the knowledge of physic has been lost, he cautions against the excessive use of a beneficial herb, lest it creates an imbalance to the humours of the blood. By contrast, the judicial use of a poisonous herb can be very beneficial to counter a disease.

> *Within the infant rind of this small flower*
> *Poison hath residence, and medicine power:*
> *For this, being smelt, with that part cheers each part,*
> *Being tasted, slays all senses with the heart.*

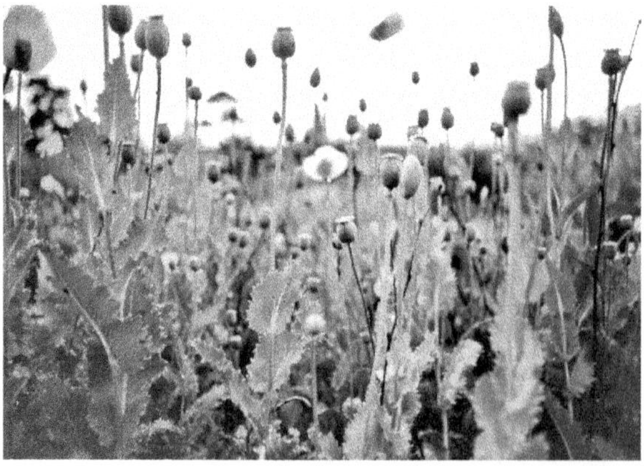

Figure 15.11: Opium poppy (*Papaver somniferum*), whose temperature has been described as cold in the 4th degree and moist in the 2nd degree

This speech is a remarkably prescient observation of herbs, which rings true with the future extraction of alkaloids, along with their increased toxicity in isolation from the physiological context of the whole herb. The paradoxical description of the herb here that *"slays all senses with the heart"* is a classic Galenic analysis of the action to a herb cold in the 4th degree, which *"mitigate desperate and vehement pains, stupifying the senses, when no other course can be taken to save life"*.

The opium poppy (*Papaver somniferum*) would fit this description. The rind here would have referred to the latex that exudes from the seedhead, which contains the hypnotic alkaloid, morphine. Bear in mind the friar here was preparing a sleeping draft for Juliet.

Two such opposed kings encamp them still
In man as well as herbs, grace and rude will;
And where the worser is predominant,
Full soon canker death eats up that plant.

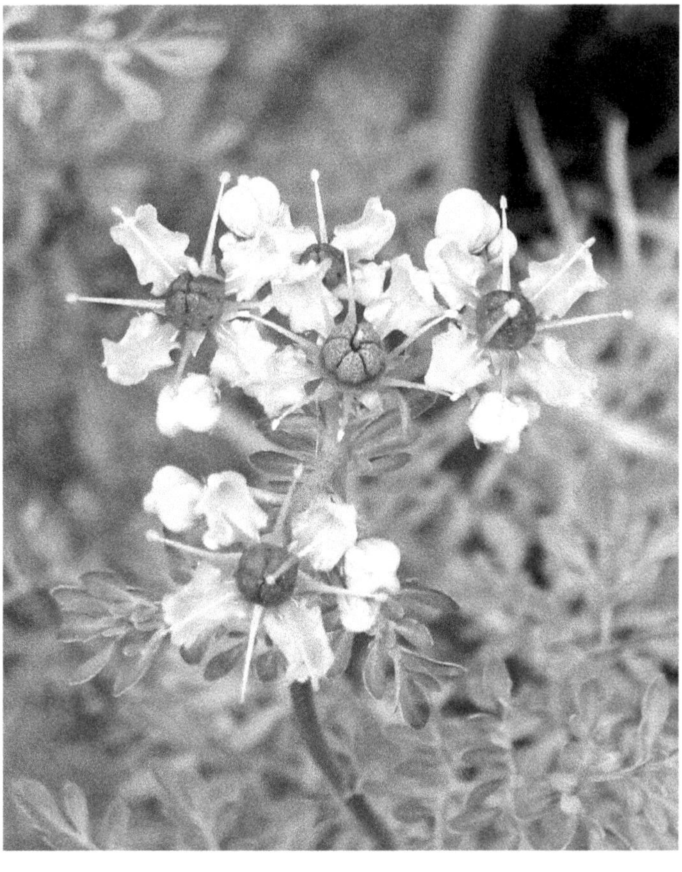

Figure 15.12: Rue or herb of grace (*Ruta graveolens*)

Shakespeare concludes the Friar's soliloquy with the example of rue as herb that embodies this paradox. He plays on its common name rue, along with its other lesser-known name, the herb of grace. Despite the striking four-fold symmetry of the flowerhead, symbolising the manifestation of the Four Elements, this Solar herb has an oil that exudes through its leaves, causing a dermatitis in sensitive individuals, making them rue their contact with it. Hence its rudeness.

Within the constraints of the literary context of his tragic play, it is remarkable how much of the metaphysical principles of physic that Shakespeare has managed to weave into this soliloquy, to communicate with his audiences, all while defying the censors.

So, both Dee and Shakespeare sought to communicate metaphysical knowledge within their work. Despite the risks involved, they attempted to make the knowledge accessible again by appealing to the imagination of their respective audiences.

With the destruction of the monasteries, access to the higher learning that they previously encouraged and contained was denied, leaving only the two principal universities in England, Oxford and Cambridge, as the remaining centres of higher learning.

They were limited in the number of students they could take in. Furthermore, prohibitive tuition fees prevented many from having the opportunity to study there. As a result, they became elitist institutions. In place of the monasteries, however, another invention started to change access to learning. William Caxton built the first printing press in Britain in 1476. Now over a hundred years later after importing the technology of printing from continental Europe, the number of presses had expanded with increasing number of books being printed. The development spurred an increase in literacy within the populace. Knowledge started to grow within society; however, it was less easy to control who had access to this knowledge.

Censorship was born. In 1603 the Company of Stationers was established, which had a monopoly of overseeing all publications, granted to it by James I. The Company was initially under the ecclesiastical control of Cambridge University. By 1632 control was additionally shared by Oxford University. All publications were brought under their scrutiny, and naturally anything that contravened the authority of the Anglican Church was banned.

Under this censorship, metaphysical knowledge was severely restricted as to what could be published. Printing or selling books that had not been seen and revised by the ecclesiastical authorities could incur corporeal punishment and all stocks of the works destroyed.

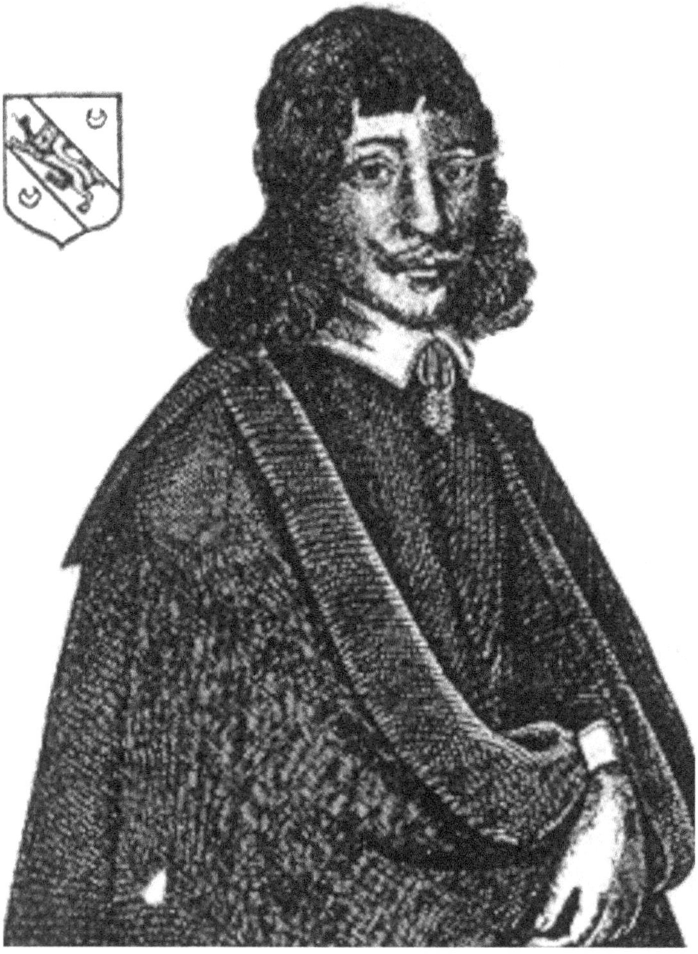

Figure 16.1: An engraving of Nicholas Culpeper

CHAPTER SIXTEEN

Nicholas Culpeper

Born in 1616, Nicholas Culpeper became Britain's best-known medical herbalist of the 17th century. Though he was a prolific writer and translator of many works, he is best remembered now, over 360 years later, for his herbal, *The English Physitian*. This book has been continuously in print ever since it was first published in 1652. It is a remarkable literary achievement, only surpassed by The Bible. Furthermore, his herbal was the first substantial medical textbook to be printed in North America.

Culpeper originally went to Cambridge University to study theology, largely at the wishes of his grandfather, the Rev. William Attersole, who wanted him to be a priest. In preparation, his grandfather had taught the young Nicholas Latin and Greek, so by the age of 11 he was proficient in both languages. His time at Cambridge was short-lived, however, as he dropped out after the first year.

He had decided theology was not for him and spent the time drinking, smoking and bathing in the River Cam. He did however get to attend medical lectures, whetting his appetite for his future vocation, but would have been prevented from studying medicine because he had not obtained his MA first.

Culpeper came from a very humble background and simply would not have had the means to spend ten years studying at Cambridge.

Following all the religious changes, from the Pope's excommunication of Henry VIII, the Dissolution of the Monasteries, and the Reformation, the high spiritual ideals of the Seven Liberal Arts had become lost. Instead in the universities, it had become an expensive intellectual obstacle course that excluded all but the students from the wealthiest families. However, Culpeper's early classical education from his grandfather enabled him to see through it. Hence the anti-elitist attitudes found in his writings.

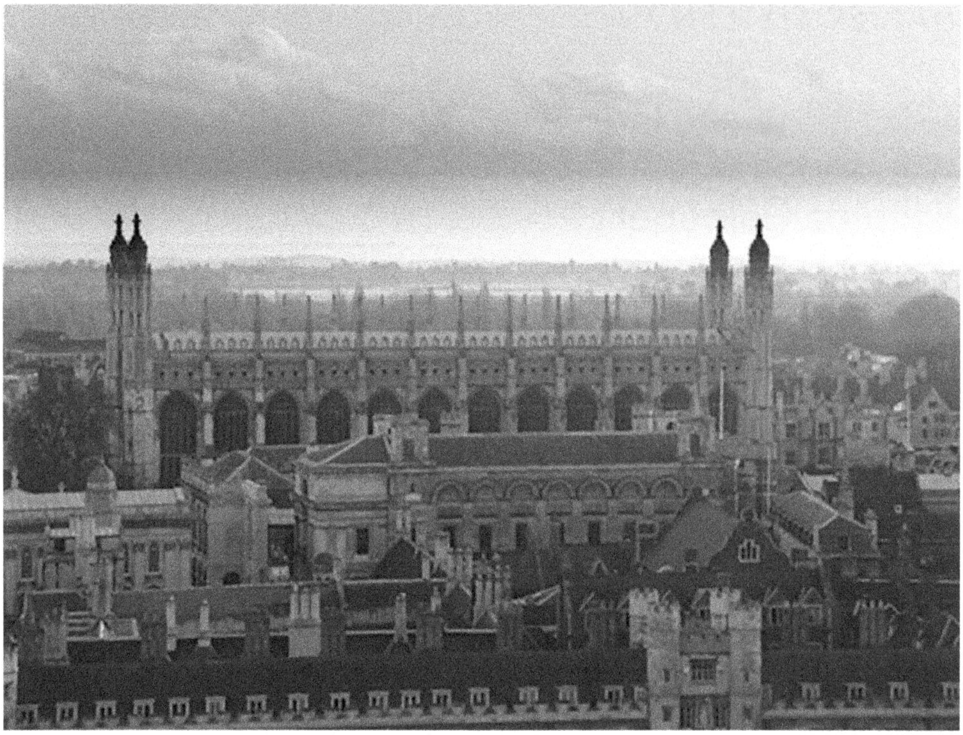

Figure 16.2: View towards King's College, Cambridge.
Photo Bob Tubbs. Public domain

Following his brief time at Cambridge he had little respect for priests, the authority of the Church and their control and suppression of knowledge:

> *Unless a man have gotten a very large estate he is not able to bring up his son to understand Latin. A dozen years of expense of time will hardly do it as they have ordered matters, in which time, whipping and cruel usage, the brains of many are too stuped that they are unfit to study. People miserably hampered by a scholastical net that they cannot get out of if they do see it. Righteous God look upon poor people and redeem them out of such Egyptian bondage.*

Having left Cambridge in disgrace, his grandfather suggested that Nicholas take an apprenticeship to become an apothecary. Culpeper became an apprentice to Francis Drake, owner of an apothecary shop in Threadneedle Street, Bishopsgate, in London. In return Nicholas is known to have taught him Latin. He was also taught *materia medica* by Thomas Johnson, editor of Gerard's *Herball* of 1633, which is why there are so many extracts of Gerard found in *The English Physitian*.

With the execution of Charles I in 1649, and the formation of the Commonwealth, the control of publications by the Company of Stationers was suspended. Consequently, the eleven-year period of the Interregnum was an extraordinary period of freedom to publish. Later that same year Culpeper's translation of the *Pharmacopoeia Londinensis* from Latin into English was published. He could see that herbal knowledge was being coveted by the Physicians. Apothecaries too were charging high prices for herbs, disguised by their Latin names, but which often grew in their own gardens and local hedgerows. Furthermore, the opening up of the New Worlds led to foreign herbs becoming more valuable than indigenous herbs, hence the apothecaries could charge more for them.

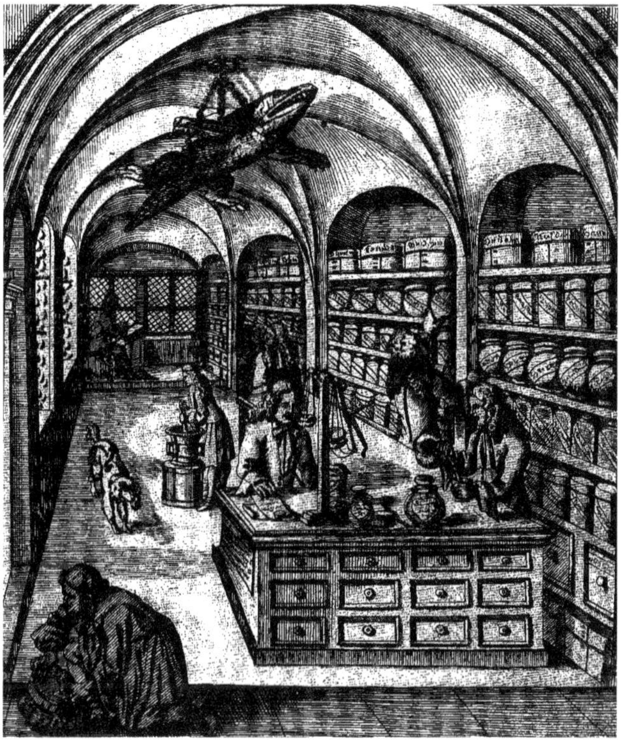

Figure 16.3: An engraving of a typical 17th-century apothecary shop

His response was this translation, of which Culpeper said:

> *I am writing for the press a translation of the physicians medicine book from Latin into English so that all my fellow countrymen and apothecaries can understand what the doctors write on their bills. Hitherto they made medicine a secret conspiracy, writing prescriptions in mysterious Latin to hide ignorance and to impress upon the patient. They* [the Physicians of the Royal College] *want to keep their book a secret, not for everybody to know.*

His uncle, Anthony Parris, cautioned Nicholas of the consequences of his translation:

> *Be careful and do not attempt an illegal translation or anything that can harm you and your family. People in high places may indict you before the* [Court of] *Star-Chamber.*

Nicholas replied:

> *The Star-Chamber has been abolished, thank God, and I am not afraid of punishment. Imagine the doctors saying, that laying medicine more open to mankind would lessen their patient's*

faith in it. The truth is that opening the book shows what jumble of obscure and costly ingredients the prescriber intends to burden our stomachs with.

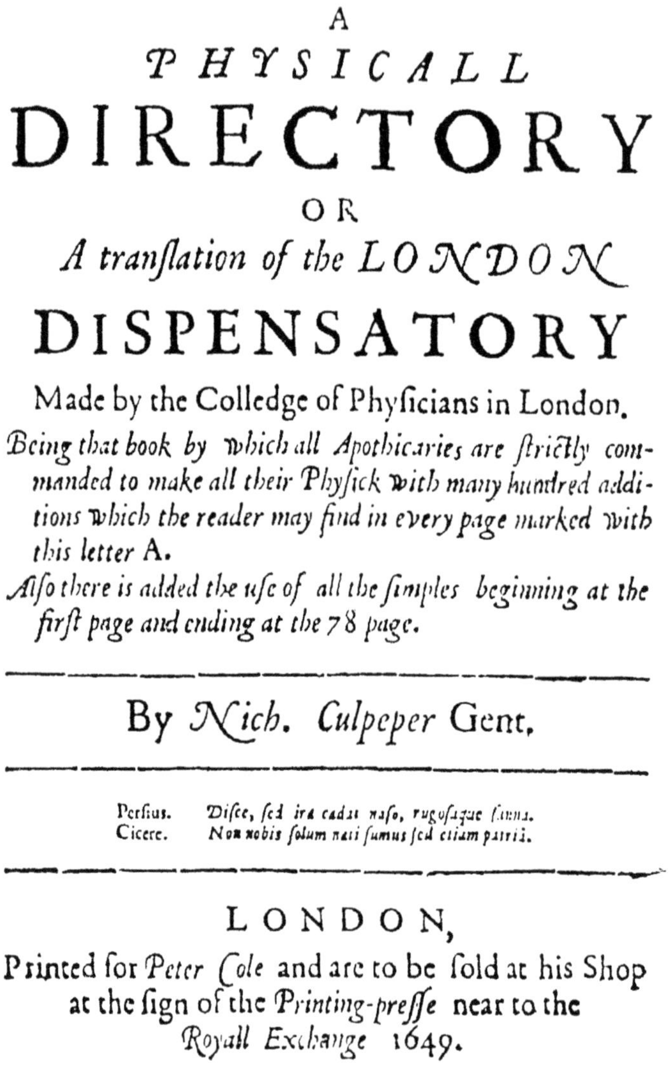

A
PHYSICALL
DIRECTORY
OR
A tranſlation of the LONDON
DISPENSATORY
Made by the Colledge of Phyſicians in London.
Being that book by which all Apothicaries are ſtrictly commanded to make all their Phyſick with many hundred additions which the reader may find in every page marked with this letter A.
Alſo there is added the uſe of all the ſimples beginning at the firſt page and ending at the 78 page.

By *Nich. Culpeper* Gent.

Perſius. *Diſce, ſed ira cadat naſo, rugoſaque ſanna.*
Cicere. *Non nobis ſolum nati ſumus ſed etiam patrii.*

LONDON,
Printed for *Peter Cole* and are to be ſold at his Shop at the ſign of the *Printing-preſſe* near to the *Royall Exchange* 1649.

Figure 16.4: Culpeper's translation of the *London Dispensatory*

The translation sparked a major controversy and the College counter-attacked in their periodical *Mercurius Pragmaticus:*

The Pharmacopoeia was done (very filthly) into English by one Nicholas Culpeper who commenced the several degrees of Independancy, Brownisme, Anabaptisme; admitted himself of John Goodwin's school (of all ungodliness) in Coleman Street; after that he turned Seeker, Manifestarian, and now he has arrived at the battlement of an absolute Atheist,

> *and by two years drunken labour hath Gallimawfred the apothecaries book into nonsense, mixing every receipt therein with some scruples, at least, of rebellion or atheisme, …*
>
> *… besides the danger of poysoning men's bodies. And (to supply his drunkeness and leachery with a thirty shilling reward) endeavoured to bring into obloquy the famous societies of apothecaries and chyrurgeons.*

What particularly excited the ire of the physicians was that Culpeper added his own commentary about the uses and virtues of each plant, hence the *"danger of poysoning men's bodies"* through the lay person not knowing how to prescribe medicines. The Physicians were clearly rattled yet there was very little they could do about it.

The College's monopoly and legal status over the practice of medicine had been granted by royal charter, yet they were unable to prosecute Culpeper owing to the abolition of Star-Chamber. Furthermore, the trying of such an outspoken supporter of the Commonwealth in the new political climate would have had very little support, since the execution of Charles I just prior to the publication of Culpeper's translation would have been a powerful blow to the authority of the College.

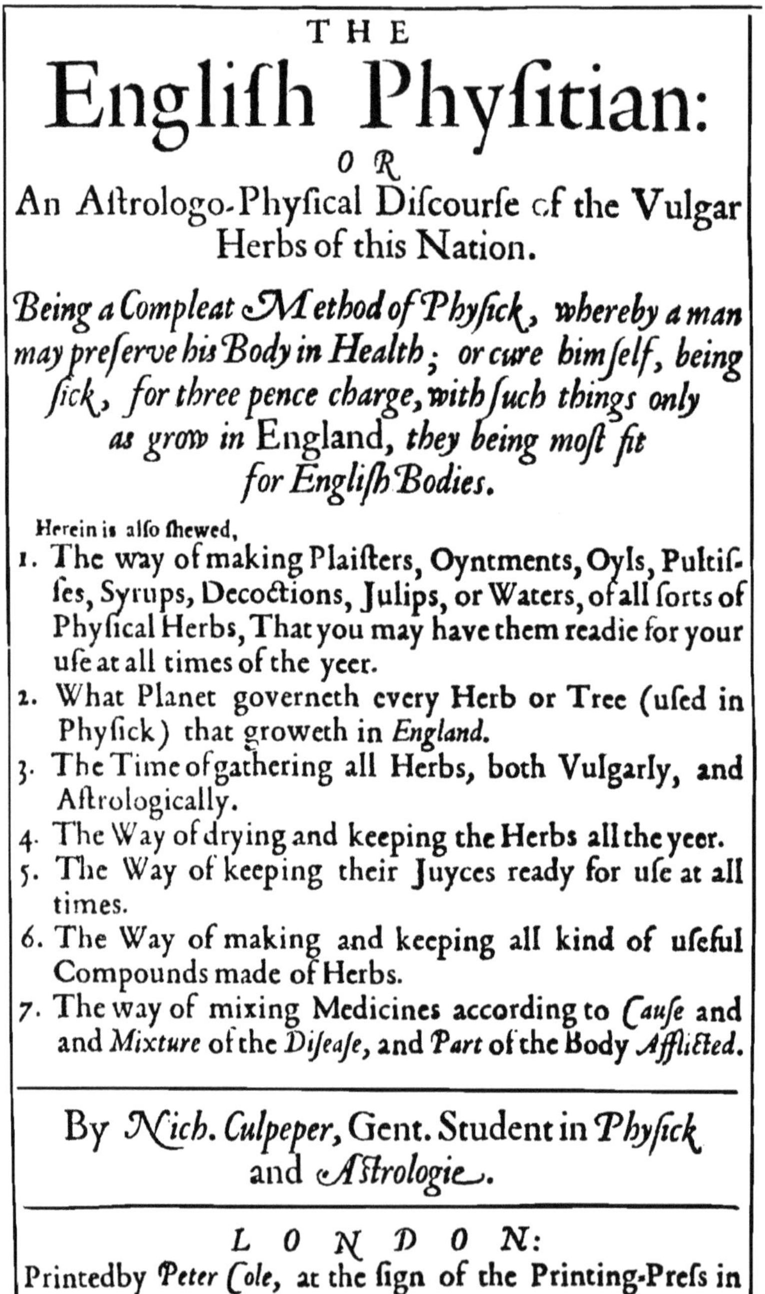

THE

Engliſh Phyſitian:

OR

An Aſtrologo-Phyſical Diſcourſe of the Vulgar Herbs of this Nation.

Being a Compleat Method of Phyſick, whereby a man may preſerve his Body in Health; or cure himſelf, being ſick, for three pence charge, with ſuch things only as grow in England, *they being moſt fit for Engliſh Bodies.*

Herein is alſo ſhewed,

1. The way of making Plaiſters, Oyntments, Oyls, Pultiſſes, Syrups, Decoctions, Julips, or Waters, of all ſorts of Phyſical Herbs, That you may have them readie for your uſe at all times of the yeer.
2. What Planet governeth every Herb or Tree (uſed in Phyſick) that groweth in *England*.
3. The Time of gathering all Herbs, both Vulgarly, and Aſtrologically.
4. The Way of drying and keeping the Herbs all the yeer.
5. The Way of keeping their Juyces ready for uſe at all times.
6. The Way of making and keeping all kind of uſeful Compounds made of Herbs.
7. The way of mixing Medicines according to *Cauſe* and and *Mixture* of the *Diſeaſe*, and *Part* of the Body *Afflicted*.

By *Nich. Culpeper*, Gent. Student in *Phyſick* and *Aſtrologie*.

LONDON:
Printedby *Peter Cole*, at the ſign of the Printing-Preſs in Cornhil, near the Royal Exchange. 1652.

Figure 17.1: Culpeper's Herbal, *The English Physitian*

CHAPTER SEVENTEEN

Culpeper's Herbal

After the Civil War, when Culpeper came to write his herbal, *The English Physitian*, he incorporated into it an astrological perspective which he called "An Astrologo-Physical Discourse". The Discourse is essentially a synthesis of Hippocratic, Galenic and Hermetic ideas. Such knowledge would have previously been only available in Latin, and much of it he had translated himself. In the spirit of the Commonwealth that followed the execution of Charles I, Culpeper wanted to make the knowledge of the principles of physic available to the common man for the benefit of everyone, rather than being the elitist preserve of the Royal College of Physicians to profit from.

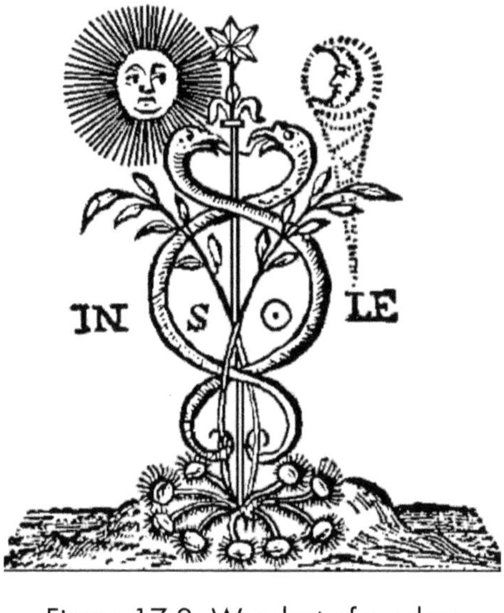

Figure 17.2: Woodcut of sundew

The herbal was written in English, not Latin, printed in a handy size, unlike John Gerard or John Parkinson's herbals, and solely focused upon the commonly available herbs found in the British countryside. In accordance with Galen's Hidden Virtues, each herb is listed with its Planetary ruler, essentially providing the key for understanding how to use the herb and when to administer it. To help explain the Hidden Virtues, and so the grasp the achievements of his herbal, we will look at the Alchemical perspective of herbs.

This 15th-century alchemical woodcut of the sundew is particularly fascinating, for it clearly recognises the amphoteric virtue of the herb as being linked to both the Sun and the Moon.

The woodcut illustrates the Hermetic cosmology, the Five Elements and the Three Alchemical Principles of Sulphur, Salt and Mercury.

The main motif incorporated into the illustration of the herb is the Caduceus, with its central stave entwined by two warring snakes—being an emblem of Mercury, the Roman god of medicine, representing the knowledge he bears.

The alchemists saw magic in the way the sundew responds to sunlight. The more the sunlight shines on it, the more the intensity of the plant as it changes its colour. The leaves and stems become much redder while the sugary secretions at the tips of the leaf hairs increase.

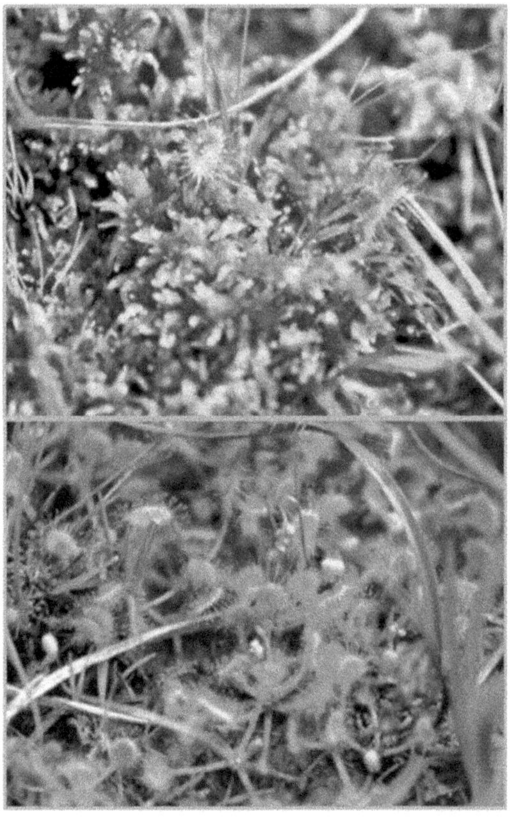

Figure 17.3: Sundew (*Drosera rotundifolia*) responding to sunlight

The upper photo shows the sundew without significant sunshine, leaving it pale and wan, while the lower photo depicts the sundew after sustained sunlight, making it robust and radiant. Consequently, it is easy to see how it has acquired the name of sundew or *ros solis*—the rose of the sun. This made the herb ideal to illustrate the principles of physic.

Of its virtue, Culpeper describes *ros solis* as a *"Herb of the Sun, and under the coelestial Crab, ... It grows on bogs in untilled places. ... It grows very low, with roundish Green leaves full of red hairs, and is fullest of dew when the Sun is hottest, whence it took its name."*

This binomial signature is revealing for it shows that Culpeper not only saw a Planet defining its virtue, but also its habitat influencing its healing energy.

Cancer, being a Water sign, is connected to boggy places: *"The Sea, great Rivers, Naviable Waterways; but in the Inland Countries it notes places neer Rivers, Brooks, Springs, Wels, Sellars in houses, Wash-houses, **Marsh grounds**, Ditches with rushes, Sedges, Sea Banks, Trenches, Cisternes."* [W. Lilly]

Furthermore. the Cancerian virtue is further reflected in the insectivorous habit of the herb. The "dew" is in fact a sugary secretion, which attracts insects to feed on it. Once the insect alights on the sticky hairs, it is unable to escape. The hairs then fold around its body, and proteolytic enzymes break down the proteinaceous exoskeleton. The amino acids and other nutrients are then absorbed into the leaf, like a primitive stomach (Cancer traditionally rules the stomach). It is how the plant has adapted to the nitrogen-poor, acidic, boggy habitat. Cancer, the crab, is notorious for once it holds something in the grip of its claws, it is unable to easily let go. Similarly, the fate of the insect is sealed once it is attached to the sticky leaf hairs.

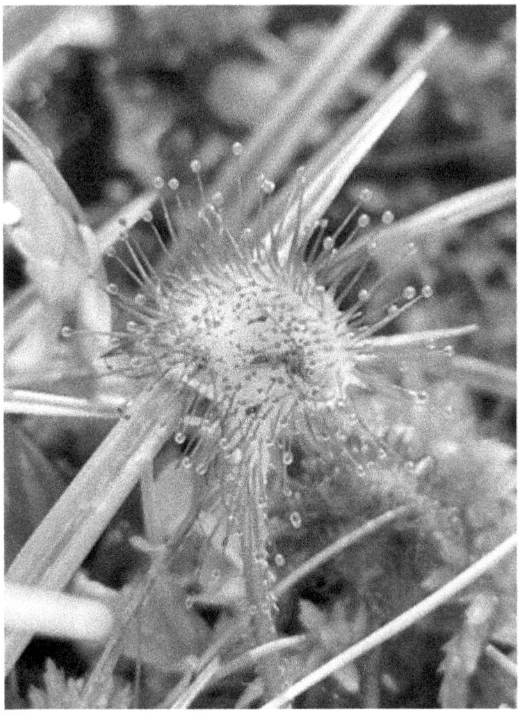

Figure 17.4: Insectivorous leaf of sundew. Photo credit Liz Downey

The alchemical woodcut clearly recognises the amphoteric virtue of the herb being linked to both the Sun (☉) and the Moon (☽) (Cancer (♋) is ruled by the Moon). The main motif of Caduceus embodies the Three Alchemical Principles or the polarity to the Vital Force. The Sulphur Principle (🜍) is represented by the left-hand snake. Its golden colour is ruled by the Sun (☉), representing Masculine, hot, expansive, sublime, rising energy. The Salt Principle (🜔) is represented by the right-hand snake. Its silver colour is ruled by the Moon (☽), representing Feminine, cold, contractive, crystalline, precipitating energy.

The central stave represents the balance or synthesis of the Mercury Principle (☿).

The silvery blue colour of the light reflected off the liquid metal quicksilver symbolises the Vital Force, ruled by Mercury (☿). The Mercury Principle represents the harmonisation of the Sulphur and Salt Principles. The three folds of the snakes from top to bottom represent the Hermetic Three Worlds: the Intellectual World, representing Spirit; the Celestial World, representing Soul; and the Elemental World, representing Matter.

At the top of the central stave is found a Fleur de Lys, which, contrary to its name, is originally a stylised version of an iris. The iris is an emblem of Mercury, and here its tripartite depiction of the flower petals is analogous to the three components of the Caduceus.

In the middle fold of the Caduceus, the word IN SO LE, the letter O has been deliberately changed to the Solar glyph (☉). The location of this glyph is significant, for the Sun represents the heart, where the soul resides and is also where the Vital Force is generated. IN SO LE here means "the Sun within". In other words, it is within the heart that the Alchemical Principles are perceived.

The woodcut contains a bit of artistic licence as the herb has been given two flowering stems, whereas a single sundew rosette of leaves typically has just one stem. The doubling of the stems is deliberate to create a symmetry to the illustration. On both stems seven flowers are depicted, alluding to the seven Planets in the Celestial World, which influence the Vital Force and describe the virtues of herbs. At the top of the central rod is a six-pointed star, which represents Ether (✡); 6 is also the number of the Sun.

As has been extensively explained in Chapter 1, within its stellate construction all the Alchemical triangular symbols of the Five Elements—Earth, Water, Air, Fire and Ether—can be found, along with their humoral correspondences. The Elemental principles of graduated materiality in relation to a plant have already been described in Chapter 10 on The Physic Garden.

The inclusion of nine leaves to the rosette of sundew underneath the Caduceus is deliberate, since 9 is the number corresponding to the Moon (☽). The Moon is symbolically the closest Planet to Earth, and is involved with mediating the different Planetary influences down to Earth, which is why the location of the Moon is so important in different alchemical operations and administration of herbs. Thus, this complex woodcut is demonstrating the Solar herb generating the Vital Force symbolised by the Caduceus along with the Alchemical Principles, Planetary and Elemental symbolism needed to understand its role in medicine and healing.

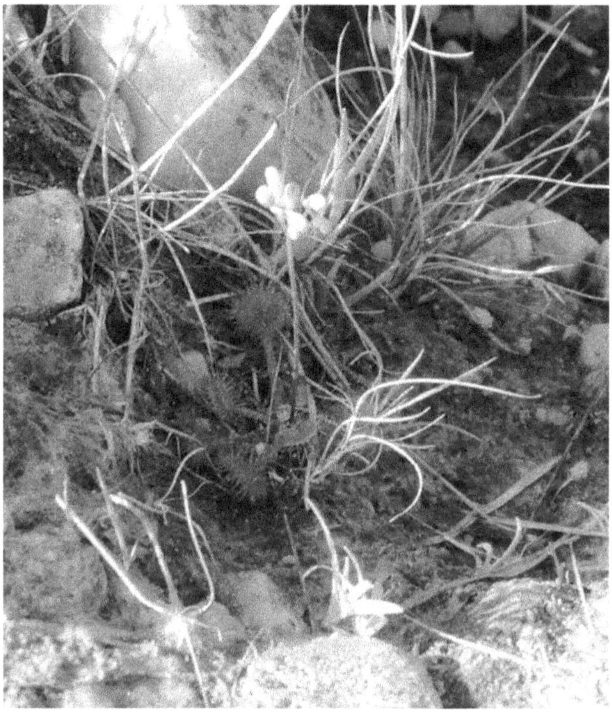

Figure 17.5: An individual sundew plant with its single flowering stem

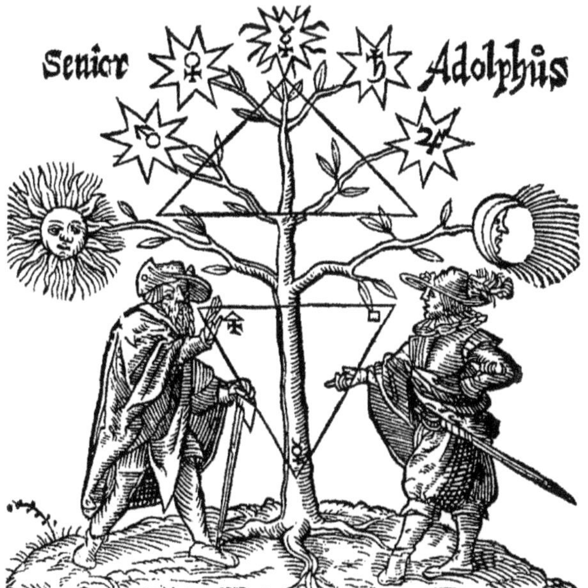

Figure 17.6: Basil Valentine's *L'Azoth des Philosophies*

This 16th-century alchemical illustration by Basil Valentine shows two philosophers discussing when to cut down a tree. The tree symbolically stands between heaven and earth. The tree has four roots (representing the Four Elements) anchoring it to the earth.

If look closely you can see the glyph for Mercury (☿) both at the roots and at the crown of the tree. Mercury corresponds to the Vital Force (Ether) in the sap rising up through the tree. This energy within the herb was known as its virtue.

As the upper triangle of the woodcut shows, the virtue of the herb was subject to the influence of the Planets: Sun (☉), Moon (☽), Mercury (☿), Venus (♀), Mars (♂), Jupiter (♃) and Saturn (♄). Each herb was thought to possess its unique Planetary rulership, which can be ascertained by looking closely at its form and structure, along with the type of habitat it prefers. The Planetary ruler then reveals their inner virtue, by linking the herb to a particular part of the body, disease and/or humour.

The lower inverted triangle of the woodcut shows the symbols of the Three Alchemical Principles, with the Sulphur Principle (🜍) on the left corner next to the Sun and the Salt Principle (□) on the right corner next to the Moon. Its apex, pointing to the roots of the tree, shows the symbol (☿) of Mercury, indicating their balance of the Sulphur and Salt principles within the virtue of the tree. The lower triangle corresponds to the manifest virtues of the herb, so that the Sulphur Principle corresponds to hot and the Salt Principle corresponds to cold, while Mercury corresponds to the relative effect the heat or coldness has on the Vital Force.

Through Mercury, herbs were thus seen to be interconnected through the realms of Spirit, Soul and Matter. The Alchemical Principles were used to connect to its temperature, whether hot, cold, wet and dry, which then describes the herb's influence on that bodily part. With these ideas in mind, herbalists interpreted the herbal kingdom around us.

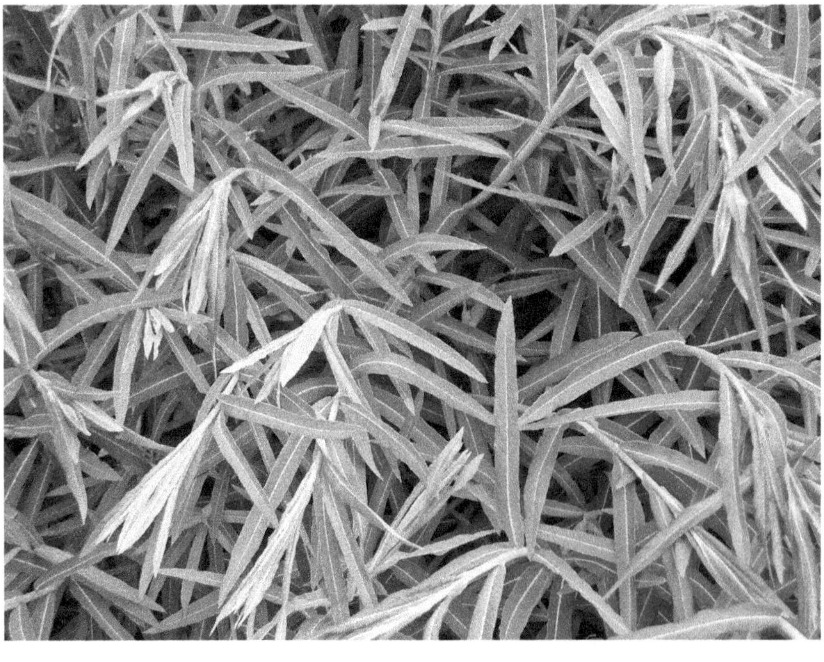

Figure 17.7: Common willow (*Salix alba*)

Taking one example to illustrate *Culpeper's Herbal* in action, consider the willow (*Salix alba*), where he says of its Planetary ruler *"The Moon doth own it."* Its Lunar signature is easily seen in how the tree loves growing beside water. This association has been made for thousands of years, for in classical Greece the tree was sacred to the Moon goddess Hecate and planted in the temple grounds. Her temple was called the Helicon from the Greek name for willow, *helix*. In the Latin tongue this became corrupted to *Salix*, forming the generic name used today.

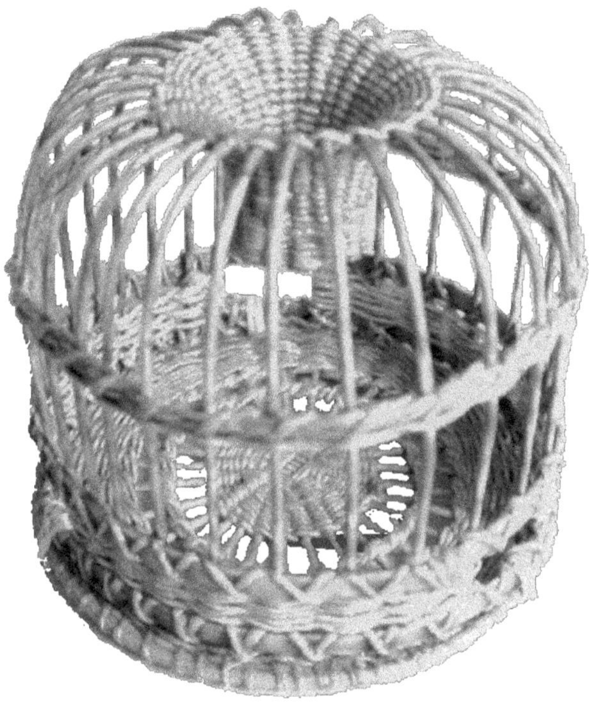

Figure 17.8: Traditional inkwell lobster pot

As has been shown, the Water Element is associated with the stem; the Lunar association of the tree emphasises their suppleness. Willow is linked to the art of wicker, where the stems or withies are woven into baskets and other items. Traditionally the withies were made into "inkwell" lobster pots. Willow wood has the quality of being resistant to rotting in saltwater, making it an ideal renewable and environmentally friendly material to make these pots from. They were used to catch crabs, lobsters and crayfish. Shellfish are associated with the sign of Cancer, since the Moon rules the sign of Cancer.

In water divining too, the willow frond is one of the preferred trees for the purpose. It makes perfect sense to use a tree with such a powerful association with water in order to identify the location of where water is located.

Some 2,500 years ago, Hippocrates described willow for extinguishing the fire of a fever or pyrexia. The word "pyrexia" is derived from the Greek *pyros*, meaning "a fire". He identified the virtue of the herb as having an affinity with the

Phlegmatic humour, which needed strengthening to counter when there is an excess of choler, as in a fever.

The contemporary use of the herb as an anti-inflammatory remedy in arthritic and rheumatic conditions still embodies these humoral ideas, for "inflammation" comes from the Latin meaning the "flames within". By contrast a "rheum" is a medieval name for phlegm, which in humoral physiology has its "seat in the lungs".

Culpeper describes willow for the ravaging fever of consumption, as pulmonary tuberculosis was described then. Of the Hidden Virtue of the herb, its Lunar virtue would have an affinity with the Phlegmatic humour and, as Hippocrates commended, would help antipathetically to extinguish the fever.

Of its Manifest Virtue, willow is described as being cold and dry in temperature. Considering the herb's affinity with the Phlegmatic humour, this would help dry out the copious quantity of mucus generated in this lung infection.

Willow is well known for being one of the source herbs for salicylic acid, in its glycosidal form salicin, which is a known antibiotic against the tubercular bacillus. Centuries before a microbiological perspective of disease, these humoral ideas led herbalists to an effective herbal remedy for the treatment of tuberculosis.

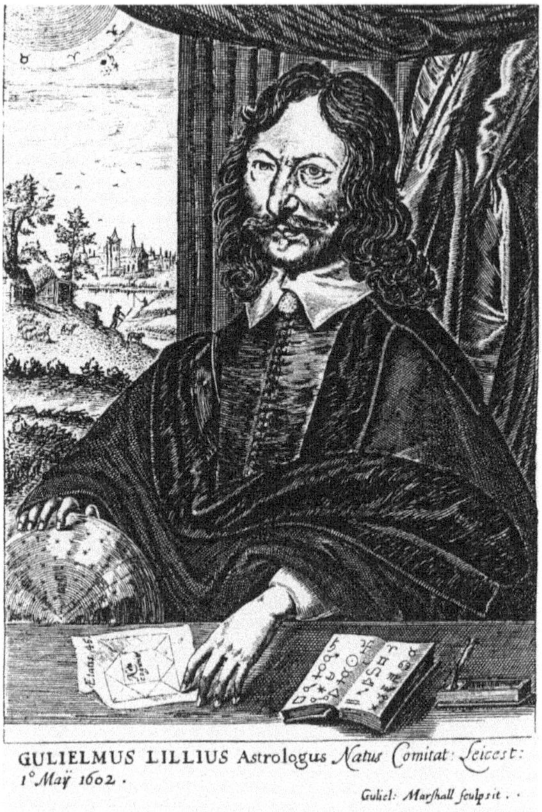

Figure 18.1: An engraving of William Lilly from his *Christian Astrology*

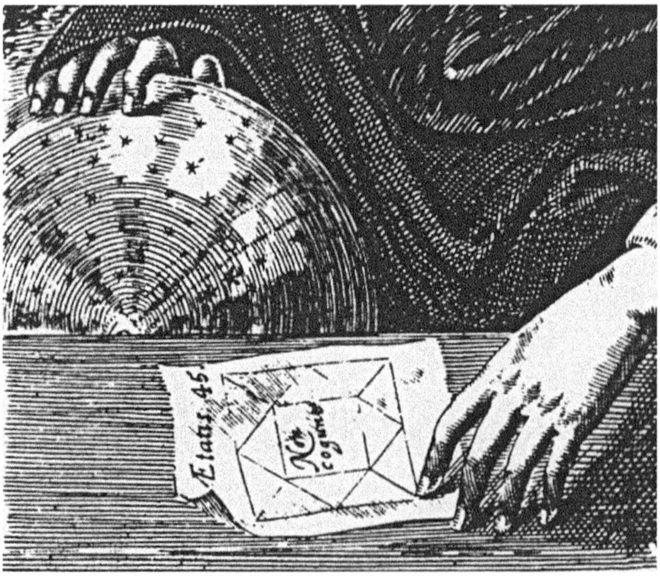

Figure 18.2: Detail from William Lilly's engraving

CHAPTER EIGHTEEN

Culpeper's Astrology

While a young apothecary, Nicholas Culpeper had the opportunity to meet the foremost astrologer of his day, William Lilly. Lilly introduced Culpeper to astrology and its importance to the practice of physic. He was able to provide Nicholas access to medical astrology works from his personal library. Lilly had a profound influence on Culpeper whose astrological skills flourished under Lilly's tutelage, and they became good friends, both supporting the Parliamentarian cause during the Civil War.

In many respects, astrology was the summation of the teachings within the structure of the Seven Liberal Arts, and the publication of astrological works enabled the knowledge that previous been secreted away in monastic schools and the universities to become available to the common man, with the increasing literacy of the populace.

Arguably, the most important of these works was Lilly's *Christian Astrology* (1647). This encyclopaedic work was the definitive astrological textbook of the 17th century. In the last thirty years or so interest in this text has grown enormously as modern astrologers are keen to reconnect with their traditional roots.

The accompanying engraving of Lilly deserves a closer inspection, for it encapsulates the role of the astrologer in this formal depiction of him.

Cheiromantical clues provide the key to unlocking its deeper meaning. Thus, the index finger of Lilly's left hand points to the third house cusp of a blank astrological chart, which corresponds to "studies and writing".

The chart, together with the adjacent open text of Planetary and Zodiacal glyphs, indicates that Lilly is indicating to the reader how to study his book. Traditionally, Jupiter is symbolically connected with the index finger, while the third house is ruled by Gemini (♊), the sign specifically ruling the arms and hands in the body.

Lilly's right hand rests on a celestial orb showing some of the signs of the Zodiac with the stars in the heavens. Closer inspection reveals that Gemini is specifically shown to "rise" above the "horizon" of the table edge.

Mercury (☿) rules Gemini (♊), making it "Lord of the Ascendant" or, in this case, ruler of the engraving. With Hermes being the Greek equivalent of Mercury, it is apparent that Lilly, the astrologer, is shown communicating Hermetic teachings. This perspective is confirmed by the Hermetic maxim "as above, so below" for, at his right hand, Gemini (♊) is shown rising in the heavens "above", while his left-hand Jupiter finger points to the third house cusp, of which Gemini (♊) is a co-significator, in the chart "below". Thus symbolically, the engraving indicates that the role of the astrologer is intermediary between the Intellectual World "above" and the Elemental World "below".

CULPEPER'S
ASTROLOGICALL
JUDGMENT
OF
DISEASES
From the Decumbiture of the ſick
much Enlarged.
1. From Aven Ezra by way of Introduction.
2. From Noel Duret by way of Direction.
Wherein is laid down,
The way and manner of finding out the Cauſe, Change, and End of the diſeaſe. Alſo whether the Sick be likely to live or die; and the Time when Recovery or Death is to be expected.
With the Signs of Life or Death by the body of the Sick party, according to the judgment of Hippocrates.
Whereunto is added,
A Table of Logiſticall Logarithmes, to finde the exact time of the Criſis Hermes Treſmegiſtus upon the firſt Decumbiture of the ſick: ſhewing the ſigns & conjectures of the diſeaſe, and of life and death, by the good or evil poſition of the Moon at the time of the Patients lying down, or demanding the queſtion: Infallible ſigns to know of what complexion any perſon is whatſoever: With a compendious Treatiſe of Urine.

By NICHOLAS CULPEPER, Gent.
Student in Phyſick and Aſtrologie.

Diſce, ſed ira cadat naſo, rugoſaque ſanna. Perſius.

London, Printed for Nath. Brookes at the Golden Angel on Cornhill, neer the Exchange. 1655.

Figure 18.3: Nicholas Culpeper's *Astrologicall Judgement of Diseases*, from *Decumbiture of the Sick*

Nicholas Culpeper's work *Astrologicall Judgement of Diseases*, from the *Decumbiture of the Sick* was published posthumously. It was drawn from writings of the Spanish-Jewish philosopher Aven Ezra and the French Astrologer Noel Duret.

The original edition of *Culpeper's Herbal* contained this decumbiture or astrological chart, which significantly was omitted in later editions. Culpeper deliberately included it to illustrate the therapeutic principles used to select the appropriate herbs for the patient, showing how the herbal was intended to be used.

Decumbiture is the form of medical astrology that is based upon the time when a patient gives in to their illness and has to lie down. The word "decumbiture" is derived from the Latin meaning "to go to bed". Understanding the symbolic principles of decumbiture is important for it reveals that a huge amount of herbal philosophy is contained within it.

It is a specialised branch of astrology, with the chart largely focusing on just five of the 12 houses. These need to be considered in detail, for it also has much to reveal about the way medicine is practised today.

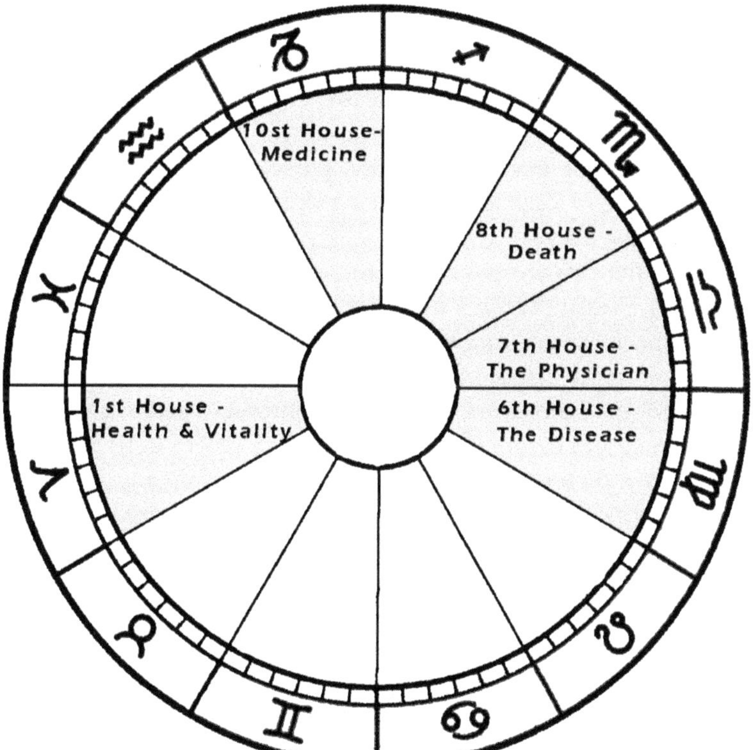

Figure 18.4: The Principal Houses of *Decumbiture*

The first house

The first house reflects the patient's physical constitution, health, temperament and vitality. It is important to note the Zodiacal sign at the Ascendant, along with its Elemental qualities. For example, if Pisces is rising at the Ascendant, then the Water Element will be a strong indicator here.

It is important to note the Planet that rules the Zodiacal sign ruling the Ascendant, for its qualities, where it is placed, and how much dignity it has, describe the condition of the person's health. In this hypothetical example of Pisces (♓) rising, this makes Jupiter (♃), with its links to the Sanguine humour, Lord of the Ascendant.

If Jupiter (♃) is placed in Sagittarius (♐), which it also rules, that would indicate that the person's health and vitality is generally robust with an abundance of Vital Force. By contrast, if it is placed in Virgo (♍), the opposite sign to Pisces (♓), where Jupiter (♃) is in detriment, that would indicate that the person's health is compromised, and their Vital Force impoverished.

The sixth house

It is important to see the nature of the disease as separate from the patient's health, which is ascertained from the sixth house. Again, note the Zodiacal sign at the sixth house cusp and its Elemental qualities. For example, if Capricorn (♑) is the sign at the sixth house, then the Earth Element, with its links to the Melancholic humour, will be a strong indicator here in the nature of the disease.

Again, note the Planet that rules the Zodiacal sign of the sixth house cusp, its qualities and where it is placed, for that describes the person's disease and often where it is located. In this example of Capricorn (♑) ruling the sixth house, it is Saturn (♄) that is the significator for the disease.

Further consideration involves whether the sixth house is aspected by the malefic Planets, Mars (♂) or Saturn (♄). This means if either of these two Planets is present in the sixth house, especially conjunct its cusp or makes an aspect with the ruler of the sixth house. Their influence colours the character of the disease.

This is the true origin of the terms "acute" and "chronic" used in both diagnosis of the duration of the disease and to describe histological differences in tissue states in the diseased organs. The term "acute" comes from the Latin *acutus*, meaning "sharp". Mars (♂), being a god of war, is associated with sharp instruments as found in weaponry and the Fire Element. An acute illness is one of a sudden onset, often with intense burning pain, inflammation and fever, which then quickly resolves—not necessarily for the good, for it may well be fatal.

By contrast, chronic illness is linked to Saturn (♄). The term "chronic" is derived from Kronos, the Greek equivalent to Saturn. Imagine the dark depths of the Winter Solstice, when the cold gets into the body and energy becomes sluggish. A chronic illness starts gradually, progressively gets worse and gets trapped in the body. It has a slow, debilitating effect compromising tissue function, which if it is not resolved ultimately can become fatal.

In decumbiture charts, the Moon (☽) is a co-significator for the disease. Her motion is used to describe the progression of the disease, its course, healing crises and judgmental opportunities. In charts where the same Planet is the significator for both the patient's vitality and disease, then the Moon is used to signify the disease in contrast to the ruling planet representing the patient's vitality.

The relationship of the first and sixth houses in decumbiture teaches the importance of not only seeing but also assessing a person's health and vitality as separate from the disease. An important a maxim of healing is: *"There are no diseases only sick people!"* In other words, without the person's body, the disease cannot exist.

Micro-organisms, whether viral, bacterial, fungal or protozoan, are not in themselves diseases, but only cause disease when they get inside people's bodies and overwhelm their immune systems. With disease being the marketplace of the pharmaceutical industry, the two are deliberately conflated to encourage people to visit their doctor. Furthermore, people are intentionally defined by their illness. Hence in medical circles patients are referred to as an "MS patient" or "angina patient". Their temperament and vitality are not even mentioned yet alone seen as a factor that may be contributing to their disease.

The seventh house

The seventh house is connected to the Physician and the Astrologer. In medieval times the two roles were synonymous, for to study medicine the student had to first complete the Seven Liberal Arts. Culpeper too was keen to point this out to his students, for in his Epistle to the Reader, which prefaces his herbal, he says, *"To such as study Astrology, who are the only men I know that are fit to study physic, physic without astrology being like a lamp without oil."* As was demonstrated in Lilly's engraving, where the astrologer was seen to link heaven and earth, so too was the physician. A quote by Culpeper is particularly revealing here:

> *Many a times I find my patients disturbed by trouble of conscience and sorrow and I have to act the divine before I can be physician. In fact our greatest skills lies in the infusion of hopes, to induce confidence and peace of mind.*

The first and seventh house axis in a decumbiture chart concerns the therapeutic relationship between the herbalist and the patient. Essentially, it shows the role of the therapist in the clinical situation: is he/she in a position to help the patient or not?

It is important to have this honesty, as there are times when a herbalist is unable to help a person. To prescribe under such circumstances at best will be ineffectual, while at worst, failure to fully comprehend the gravity of their illness will make their condition worse.

There are a number of astrological indicators that help understanding in the context of the clinical situation. For example, if Saturn (♄) is present in or aspects the seventh house, it is an indication that judgment may be blocked, in not being receptive and listening to the patient's needs.

The eighth house

The eighth house of a decumbiture chart is connected to the potential death of the patient. It has obvious importance in the prognosis in any disease, even for it to be excluded in most decumbiture charts.

How does the Planet that is the significator of death relate to sixth house of illness? Does it make an aspect to the Planet that rules the sixth house?

For example, is the significator for death also linked to the sixth house or located in it? Sometimes the same Planet rules both the sixth house of disease and the eighth house of death. In this case it is an indication that the illness has the potential to be fatal.

The tenth house

Traditionally the tenth house in a decumbiture chart is linked to the medicine. The cusp of the tenth house is the mid-heaven, where the Sun reaches its zenith in the sky. As has been shown, the Sun (☉) is symbolically linked with Apollo and his son Asclepius, the Greek god of medicine. The prevailing medicine for the many centuries since the time of Galen when decumbiture was used was physic or herbal medicine.

Plant photosynthesis reaches its peak at midday, when the maximum amount of sunlight reaches the Earth, sustaining all life, especially plant life, on the Planet. Just as light passing through a prism splits up into the colours of the spectrum, so too the healing power of the Sun (☉) was seen to be taken up by plants and manifest as the spectrum of healing virtues of the different herbs. The tenth house, then, is symbolic of the healing power of the Sun (☉), via the virtues of herbs strengthening the vitality of the patient. The word "medicine" comes from the Latin *medicio*, meaning the "art of healing", implying there is skill in understanding the virtues of the different herbs and how to make medicines from them.

"The way of mixing medicines according to the cause of the disease, and parts of the body afflicted"

Here Culpeper outlines his astrological principles, which are derived from the Paracelsian concepts of sympathy and antipathy.

1st principle: *"Fortify the body with herbs of the nature of the Lord of the Ascendant, tis no matter whether he be a Fortune or an Infortune in this case."*

By choosing herbs that are of the same nature as the lord of the Ascendant the patient's health and vitality are sympathetically strengthened. When the strength of their vitality exceeds the strength of their disease, they will be able to overcome it.

2nd principle: *"Let your medicine be something antipathetical to the Lord of the 6th."*

By choosing herbs that are opposite in nature to the lord of the sixth house the disease is antipathetically weakened. By weakening the disease, it helps the patient's vitality in overthrowing it. Once the patient's vitality is stronger than the disease, healing and recovery will occur.

3rd principle: *"Let your medicine be something of the nature of the sign ascending."*

Though similar to the first principle, choosing herbs that are of the same nature as the sign of the Ascendant sympathetically enhances the patient's physical constitution.

4th principle: *"If the Lord of the 10th be strong, make use of his medicines."*

If the lord of the tenth house of medicine is well dignified, choosing herbs that are of the same nature as the lord promotes healing generally.

5th principle: *"If this cannot well be, make use of the medicines of the Light of Time."*

If the lord of the tenth house lacks dignity so that herbs of the same nature cannot be used, then use Solar herbs by day or Lunar herbs by night. Again, these will enhance healing generally.

6th principle: *"Be always sure to fortify the grieved part of the body by sympathetical remedies."*

Thus, if a knee is injured, then using herbs of Saturnine or Capricornian nature will sympathetically strengthen it, so enhancing its healing.

7th principle: *"Regard the heart, keep that upon the wheels, because the Sun is the foundation of life:* [therefore solar remedies] *cure all diseases by fortifying the heart."*

The heart generates the Vital Force. In cultivating the patient's health and vitality it is important to ensure the sustained supply of vital energy. Accordingly, the use of Solar or cordial herbs strengthens the patient's vitality and tonifies their body.

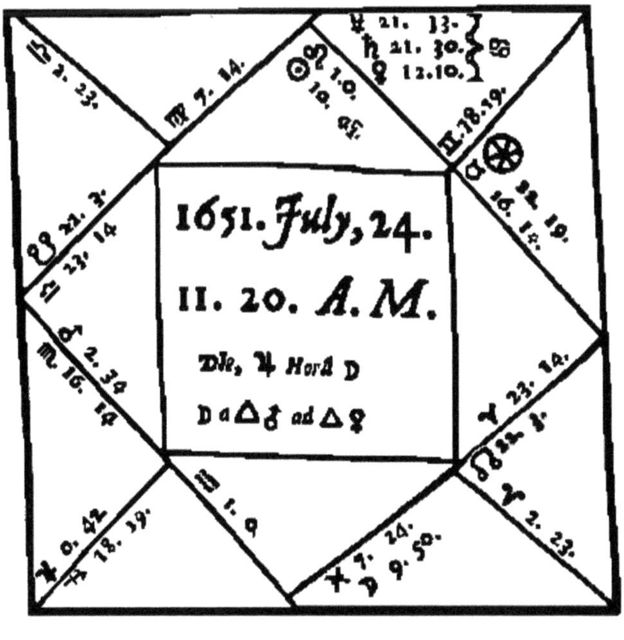

Figure 18.5: Nicholas Culpeper's *Decumbiture* from *The English Physitian*, 1652

Culpeper used this chart in his herbal to illustrate the therapeutic principles used to select the appropriate herbs for the patient. The following occasion concerns a lady friend of one of Culpeper's students and was written in a letter responding to his student's request. His diagnosis was as follows:

> *Venus, Lady of the 12th, and the Ascendant, and 8th, shows her always to be her own foe in respect of Health; and truly I believe the origin of the Disease was a Surfeit either by eating moist Fruits, or else by catching wet in travelling; … Venus with Saturn, who is quartile to the Ascendant troubles her Breasts with tough Flegm and Melancholy.*

Culpeper's judgment that the woman was *"her own foe in respect of health"* is taken from the fact that Venus rules the 12th house of "self-undoing" as well as the Ascendant.

Diseases for Venus (♀) in Cancer (♋): *"shows the stomach is much afflicted with cold, raw undigested humours, many times with surfeit."*

Venus (♀) rules fruits and berries generally, especially sweet ones, while her placing in the water sign of Cancer (♋) leads to the idea of *"eating moist Fruits"*. Such a moist Venus (♀) in the ninth house of *"long journeys"* invokes the idea of her *"catching wet in travelling"*. Before waterproof clothing this was a common risk.

Venus (♀) co-rules the Phlegmatic humour, which has its seat in the lungs; Cancer (♋) signifies the chest—hence the signification specifically indicates a phlegmatic condition of the lungs, *"troubles her Breasts with tough Flegm and Melancholy"*, since the cold and dry influence of Saturn (♄) causes the phlegm to congeal.

Saturn (♄) is square (90°) to the Ascendant, indicating the depression of her vitality leading to "melancholy", which is worsened by the approach of Venus (♀) to Saturn (♄). The modern diagnosis of this condition would be chronic bronchitis.

From the Moon (☽) Culpeper notices: *"… a most forcible reception between the Moon and Venus from fruitful signs, I question whether she be with Child or not, the Moon being in the 5th House."*

The mutual reception allows Venus (♀), a natural significator for the womb, as well as the woman, to be received into the fifth house "of Children" while the fruitful (Water) sign of Pisces (♓) on the fifth house cusp strengthens the possibility of pregnancy.

From the sixth house of disease Culpeper notes:

> *Mars, Lord of the Disease, really in the Scorpion, and accidentally in the Ascendant, together with Aries on the 6th; show the Disease keeps his court in the Womb, and accidentally afflicts the Head from thence, so that the heat of the Womb must needs be the cause of the present distemper, and Mars in a moist Sign in the first* [house] *next to the second may well denote heat and breaking out about her Face and Throat.*

Mars (♂), lord of the sixth house located in Scorpio (♏), indicates that the disease is some sort of inflammation affecting her reproductive organs. The modern blanket term would be "pelvic inflammatory disease".

Interestingly, Culpeper also sees the location of Mars (♂) in the first house, together with Aries (♈) on the sixth house cusp—both corresponding to the head—as indicating a secondary manifestation of the disease affecting the head. More directly he sees Mars (♂) in a Water sign as indicating some sort of eruptive, acne-like, skin disorder. With Mars near the second house cusp, it indicates that the skin disorder is located on her body in the region between her head and neck.

Next Culpeper considers prognostic considerations:

> *... Whether she will be Curable or not, or how, or when the Disease will end, is our next Point? Truly I can see no danger of Death, the Moon being strong in her Wain, and applying by trine with a strong reception to the Lady of the Ascendant.*

Culpeper clearly had the following aphorism in mind:

> *The Lord of the eighth house in conjunction, square, or opposition of the Moon at the Decumbiture, threatens death unless there be a reception between them.*

Here the Moon (☽) is applying to the trine (120°) of Venus (♀), Lady of the eighth house. Furthermore, there is a powerful mutual reception between them, hence he saw no danger of death.

> *... yet this is certain, Mars is strong in a fixed sign, will maintain the Disease stoutly, her hopes will be but small when Venus comes to the body of Saturn, viz August 2, for she will be overpressed with Melancholy.*

The sixth house ruler, Mars (♂), situated in a fixed sign (♏), indicates an illness of long duration. This is compounded by Saturn (♄) afflicting both Venus (♀) and the Ascendant, indicating a chronic illness by the depression of the patient's vitality. Culpeper observes this will be particularly intense when Venus (♀) makes her partile (exact) conjunction with Saturn (♄).

> *... the time I suppose of her Cure may be (if good courses be taken) when Mars leaves the Sign he is in, and comes to the place where the Body of Jupiter is, or then may at least turn to another Disease more propitious.*

While Mars (♂) remains in his own sign (♏) the disease is strongly maintained. When he ingresses into Sagittarius (♐) his dignity, and consequently the woman's disease, weakens.

However, the most favourable indication is the future conjunction with Jupiter (♃). Jupiter, the author of temper, responsible for the balance of all the humours in the blood, counters the maleficity of Mars (♂), restoring temper to the humours.

Of her treatment Culpeper notes:

> *the Sun so strong in the 10th shows she may be cured by Medicine, and being exalted in the Seventh, and Caput* [North Node] *there, I do not know but you are as likely a man to do it as any.*

The Sun (☉) is dignified in its own sign of Leo (♌), implying Solar medicines are appropriate for treatment. Furthermore, in recognising the Sun (☉) is exalted in Aries (♈) on the seventh house cusp of the physician, Culpeper sees the medicine as working well through the hands of his student.

Commenting on the curative indications he observes:

> *… it is confessed here, that the Sun being exceedingly strong in the 10th House should naturally signifie the Curative Medicine, and as true that the evil of Mars, viz. Heat of the Womb, and a salt* [Water] *humour in the blood ought to be removed before you meddle in the tough flegm in the Breast; …*
>
> *… but yet seeing the Disease seems rather to participate of offending heat than any other simple quality, you must have a care of hot Medicines lest you go about* ignem olea extifugere [lighting oil and putting to flight to the principal organs of the body]:

He concludes:

> *The Medicines must first be Cool: Secondly, strengthening* [to] *the Womb: Thirdly repressing the vapours; Forthly of the nature of Sol and Venus.*

Cooling medicines generally remove heat from the body, reduce inflammation and calm the nervous system.

The instruction that medicines need to be *"strengthening* [to] *the Womb"* is given because this is where the disease is located, as shown by the position of the sixth house ruler—Mars (♂). For a disease to become located in a particular organ, the vital energy of the organ itself must have become weakened and consequently needs to be strengthened.

The term "vapours" refers to the Vital Force. Mercury (☿) symbolises the Vital Force flowing through the nervous system. When quicksilver is heated, the liquid metal gives off a heavy vapour. By analogy "vapours" symbolise the excessive functioning of the nervous system, such as when it becomes over-stimulated by stress or pain. Thus, a medicine that *"represses the vapours"* is essentially a sedative that calms the nervous system.

The final instruction that medicines need to be of the *"nature of Sol and Venus"* utilises the principles of physic within decumbiture. Venusian herbs will fortify the woman's health and vitality since she is lady of the Ascendant. These herbs will also counter the disease since Venus (♀) is antipathetic to Mars (♂), lord of the sixth house. Finally, they will sympathetically strengthen the womb, since Venus naturally rules this organ.

Solar herbs are indicated since the Sun (☉) is lord of the tenth house and strongly dignified in its own sign. Their virtues oppose the influence of Saturn (♄) and generally strengthen the Vital Force.

Bearing these principles in mind, Culpeper then recommends the following herbs:

> *To this intent I first commend unto you stinking Arrach, a pattern whereof I have sent you here enclosed; you may find it upon dunghils, especially such as are made of Horse-dung. It is cold and moist, an Herb of Venus in the Scorpion:*

The Venusian (♀) signature clearly has been identified from the arrach's vulval-shaped leaf, which is reflected in its specific name *vulvaria*. The choice of this Venusian herb is because it is antipathetic to Mars (♂), which rules her disease. The herb is particularly appropriate as its virtue is associated with Scorpio (♏), ruling the womb.

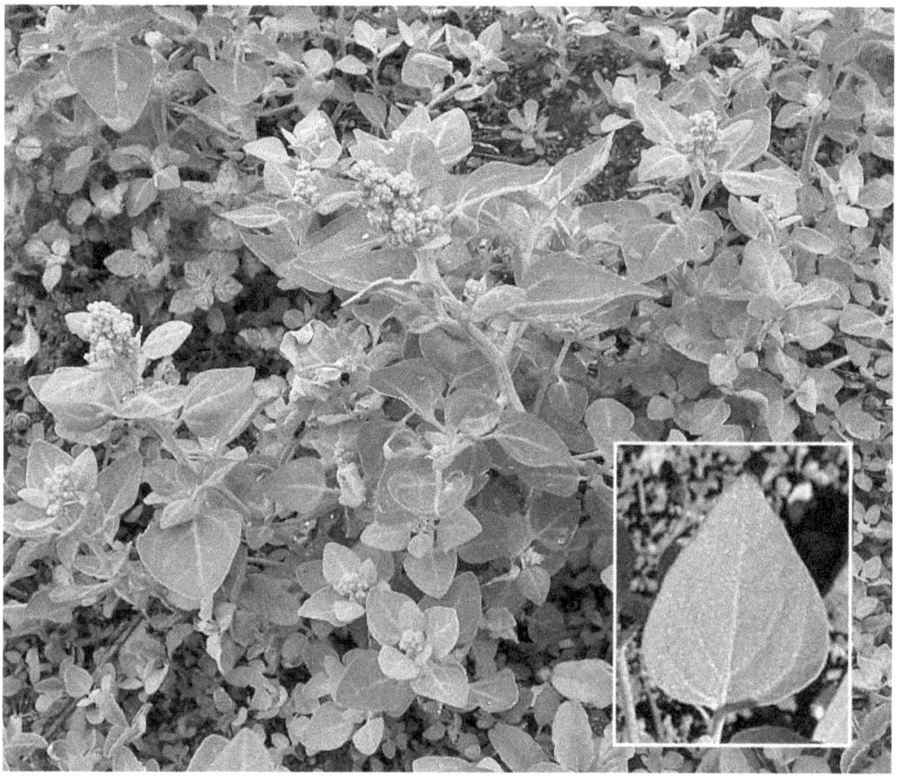

Figure 18.6: Stinking arrach (*Chenopodium vulvaria*)

This listing of the herb again illustrates that the virtue of a herb is also influenced by the Elemental energy of the place in which it grows. Dung heaps are linked to Scorpio (♏), since they are largely composed of the excrement from the Scorpionic region of various animals, which rots and decomposes. In so doing the heaps create warmth (Mars ruling Scorpio).

Incidentally, one of the reasons for the decline of Britain's snakes—ruled by Scorpio—is that they frequently laid their eggs in dung heaps, so that the heat from the decaying organic matter incubates them. With the increased use of fertiliser replacing the need for dung heaps, snakes have had reduced opportunity to incubate their eggs, leading to a marked decline in their numbers.

> *... also Ros Soils, an Herb of the Sun and under the coelestial Crab, may do very well, and the better because Venus is in Cancer: It grows on bogs in untilled places, and is in flower about this time: It grows very low, with roundish Green leaves full of red hairs, and is fullest of dew when the Sun is hottest, whence it took its name;*

Cancer (♋) rules the chest and stomach. Venus rules the Phlegmatic humour, which has its seat in the lungs, being conjunct Saturn describes tough phlegm and melancholy afflicting her chest, such as would be described as chronic bronchitis today. *Drosera* directs its Solar (☉) virtue to these areas, hence it is used for melting away chronic catarrhal conditions of the chest and chronic gastritis.

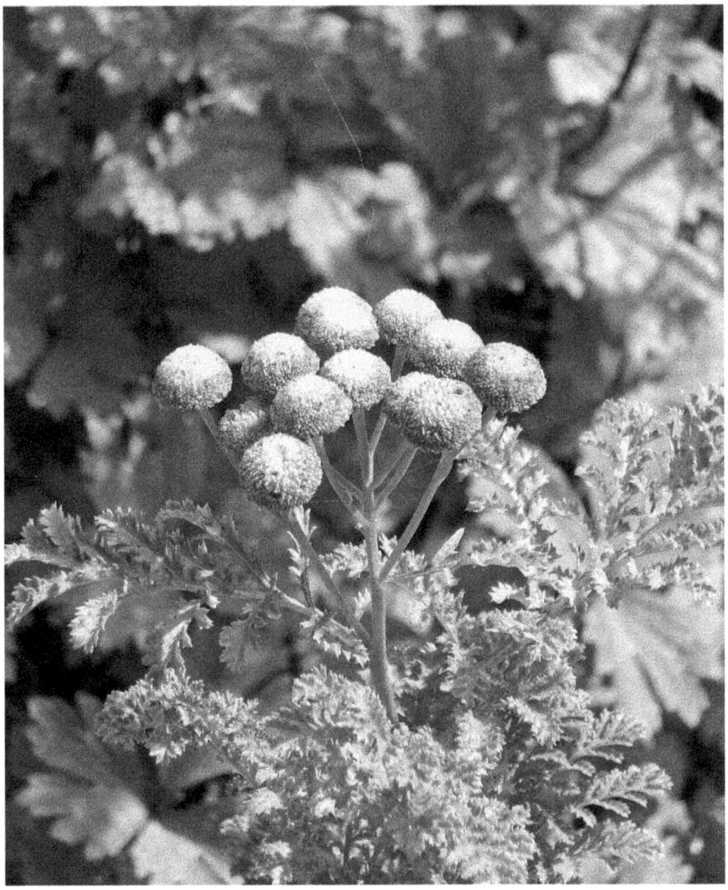

Figure 18.7: Tansy (*Tanacetum vulgare*)

... to these you may add Tansie, which I take to be a herb of Venus in Libra,

The sign of Libra (♎) is associated with balance. In the morphology of tansy, its structure displays a remarkable symmetry. Just as the architecture of the plant displays this balance, so the herb was seen to confer this balance and harmony to the body.

Here, Culpeper suggested the use of tansy for sympathetically strengthening the patient's health and vitality, antipathetically countering the Martian (♂) disease and activating the mutual reception between Venus (♀) and the Moon (☽).

... also Orpine, another Herb of the Moon is very good in this case.

Orpine is a long-forgotten healing vulnerary herb, whose cooling and soothing energy has been used to counter inflammation and pain in the body. Here Culpeper chose it to further evoke the Venus (♀) and Moon (☽) mutual reception, thereby enhancing the healing process.

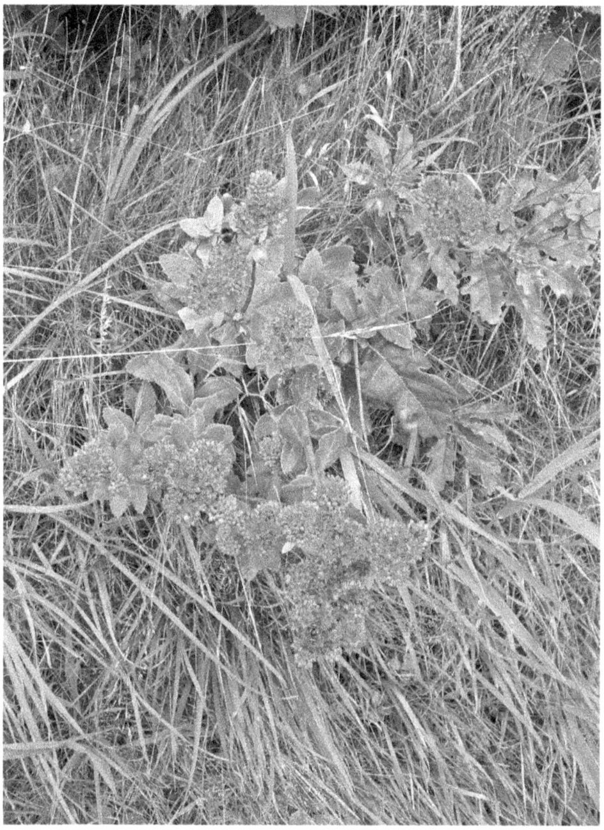

Figure 18.8: Orpine (*Sedum telephinium*)

Hopefully, this account will illustrate the importance of Nicholas Culpeper in making the principles of physic freely available to humanity once more. Culpeper died shortly after his herbal was published and never got to see the full extent of the success of his life's work.

CHAPTER NINETEEN

The age of enlightenment

Following the restoration of Charles II to the throne in 1660, less than ten ten years after Nicholas Culpeper had made the principles of physic accessible for the lay person in his *The English Physitian*, the climate towards metaphysical knowledge dramatically chilled. Censorship had returned while astrology in particular, which had been used as a powerful propaganda weapon to predict the outcomes of battles in the Civil War, was a notable target. William Lilly had been the astrologer for the Parliamentarian forces, while his friend George Wharton had been the astrologer for the Royalist forces. With echoes of the witch hunts following the Black Death, astrology in intellectual circles started to be looked down upon and discouraged as a serious study.

The renowned natural philosopher Robert Boyle (1627–91), for example, eschewed his former astrological ideas when writing his book *The Sceptical Chemist* (1661). Boyle's radical ideas made him one of the patriarchs of modern chemistry, for in it, he destructively criticises the Four Elements—Earth, Water, Air and Fire—along with the Three Alchemical Principles—Salt, Sulphur and Mercury.

In his work, Boyle explained how his doubts developed from being unable to equate experimental findings in his laboratory, where he had been combusting a range of different substances, with his attempt to understand the nature of the Elements and Alchemical Principles. Though he never succeeded in identifying a single chemical element in his lifetime, his experiences led him in this work to define a chemical element in terms of a substance incapable of being decomposed into simpler constituents:

> *I now mean by Elements, as those Chymists that speak plainest by their Principles, certain Primitive and Simple, or perfectly unmingled bodies; which not being made of any other bodies, or of one another, are the Ingredients of which all the perfectly mixt Bodies are immediately compounded, and into which they are intimately resolved.*

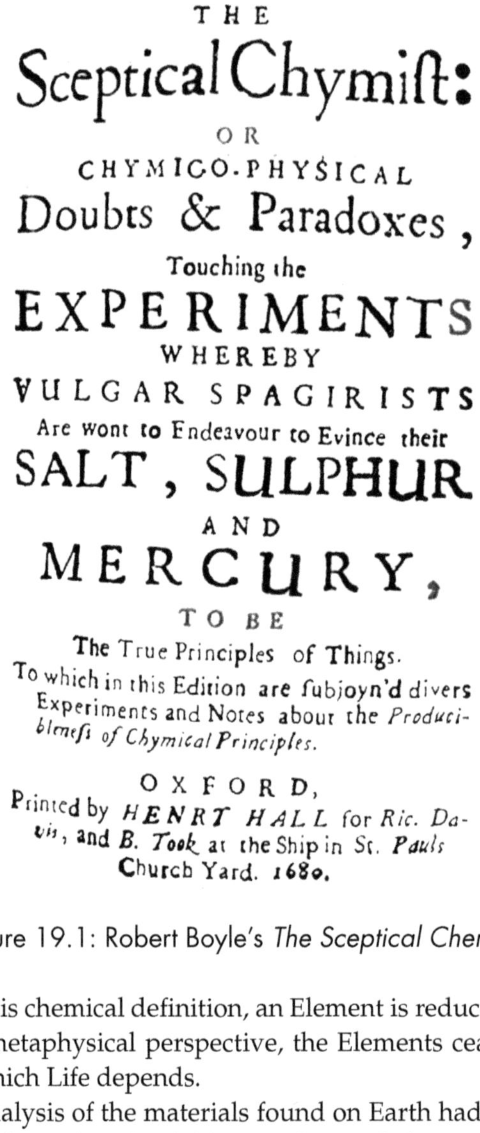
THE
Sceptical Chymiſt:
OR
CHYMICO-PHYSICAL
Doubts & Paradoxes,
Touching the
EXPERIMENTS
WHEREBY
VULGAR SPAGIRISTS
Are wont to Endeavour to Evince their
SALT, SULPHUR
AND
MERCURY,
TO BE
The True Principles of Things.
To which in this Edition are ſubjoyn'd divers Experiments and Notes about the *Producibleneſs of Chymical Principles*.
OXFORD,
Printed by *HENRY HALL* for *Ric. Davis*, and *B. Took* at the Ship in St. *Pauls* Church Yard. 1680.

Figure 19.1: Robert Boyle's *The Sceptical Chemist*

In other words, in this chemical definition, an Element is reduced to a unit of material composition. From a metaphysical perspective, the Elements ceased being seen as the Universal Forces on which Life depends.

Boyle's imperfect analysis of the materials found on Earth had revealed that they are potentially composed of a multitude of different chemical elements. Over a century later, the science of chemistry started to gain momentum with the French chemist Antoine Lavoisier (1743–94). Building on Boyle's definition, in 1787 Lavoisier showed in his combustion experiments that water was composed of hydrogen and oxygen. Lavoisier even named the gas "hydrogen", meaning "water producer", after his observation that when it burnt with a blue flame in air, it formed water droplets; he called the other gas "oxygen", meaning "acid producer", from his other combustion experiments with burning non-metals such sulphur and carbon in air. The resultant gases, sulphur dioxide and carbon dioxide respectively, then dissolved in water to form the weak sulphurous and carbonic acids respectively, hence his naming of the gas.

Lavoisier's combustion work revealed that air too was composed not only of oxygen, but also another portion that did not support combustion. He then named this portion "azote", because he noted in a mouse experiment that when the oxygen from the air had been removed by combustion, it did not support life. The poor mouse had died. The name "azote" is derived from the Greek, meaning "absence of life". Later chemists would analyse azote further to find it is largely composed of nitrogen, with lesser amounts of carbon dioxide and the rare earth gases.

Also, Lavoisier noted that fire, the agent used to destructively analyse the other elements, could not exist without oxygen, so also failed the chemical definition of an element.

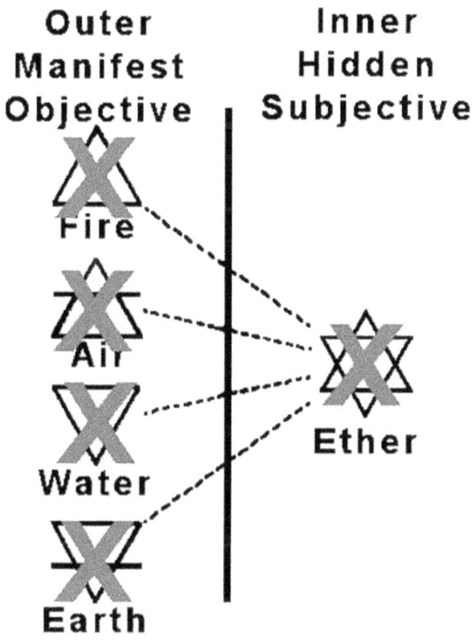

Figure 19.2: The impact of the chemical definition on the five elements

With the four material Elements failing to match Boyle's definition of a chemical element, Ether, the quintessential immaterial Element, stood no chance of fulfilling this definition. The concept of Ether, representing the Vital Force animating the four material Elements, seemed equally untenable, leading Isaac Newton to declare at the time "it did not exist".

However, from an alchemical perspective, with Ether representing Consciousness, the decline of Elemental knowledge led to the removal of consciousness from matter and the development of the mind/body split that has characterised Western thinking since the Age of Enlightenment. Chemistry became separated from Alchemy; Astronomy became separated from Astrology; Materialism usurped Symbolism; the pragmatism of Empiricism took over from Vitalism.

The birth of chemistry is responsible for the loss of awareness of the interrelationship of consciousness with matter, which had an enormous impact on the practice of physic, and ultimately led to the separation of pharmacology from the Galenic Virtues and Temperatures.

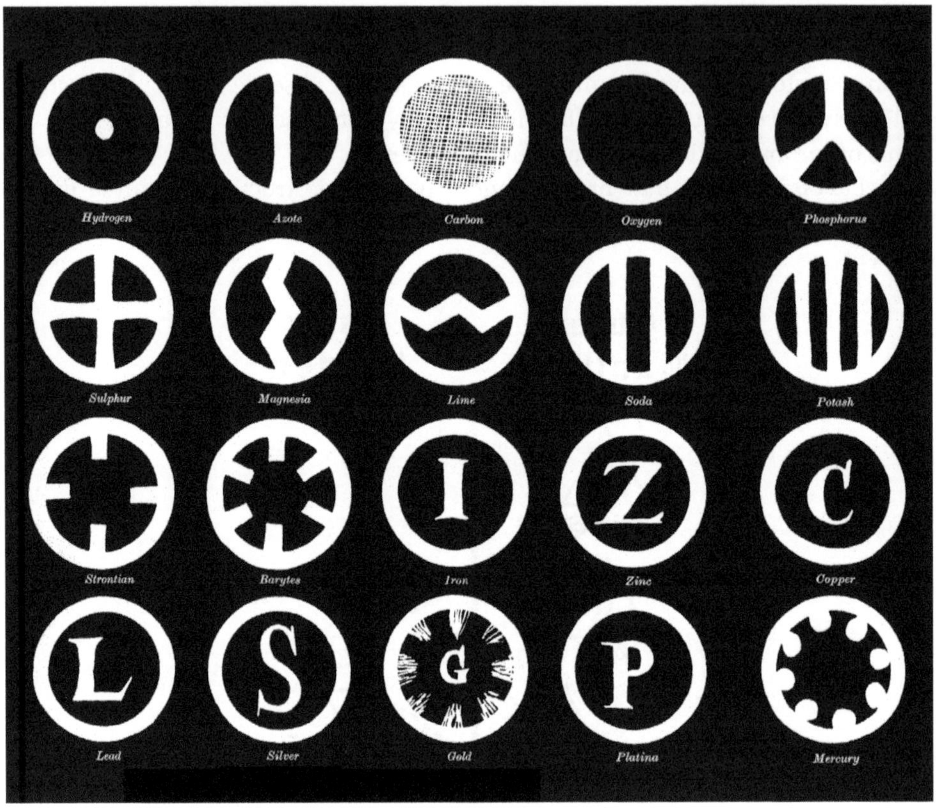

Figure 19.3: John Dalton's symbols for his chemical elements

In the early 19th century John Dalton proposed his atomic theory, in which all elements were composed of indivisible spheres of matter, which he called "atoms", a term derived from the Greek *a* + *tomos*, meaning "that which cannot be cut".

The diagram shows Dalton's 20 symbols for the known elements of his day. It is notable that this list contains a number of salts—soda, potash, lime, magnesia, strontian and barytes—rather than true chemical elements.

However, Sir Humphry Davy, in 1807, started to separate metals from these salts, isolating sodium, potassium, calcium, magnesium, strontium and barium respectively using electrolysis. Matter thus became "visualised" as tiny solid balls existing quite separately from the person observing them. Chemistry became essentially an abstracted, avitalistic conception of matter, removed from the context of the nature.

The birth of the pharmaceutical industry

With the increasing momentum of the reductionist ideas through the 19th century, in 1826 Italian chemists identified the glycoside "salicin" to be the "active ingredient" of willow bark, and possessing the antifebrile and anti-inflammatory actions of the herb, described in the Hippocratic writings. The sugar component of the glycoside was removed, leaving the refined salicylic acid. Early uses of salicylic acid, however, revealed that it was very corrosive to the stomach, causing ulceration and bleeding from the organ's mucosal lining.

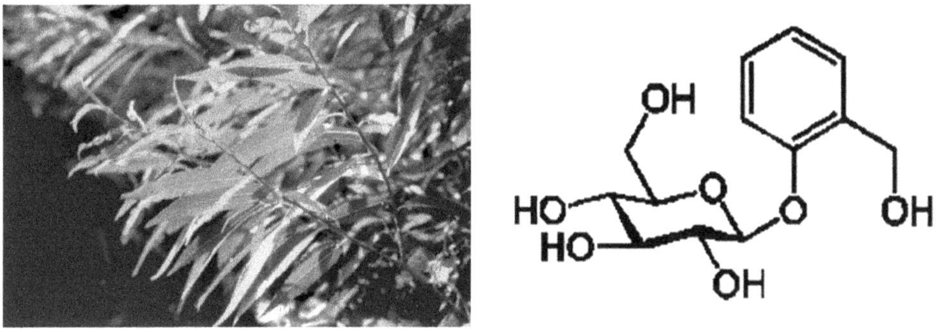

Figure 19.4: The leaves of the common willow (*Salix alba*) together with the molecular structure of its glycoside salicin, shown right

By 1839 chemists found an additional source of "salicylic acid" in the plant meadowsweet. Here it was found in the form of its ester, acetyl salicylate. This natural form did not have the corrosive effects on the stomach of the refined salicylic acid.

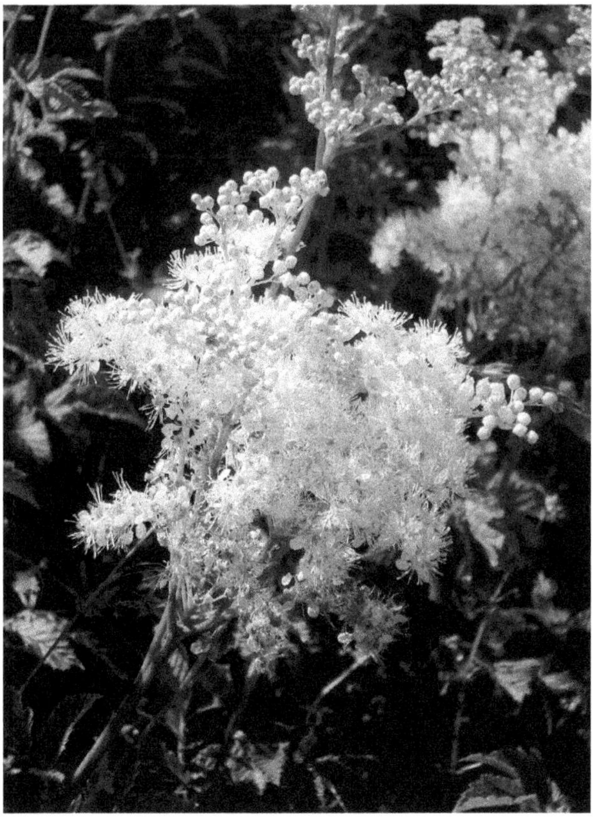

Figure 19.5: Meadowsweet or queen of the meadow (*Filipendula ulmaria*)

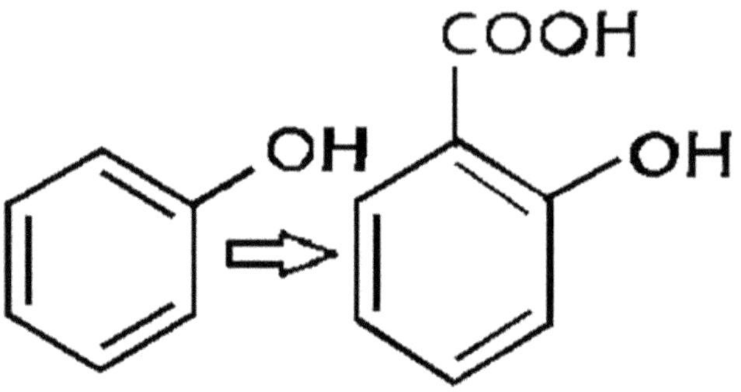

Phenol **Salicylic Acid**

Figure 19.6: Synthesis of salicylic acid

In 1899 chemists at the drug and dye firm Bayer learnt how to synthesise salicylic acid from phenol in coal tar, a by-product of the coal industry, then copying the naturally occurring form meadowsweet, and esterified it with acetic acid found in vinegar, to make acetyl salicylic acid.

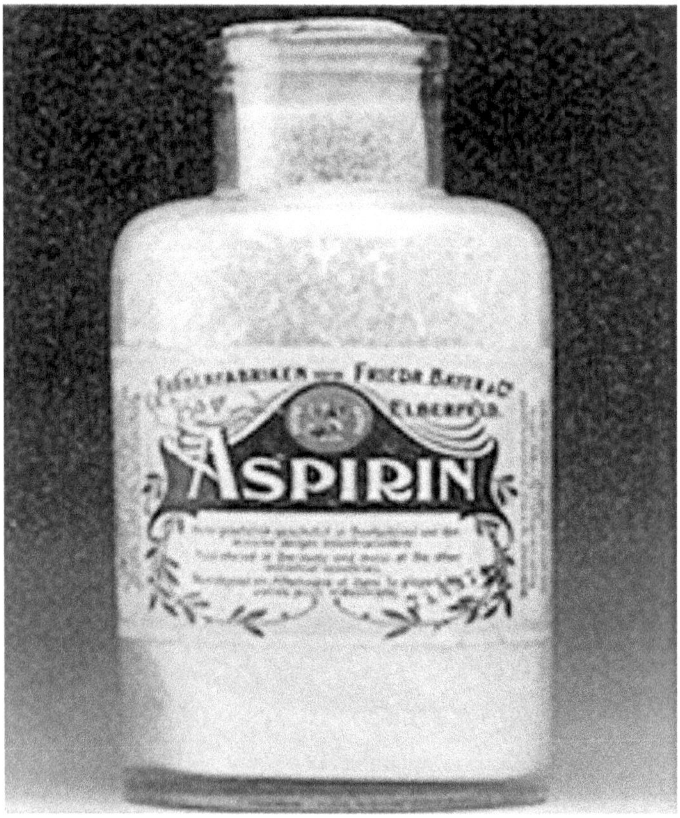

Figure 19.7: Bayer's marketing of Aspirin

Bayer then marketed the drug with name Aspirin, being derived from a corruption of *Spirea ulmaria*, the former generic Latin name for meadowsweet.

The patenting of a chemical process enabled even greater profits to be made. The synthesis of Aspirin by Bayer proved to be a watershed in relation to herbal medicine, for it "proved" from an economic perspective that synthetic medicine is superior to herbs. In the case of Aspirin, the abundant availability of coal tar from the coal industry meant that this medicine could be made continuously and no longer be subject to seasonable availability. This was the moment when medicine politically became increasingly dissociated from nature, leading to the decline of herbal medicine in the 20th century.

This development of the reductionist science in the 19th century drastically changed perceptions of herbs into being just collections of chemicals that could be exploited for potential medicines. This perception gained momentum when a simple quirk of chemistry led to the isolation of the alkaloids.

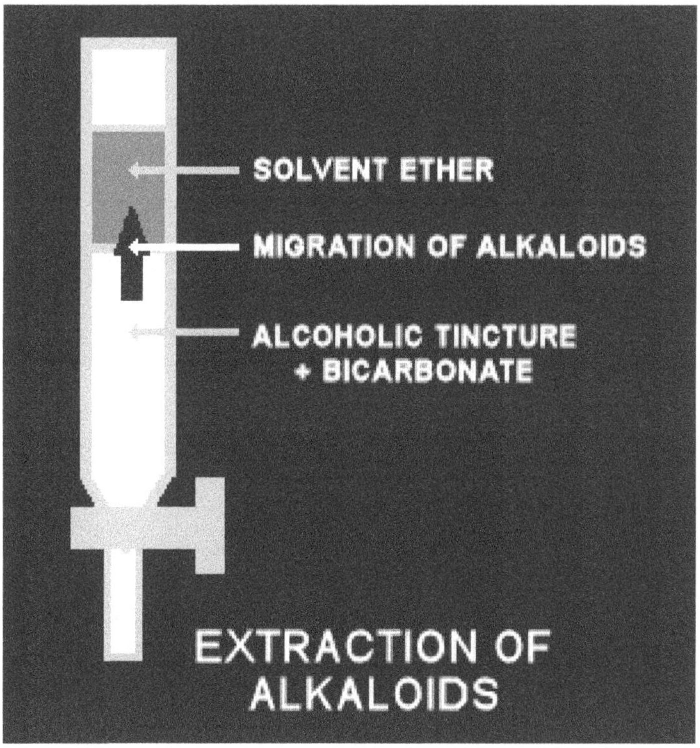

Figure 19.8: Extraction of alkaloids

Alkaloids derive their chemical name from the process of their extraction. When a herbal tincture is made alkaline, such as by adding a little sodium bicarbonate to the solution, then, when an organic solvent—such as diethyl ether—is poured on top, the alkaloids migrate from the alcoholic solution into the solvent.

As the two liquids are immiscible, the tincture can be drained below from the organic solvent. The solvent is simply left to evaporate, depositing the crystalline alkaloid.

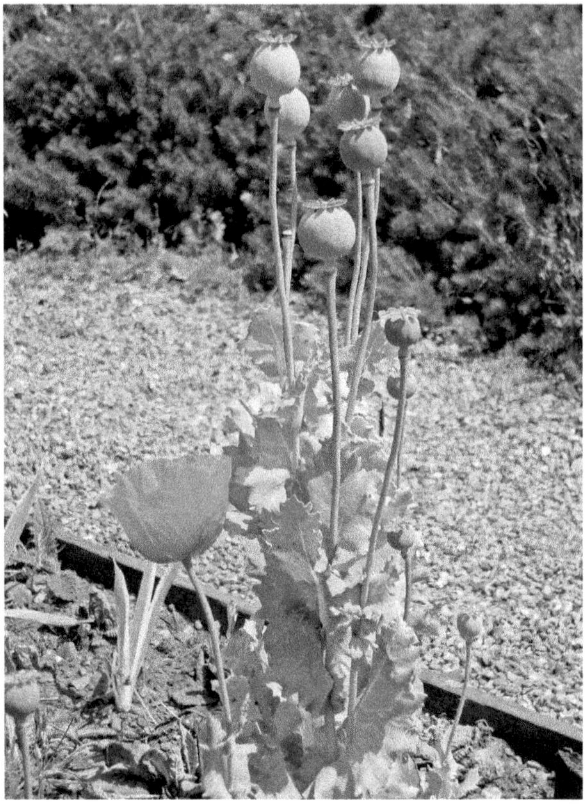

Figure 19.9: Seedheads of the opium poppy (*Papaver somniferum*)

Using this technique, very quickly a whole range of alkaloids were identified throughout the plant kingdom. The first individual alkaloid (called morphine after Morpheus, the Roman god of sleep) was isolated in 1804 from the opium poppy (*Papaver somniferum*) by the German chemist Friedrich Sertürner. The opium poppy in fact yields several alkaloids, another well-known one being codeine, the analgesic drug.

In the reductionist zeal of the chemists, alkaloids were believed to be the essence of the medicinal action of a herb. The economic potential of alkaloids came to attention of the nascent oil industry. John D. Rockefeller, the American oil magnate, immediately recognised that in future the pharmaceutical industry could become the most profitable wing of the petrochemical industry.

Their chemists decided, as in the synthesis of Aspirin, that if using the hydrocarbon molecules from the leftover tarry residue from the oil refinement, they could synthesise alkaloids to mimic the structure of naturally occurring alkaloids, and then patent them, they could make a fortune from the discarded waste.

Where synthesis from molecules found in oil was not possible, the alkaloids were extracted from plants and then patented by adding side chains, since it was not possible to patent a naturally occurring molecule. An alternative to adding side chains to the molecule was by joining two morphine molecules together to make diamorphine, which could then be patented and marketed as Heroin.

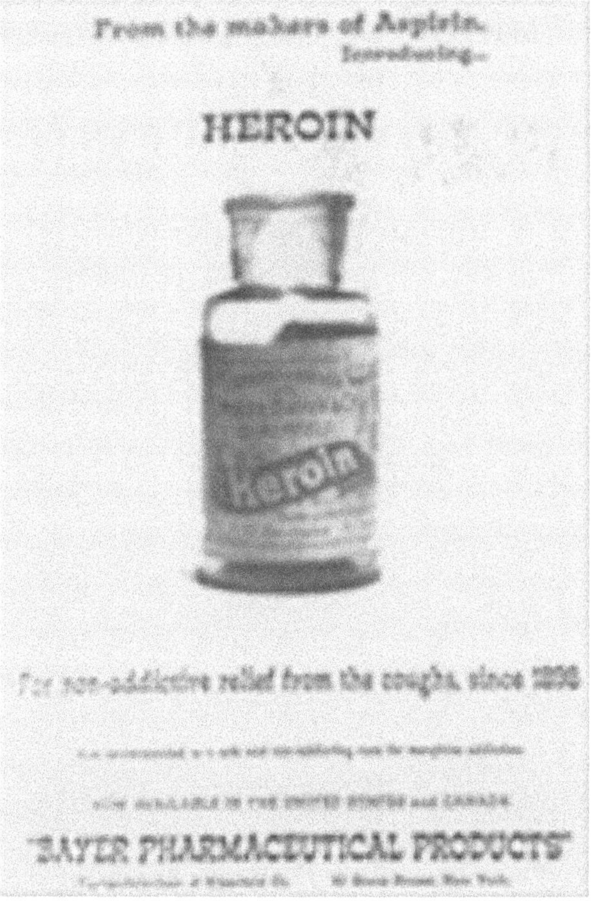

Figure 19.10: The marketing of Heroin, "For non-addictive relief from coughs, since 1896"

At the turn of the 20th century, the oil industry was in its infancy. The internal combustion engine had only recently been invented, and cars were limited in manufacture and affordability, so the market for the sale of petrol was also very limited. There were only 1,000 cars in the USA at the time! Compare that to the number of people needing medicine. But how did Rockefeller go about creating a market for these new drugs?

In the early 20th century, the American Medical Association (AMA) realised that medical education was inconsistent and often of poor quality. In 1904 the AMA formed the Council for Medical Education, to study the need for improvements in medical education. However, the AMA could not afford to do such a study. Henry Pritchett of the Carnegie Foundation offered to help finance this project and appointed Abraham Flexner to lead it.

The Carnegie Foundation, flush with money from Andrew Carnegie's hold over the steel industry and augmented by Rockefeller's hold over the oil industry, supplied millions of dollars to support this study, essentially taking over management of the Council for Medical Education.

MEDICAL EDUCATION
IN THE
UNITED STATES AND CANADA

A REPORT TO
THE CARNEGIE FOUNDATION
FOR THE ADVANCEMENT OF TEACHING

BY
ABRAHAM FLEXNER

WITH AN INTRODUCTION BY
HENRY S. PRITCHETT
PRESIDENT OF THE FOUNDATION

BULLETIN NUMBER FOUR (1910)
(Reproduced in 1960)
(Reproduced in 1972)

Figure 19.11: The Flexner Report

The Flexner Report, which was published in 1910, looked at the training of every medical school in North America. While the report helped lead to a standardisation of medical education, it was biased by the funding of the Carnegie Foundation, which came from Rockefeller and other industrialists with a vested interest in developing the emerging petrochemical industry.

Naturally, the report leaned towards the emerging opportunities of the pharmaceutical industry and was antipathetic towards natural medicines. It ultimately led to the banning of natural medicines and the various schools that taught this knowledge.

The report concluded:

> *Medical schools that offered training in various disciplines including electromagnetic field therapy, phototherapy, eclectic medicine, physiomedicalism, naturopathy and homeopathy were all told to drop these courses from their curriculum or lose their accreditation and underwriting support. A few schools resisted for a time, but eventually all either complied with the report or shut their doors.*

By 1935 the Carnegie Institute had been given the sole responsibility of accreditation of medical schools in both Canada and the USA. Consequently, all medical schools offered only pharmaceutical medicine, vaccines and surgery. Using their economic might, the pharmaceutical industry was able to pressure governments into passing legislation giving exclusive rights to the emerging industry.

Extracting and classifying a whole range of alkaloids from the plant kingdom was straightforward, but it was found that in isolation these compounds, removed from the context of the mother plant, often behaved in ways on the body that were different from the action of the whole herb. Physiological experimentation was required to find out what action they had on the body. How did they do that?

Prior to the Second World War, John D. Rockefeller massively invested in I.G. Farben, the German chemical conglomerate comprising BASF, Beyer, Hoechst and three other companies. In turn, I.G. Farben paid massive amounts of money to the Nazi party, becoming their largest donor. When his party came to power, Hitler allowed I.G. Farben to build concentration camps specifically for chemical experimentation. The camps were administered by soldiers from Himmler's SS.

Thousands of people, stripped of their basic human rights and from many ethnic backgrounds, were subjected to the indignity of being experimented on with a range of different hydrocarbon chemicals, including all the alkaloids, along with novel surgical procedures. Most died from their mistreatment, and in their postmortems their organs and tissues were microscopically examined for evidence of what pharmacological changes had been induced.

Some of these experiments were particularly gruesome, as in one trial 300 inmates all died painfully from 100 ml of phenol being injected intravenously.

After the 67th Anti-tank Division of the Royal Artillery liberated Belsen in April 1945 the scene as they arrived at the camp was truly horrific. Over 10,000 bodies were dumped up to 14 deep in places, rotting away all around the two miles of perimeter fencing. Unlike the death camps in Poland, Belsen only had one oven to cremate the bodies. It was completely inadequate to deal with all the corpses. The stench of death was everywhere, with cholera, dysentery and typhoid rife among the malnourished and exhausted inmates.

The author's father, Lieutenant John Warren-Davis, was appointed the officer in charge of the clean-up, which continued for many months after Germany had surrendered. He used the former commandant's office, which was located immediately above the torture rooms. He described how stairs led down into one large room that was fitted out like an abattoir, completely spotless, with tiled walls, channels and drains in the floor, hoses to wash it all down and a long, stainless-steel rail across the room complete with meat hooks. There were several metal tables, with surgical equipment, where the autopsies and surgical procedures had been done.

In the commandant's office, six large metal filing cabinets contained all the records of the experiments performed there, meticulously recorded with accompanying "before" and "after" photos. Some of the surgical procedures were even filmed. While it was all written in German, which he could not understand, my father said that "the photos did not leave much to the imagination". He added, "The sheer scale of the experimentation recorded in them defied belief." Being a witness to the extent of the suffering inflicted on the inmates of the camp shocked him to the core of his being. "How could man have acted to so inhumanely to his fellow man?"

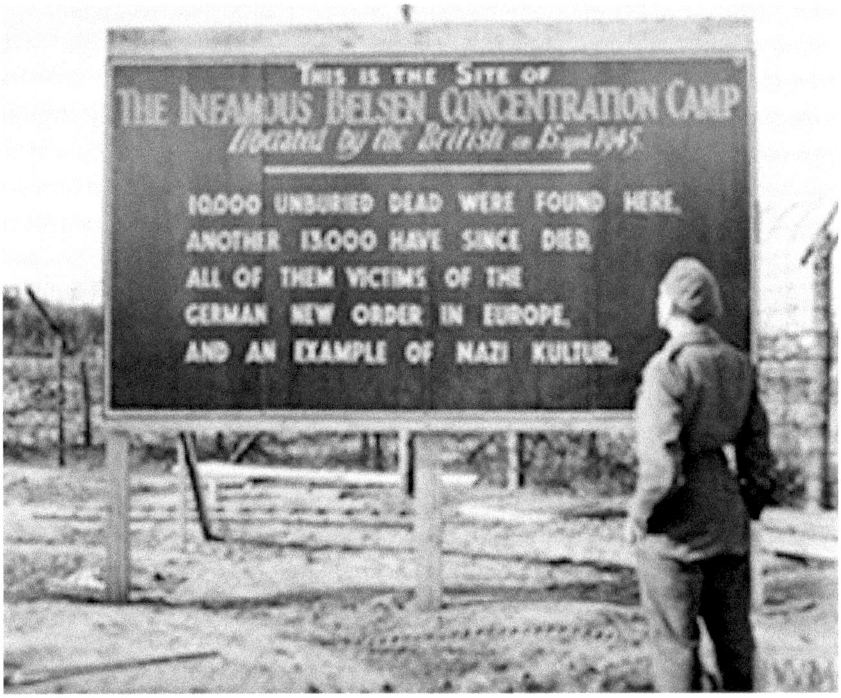

Figure 19.12: The site of Belsen Concentration Camp

Though news of the Allied advance had reached the concentration camp, leading to an attempt at burning the evidence before the British arrived, the photographic paper fortunately defied combustion, so only in just one drawer, the files were partially damaged. All of the files that were in the office were sent to the Nuremberg Tribunal as evidence of war crimes.

At the Nuremberg War Crimes Tribunal, 24 I.G. Farben board members and executives were convicted for mass murder, slavery and other crimes against humanity. While the worst offenders in the Nazi party were hanged, most of the scientists who had participated in the experimentation were only given long prison sentences. Afterwards, I.G. Farben was then split up into the six companies that had made up the conglomerate, and then the leading three, BASF, Beyer, and Hoechst (now Avantis). However, by 1952, all 24 of the convicted perpetrators had been released and then employed as executives and scientists at these companies.

The legal outcome of the Nuremberg Tribunal was the drawing up of the Nuremberg Treaty, which expressly forbids human experimentation without consent. Before giving consent, one has the legal right to understand all of the implications, health problems, and future health hazards. Most importantly, one has the legal capacity to say, "no".

While this horrendous human experimentation was being conducted in the German concentration camps, in the UK, the Pharmacy Act of 1942 passed in the dead of a winter's night, during the darkest depths of Britain's despair in the war. This act gave legal legitimacy to pharmaceutical medicine and effectively made herbal medicine illegal in the UK. Herbal medicine remained illegal till the passing of the 1968 Medicines Act restored the common law right of herbalists to practise.

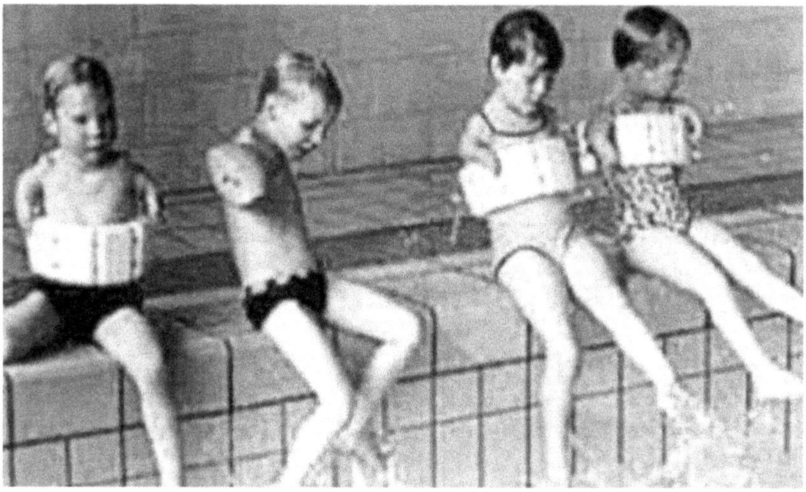

Figure 19.13: Limbless children born after their mothers were given Thalidomide, for morning sickness. Public domain

The Medicines Act was a legal response to curb the reckless practices of the pharmaceutical industry, exposed by the teratogenic tragedy of the thalidomide drug. However, the Act also provided the opportunity, thanks to Fred Fletcher Hyde, BSc, FNIMH and others, to persuade Parliament to include a special section once more restoring the common law right of herbalists, granted previously by Henry VIII.

The patenting of compounds as drugs enables vast profits to be made. Drug companies arbitrarily define their own profits, and typically they are marketed with 1,000+% markups in price. With chemotherapy drugs the markup may be even higher at 2,000% or even 3,000%. This makes the pharmaceutical industry more profitable than the banking industry. Imagine trying to pay back a loan with 1,000% interest on it!

As a rough illustration, an average week's prescription for Aspirin (its patent has long expired) costs the NHS £25. Hypothetically, if the daily dose of Aspirin is 25 mg, then that translates to 175 mg per week. This means that 1 mg = £0.14, therefore 1 g = £140, while 1 kg = £140,000. With 1 kg being the equivalent to 1 lt fluid volume, filling up a family car with 50 litres of petrol in the tank is approximately £60. If you had to pay for 50 litres of petrol at pharmaceutical prices, then you would have to fork out £7,000,000! You can see why Rockefeller foresaw that the development of pharmaceuticals would be the most profitable part of the oil industry.

With vast profits so easily generated, pharmaceutical companies are seen as sound places to invest money. The pharmaceutical industry is essentially an investment industry, driven by making profits for its shareholders, not necessarily for improving human health.

By conflating financial success with the pharmacological benefits of a drug, the marketing of these new compounds could now be sold as another triumph of science over the superstitions of the past, even though in the long term the specific drug may not even be beneficial to the body. This is not to mention the effects of addiction, which though denied, have definitely been commercially advantageous to exploit.

Disease is the marketplace for the pharmaceutical industry, which has sought to define its market by the treatment of disease symptomatically. This prolongs the existence of the disease and consequently the need to keep taking the drugs, serving to perpetuate the industry's profits.

The pharmaceutical model is not a therapeutic system; it does not seek to make people whole again, as was shown in the conclusion of the Flexner Report. To capture their market, the industry has a vested interest in not allowing people to understand how their body functions, thereby taking responsibility for their own health. Likewise, it is antipathetic to all forms of natural medicine that can heal patients from their conditions, as this reduces their market scope and detracts from their profits.

They plough a portion of their profits back into academic institutions and medical schools, such that much of what doctors are taught is heavily biased towards maintaining the market of the pharmaceutical industry. Vast amounts of money too are spent on advertising, capturing the influence of the media, which consequently is solely supportive of pharmaceutical medicine, lest they lose their advertising revenue. As a critic put it, "The Hippocratic maxim has been subverted to—First do no harm—to the profits of the pharmaceutical industry!"

This premise of extracting the "active chemicals" out of herbs does not always work—as shown by the resounding failure of Tamiflu. The development of this drug embodies the very exploitive principles that Culpeper railed against: choose a foreign herb, extract a chemical out of it, modify it by a patentable process and sell it to as large a market as possible.

The drug was synthesised from shikimic acid, a constituent of star anise (*Illicium verum*). It was promoted as an "antiviral drug" to protect people from the H1N1 "Swine 'Flu". Governments spent huge sums of money on stockpiling it, but when it was put to use, it was found to be ineffectual and, far from preventing flu, it typically made people taking it have an even worse experience.

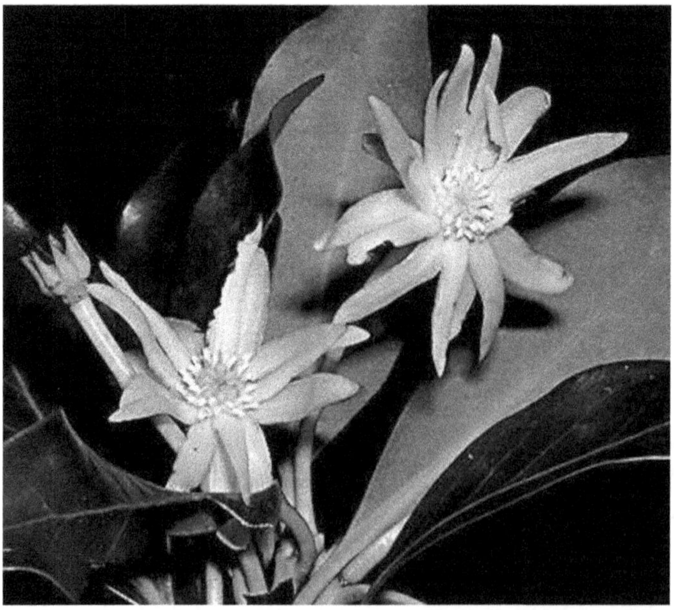

Figure 19.14: Star anise (*Illicium verum*)

Tamiflu proved to be unable to counter H1N1 influenza virus, and instead of freeing up the secretions from the lungs so that the chest can be naturally clear, it caused a blockage of these secretions with subsequent respiratory distress.

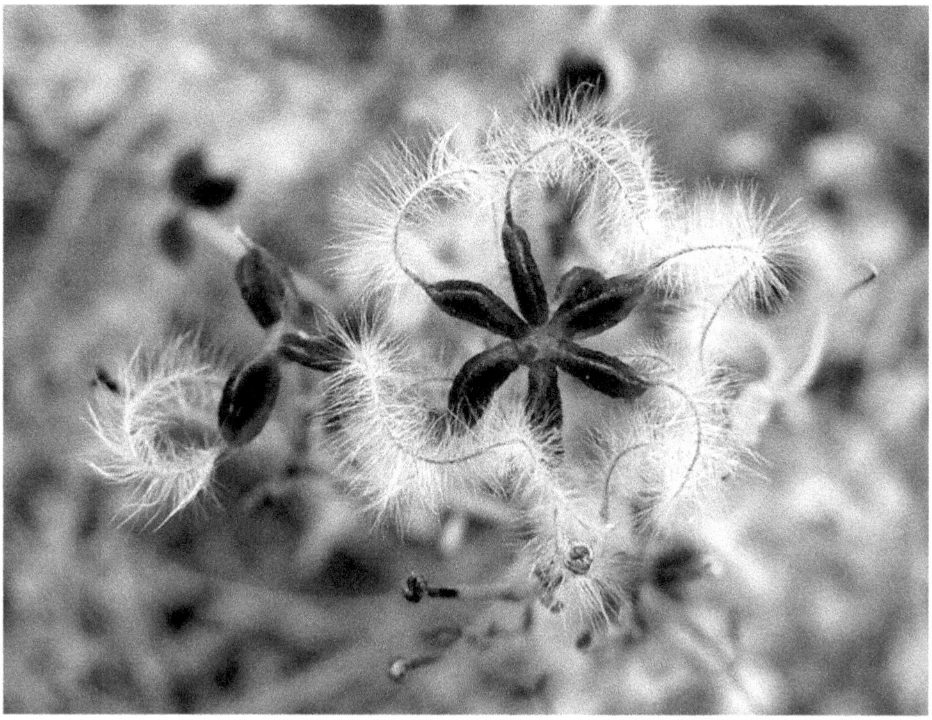

Figure 19.15: The familiar seedpods of star anise

Star anise is used in Chinese and Vietnamese medicine to relieve the congestion of 'flu and other respiratory disorders. The whole herb clearly would have been better than the drug. It is even readily available in UK supermarkets as an ingredient for Asian cuisine. But people were not told about it.

However, how about using a herb that is more local? A simple tea made from elderflowers has worked well for centuries for relieving colds and chest infections. Called *Blodau yr Ysgawen* in Welsh, elderflower was used by the Physicians of Myddfai, as shown in their writings, for treating phlegmatic conditions.

Why go to all that expense of developing Tamiflu when these native herbs work wonderfully? We should be using the philosophical principle of Ockham's Razor: If you can do something simply or a more complicated way, it is always better to choose the simpler option.

Clearly, promoting Tamiflu required populations of people being ignorant of these simple remedies. Despite it not being effective, even counterproductive for some, millions of pounds profit was made out of the drug by selling it to governments around the world. So, purely from a profit point of view, it was highly successful.

CHAPTER TWENTY

Physic in the 21st century

As science has evolved in the last three centuries, herbal medicine has acquired two contrasting perspectives of herbs: the metaphysical and the pharmacological. The former perspective, which has been demonstrated in the previous chapters, explains how 90% of the uses of herbs have evolved through the last 2,500 years, while the latter has only been applied to herbal medicine in the last 125 years.

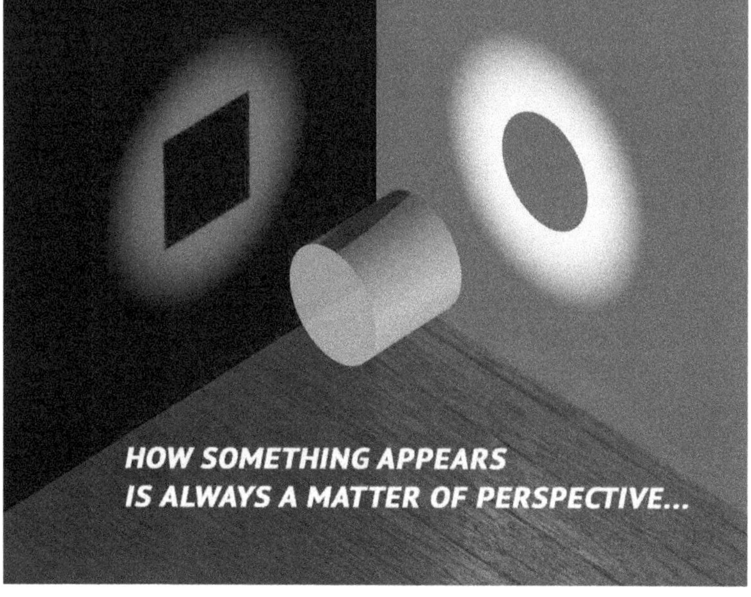

Figure 20.1: Matter of Perspective AI

Both perspectives have their own discipline and methodology. The former connects with a profound respect and intuitive understanding of nature. The latter is largely a reductionist superimposition onto the herbal kingdom, having derived chemical insights into the specific actions of herbs.

The big problem of the pharmacological perspective for herbalists, as has been historically shown, is that it is the language of the exploitation of herbs and disease for profit. The funding for research into the actions of herbs is largely derived by the pharmaceutical industry's continual quest to identify compounds from which to develop new drugs, not to further the benefits of herbal medicine.

This latter perspective is largely a response to the 1942 Pharmacy Act, where herbal medicine was unceremoniously dumped, not because herbs do not work as a healing modality, but because its very success detracts from the marketplace of the pharmaceutical industry and limits its profits. Furthermore, herbalists, in helping patients resolve their health issues and regain their autonomy, detract from the profiteering of the pharmaceutical medicine. Patients have often said, "Why do doctors not tell you the advice you need to get better, instead of just doling out drugs?"

However, despite being seemingly diametrically opposite perspectives, both can learn from each other, to achieve an even greater understanding of the enormous therapeutic potential of herbal medicine.

How this synthesis can be achieved requires a conceptual understanding of how metaphysical knowledge was lost in the chemical redefinition of an element as a unit of material composition. When the classical understanding of the Elements as the universal forces on which life depends is restored, it can still be seen to hold sway in the clinical situation.

Arguably, nowhere is the importance of the Five Elements better shown than in the principles of first aid. There is a mnemonic that emphasises the importance of preserving life in the body: 3 minutes without Air, 3 hours without heat (Fire), 3 days without Water, and 3 weeks without food (Earth). Add 3 months without sunshine to this list and you have here the basic tenets of Hippocratic medicine.

To prevent this from happening a second mnemonic, "Dr ABC", comes into action. Once the body is removed (R) from immediate physical danger (D), it is primarily important to check that the airways (A) are not obstructed, that breathing (B) is happening and that the heart is beating (C). If the heart is not beating and/or breathing is not happening, then administering CPR (cardiopulmonary resuscitation) is vitally important to ensure or restore the supply of oxygen to the cells. Then the body is manoeuvred into the recovery position, and kept warm and hydrated.

Instead of seeing the chemical definition of matter as replacing the metaphysical understanding, it is important to see the two perspectives coexisting. This facilitates looking at the reductionist discoveries of anatomy and physiology in the body as a part the greater metaphysical context of the Five Elements.

To achieve this, there is an obstacle with pharmaceutical medicine as it is deliberately stuck in the 19th-century, Daltonian conception of solid atoms. The idea that a drug or molecule has a particular action/s becomes a nonsense with a post-nuclear conception of an atom. The principal revelation of the nuclear conception is that the structure of an atom is 99.9999999999% space. All its mass is located in the nucleus, which makes up less than 0.0000000001% of its total structure. So, the conception of the atom or molecule in a drug "possessing" its action cannot be true, as there is to all purposes nothing there to possess anything. At the very least, it makes the patenting of drugs highly questionable.

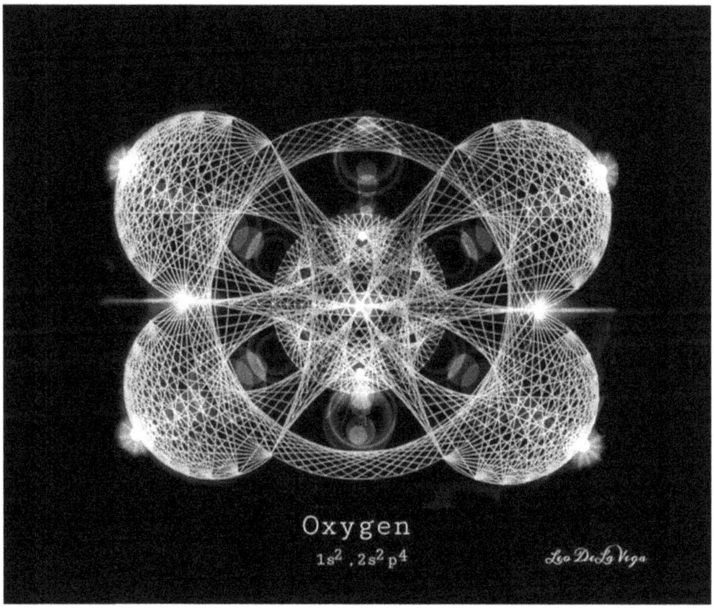

Figure 20.2: Structure of an oxygen atom. Image Leo Delavega

The relatively vast space inside an atom is taken up by electrons travelling at the speed of light, held in their orbits by the electrostatic pull of the positrons in the nucleus. The sum total of all chemical properties and reactions between atoms lies in the number and orbital configuration of the electrons, along with the energy they possess.

As Werner Heisenberg observed, the movement of the electrons is subject to the consciousness of the observer. In the subatomic realm, he realised that the influence of the observer changes the outcome of the experiment, leading to the statement of his Uncertainty Principle: *"What we observe is not nature itself, but nature exposed to our method of questioning."*

The medical counterpart to the Uncertainty Principle is the placebo phenomenon, whereby just the belief that a drug will benefit you has the desired effect, despite the drug being a physiologically inert substance. This phenomenon, and its inverse, the nocebo phenomenon—the belief that the drug will have a negative outcome—both show that the consciousness of the patient can powerfully influence the physiology of the body.

But how?

As we have already seen, Plato regarded his geometric solids as fundamental building blocks of matter. The NASA space scientist and professor of mathematics at the University of Chicago, Dr Robert Moon, inspired by ideas that Johannes Kepler had of the Planets' orbits being arranged around the Sun like Plato's Solids nestled within each other, suggested that the space in the nucleus of an atom is quantised, with the protons and neutrons being arranged in accordance with Plato's geometric shapes.

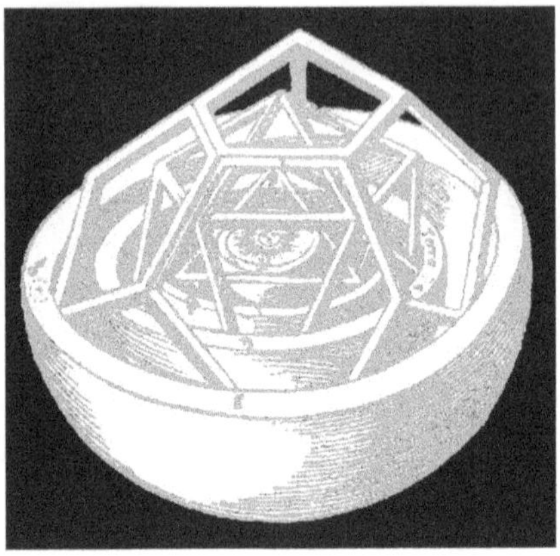

Figure 20.3: Johannes Kepler's vision of the Planets' orbits being arranged around the Sun like Plato's Solids nestled within each other

The configuration of the protons electrostatically holds the electrons in their "shell like" orbits. It is very probable that the configuration of the nucleus is not permanently rigid, but highly malleable—like a Rubik's Cube. Subtle changes in the configuration of the protons will have powerful effects on the orbiting electrons and the chemical reactivity of the atom.

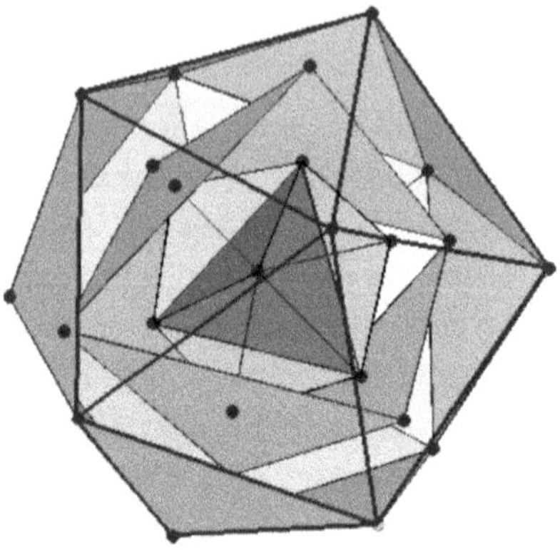

Figure 20.4: Arrangement of protons within the nucleus of an Iron atom, in accordance with Dr Robert Moon's postulation

The atoms composing the body are subject to the control of the individual's consciousness, so that when a person applies their will, their intent changes the nuclear configuration, activating the biochemical reactions that make up the physiology of the body.

As the father of quantum physics, Max Planck, said, *"I regard consciousness as fundamental. I regard matter as a derivative from consciousness. We cannot get beyond consciousness."*

In the language of chemistry just how consciousness influences the body is hard to explain. However, if Dr Moon's hypothesis of the protons in the nucleus being arranged in two Platonic geometric shapes is correct, then if the interaction of consciousness affects the smallest movement of one geometric shape in relation to the other in the nucleus, that has a dramatic effect on the orbiting electrons and their chemical interactions with other chemical elements.

In quantum physiological terms, then, it is consciousness that permeates every atom of the body, controlling every biochemical process, maintaining its structure against its entropic dissolution. So, the mapped-out physiological pathways of cellular metabolism are patterns of consciousness, just as patterns in iron filings on a card map out the magnetic fields of a magnet underneath.

The fact that, excluding the microbiome, the adult body has some 7 trillion cells within its structure, which developed from just two cells, and are maintained over a lifetime, is an astonishing feat of engineering. Chemistry focuses on the structure of matter but does not see how intricately consciousness can organise matter.

Nowhere is this more readily seen than in deoxyribonucleic acid (DNA). Biochemists have looked at the double helical structure of DNA for the greater part of a century, largely focusing on the sequencing of the purine and pyrimidine bases that make up the genes. Less attention has been paid to the spatial arrangement of the double helix, other than its ability to unzip and zip up in cellular division and protein synthesis.

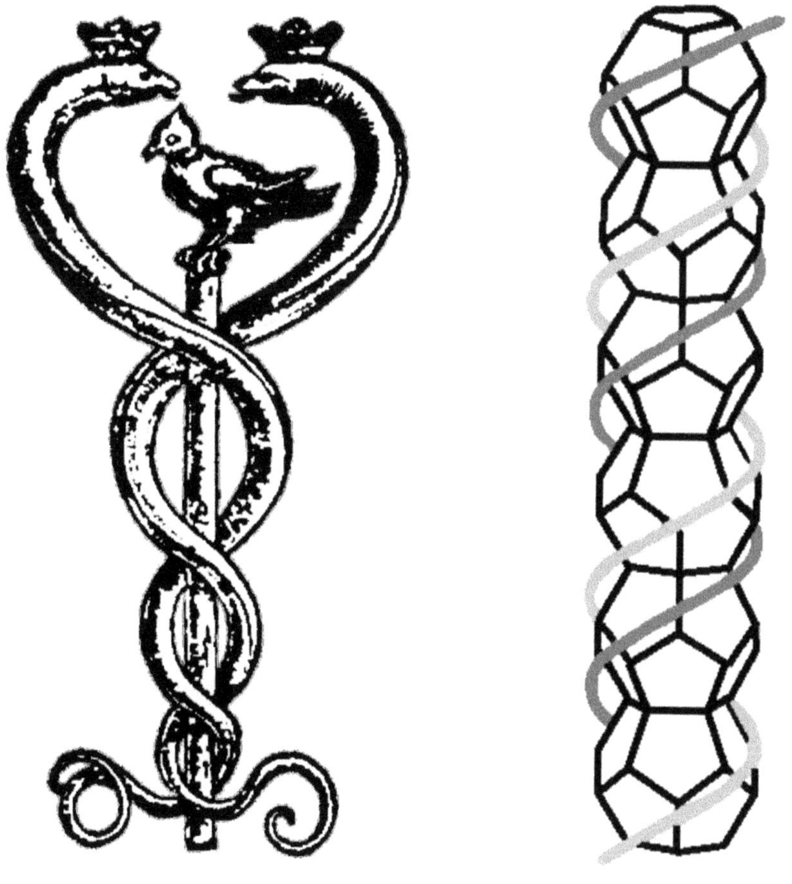

Figure 20.5: Comparison of the structure of DNA and the Caduceus, after Holbein

Many people have noticed the double helical structure of DNA is analogous to the two entwining serpents around a central staff that makes up the Caduceus, the emblem of Mercury. Furthermore, when the space encapsulated by the dodecahedron is understood symbolically as corresponding to Plato's Ether, then it can be seen how the structure of DNA is organised by consciousness. The pentangular coiling of the helical spirals is affected by the 5-carbon monosaccharide, ribose.

This link between Ether and space inside the DNA is important, for genes code for the sequence of amino acids that make up a protein, which is then assembled on the ribosomes, but *not* its function. The original concept of primacy of the gene theory, that the nucleus is in control, is now disproven, for a protein is not complete until it is correctly glycosylated, where monosaccharide sugars are inserted into the amino acid sequence to create the tertiary or spatial structure needed to fulfil its function. Glycosylation happens in the endoplasmic reticulum, in a separate and parallel cellular process that is not subject to genetic control, after the peptide sequence has been assembled on a ribosome.

The birth of the science of glycobiology evolved from research into one of the most important healing herbs in the Western *materia medica*, aloe (*Aloe vera* and *A. barbadensis*). Aloe has an almost legendary reputation as a healing vulnerary herb, that is, for wounds, especially for burns, where its cooling and moistening gel soothes inflammation and enhances healing.

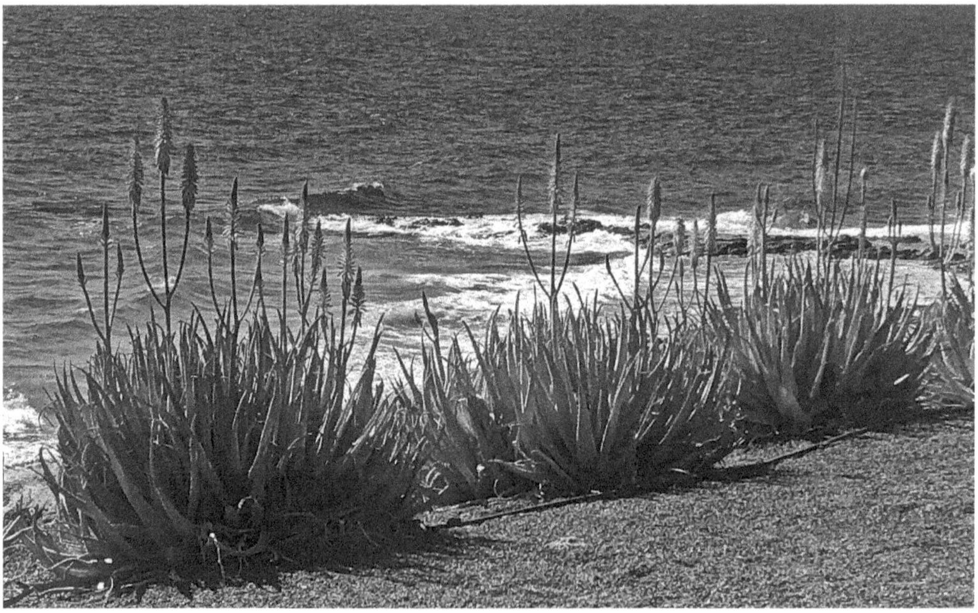

Figure 20.6: *Aloe barbadensis* growing by the sea in Lanzarote

In Arabic medicine aloe gel has been used for treating sunburn for centuries, and today the gel is commonly used as the principal ingredient for "after sun" products.

In 1960s stories among the hippie communities in the USA suggested that aloe was good for radiation burns. This time was the height of the Cold War with the USSR, and the American military took these anecdotes seriously, stockpiling drums of the gel as a part of their defence strategy.

Having stored the gel for months, they decided to test its healing properties. The results showed that it now had none. The military subsequently approached a young PhD biochemical student, Bill McAnalley, and asked him to find out why the gel lost its potency, so that it could be preserved.

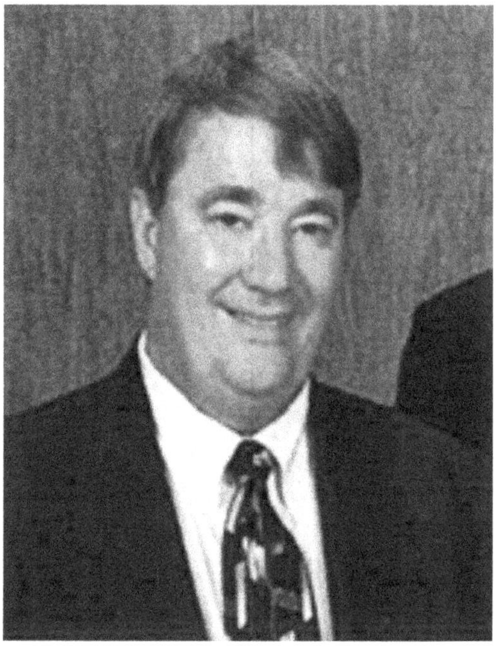

Figure 20.7: Bill McAnalley, PhD

This raised the question, what substance in the gel had the healing power? Without knowing that, preserving the effectiveness of the gel would have been a stab in the dark. After months of research the principal ingredient was found to be acemannan, a complex polymer of the monosaccharide sugar mannose. At first mannose created disbelief, for at the time sugars were just considered to have no physiological role other than a source of energy, such as glucose. How could it possibly have this effect?

McAnalley proved, by radio tracing, that mannose, rather than being broken down to create energy actually became incorporated into the cell membrane, but why? He was able to show that when the juice was stored, the mannose component was rapidly broken down. Hence the juice lost its healing property. But his research did not explain how the mannose was so important to the herb's healing action.

This discovery dovetailed with the work of Günter Blobel, who in the 1960s asked the question: how do newly synthesised proteins find their correct destinations within a cell? He discovered in his research that after a protein is synthesised, it is tagged by a short sequence of sugars, which act as a post code of where it was to perform its function in the body.

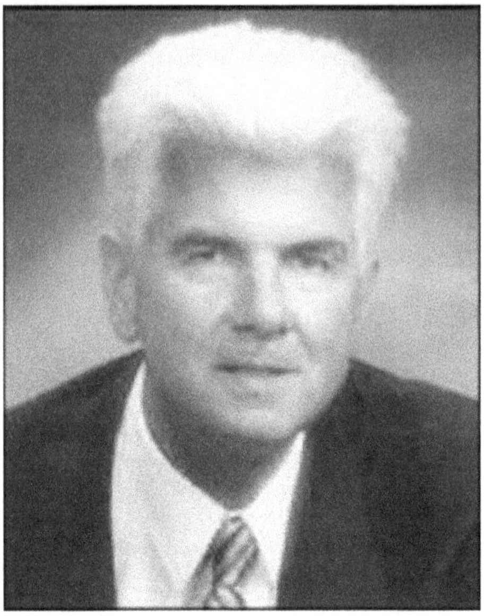

Figure 20.8: Günter Blobel won the 2000 Nobel Prize for Medicine and Biochemistry after 20 years of research

Furthermore, Blobel's research demonstrated that this information was coded with the monosaccharide sugars composing the tags, in a homologous way to the coding of genetic information with the purine and pyrimidine bases within DNA.

Following this breakthrough discovery, it was now possible to understand the function of the glycoforms—the sugary projections covering every cell in the body. This has been a mystery ever since they were first seen by electron microscopy as tiny "furry" projections. Since information was coded in the structure of a protein by these monosaccharides, then it was realised that these glycoforms too were cellular messages. All these messages were composed of just eight monosaccharide sugars.

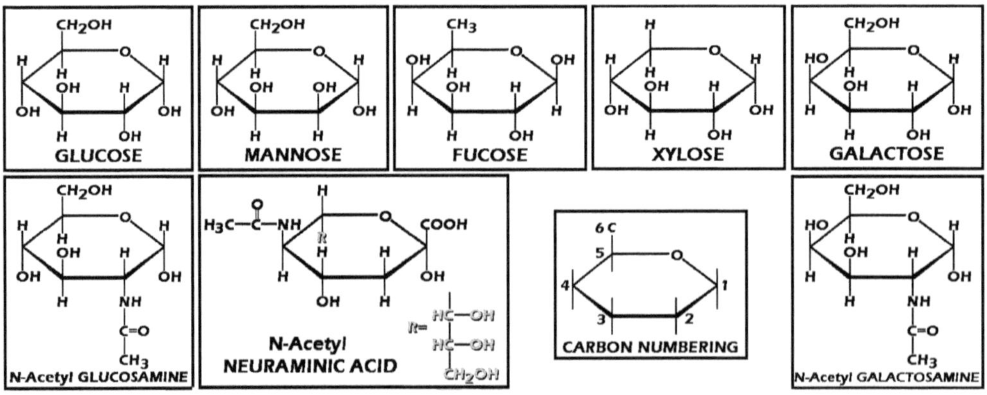

THE RELATIVE CHEMICAL STRUCTURES OF THE EIGHT ESSENTIAL SUGARS

Figure 20.9: The eight essential monosaccharide sugars

These sugars were defined in *Harper's Illustrated Biochemistry* in 1996 as: glucose, galactose, mannose, fucose, xylose, N-acetyl glucosamine, N-acetyl galactosamine and N-acetyl neuraminic acid (also called sialic acid).

Every cell in the body is essentially covered with tens of thousands of glycoforms. Each glycoform is a message from the cell and is composed of differing combinations of the eight essential sugars.

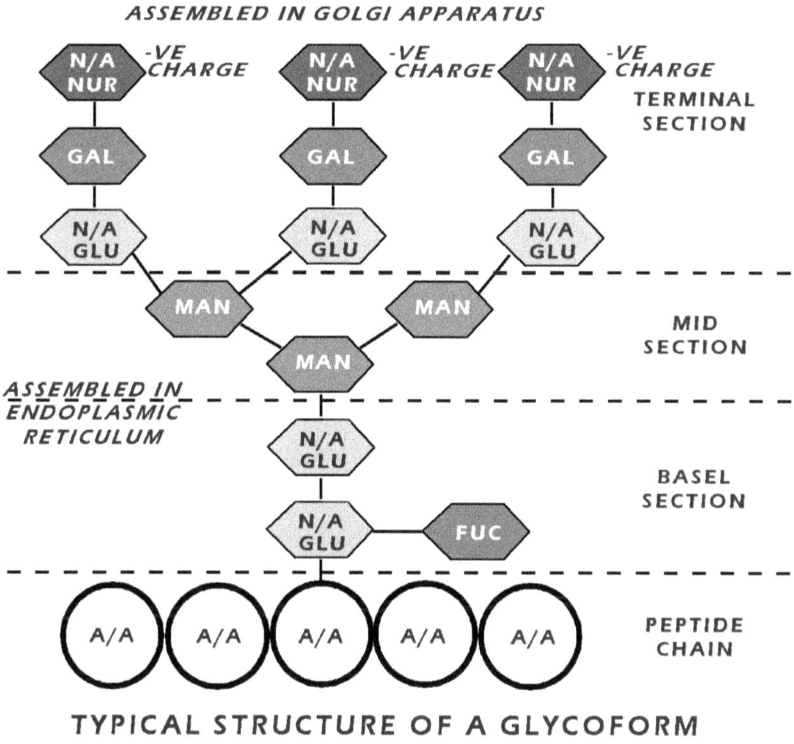

Figure 20.10: Typical structure of a glycoform

With the monosaccharide sugars forming the letters of each message, if any sugar is missing, then cellular communication is compromised, particularly if it is incorporated in the foundation of the glycoform, so the rest of glycoform cannot be assembled. Note the position of mannose (MAN). Note also that the N-acetyl monosaccharides have a negative charge, so the sugars in terminal section repel each other and spatially adopt a triangular relationship.

Here we can introduce the molecule dolichol, which acts in a parallel way to transfer RNA, collecting amino acids from the cytoplasm. Instead, it collects free monosaccharides, also from the cytoplasm, then starts building them into a glycoform template, which it then delivers to the endoplasmic reticulum.

The enzyme oligosaccharyltransferase (OST) detaches the glycoform structure from the dolichol molecule and attaches it to just three specific amino acids in a peptide chain: serine, threonine and asparagine.

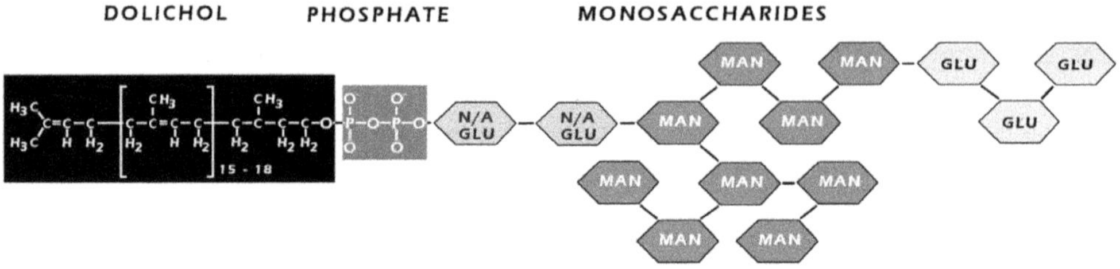

DOLICHOL STRUCTURING PROTO-GLYCOFORM

Figure 20.11: The structure of dolichol forming a glycoform

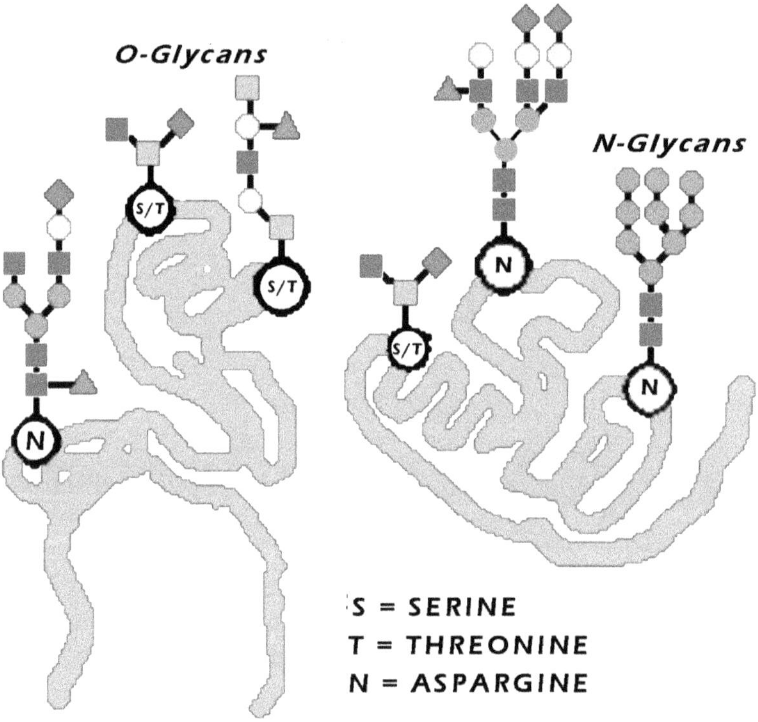

Figure 20.12: Insertion points of glycoforms in a peptide

Firstly, the glycoforms, with their electrostatic charge, are added to "bend" the peptide chain spatially into the right shape for its function—called its tertiary structure—as shown by the precision of enzymes fitting their substrates.

Secondly, as Günter Blobel discovered, a little tag of sugars is added to act as a "post code" to direct the protein to where it is needed.

Thirdly, sugar chains may be incorporated into the peptide structure to confer specific properties of the monosaccharides into the protein. An example is the protein crystalline, which makes up the lens of the eye. Generally, peptides are opaque, but by incorporating the crystalline properties of the monosaccharides into the structure they become translucent.

In the final stages of protein development, it is transferred from the endoplasmic reticulum to the specific layers of the Golgi apparatus, where more monosaccharides are added or substituted into the original glycoform template, and the terminal N-acetyl sugars attached. The cis layer of the Golgi apparatus is where the proteins are completed for external cellular secretion, such as the peptide hormones. The trans layer is where the proteins are completed for internal secretion, such as the proteolytic enzymes for the lysosomes. These two mid layers are where the glycoforms are made for cellular communication.

It is estimated that a gene, coding for a single peptide, by insertion of these eight monosaccharides, can be adapted into the structures of up to a thousand different proteins. This explains the conundrum of the apparent insufficient number of genes on our chromosomes to makes all the proteins of the body. The number of genes in our genome has currently been revised down to just 19,000, about half the number of the genes of a banana!

This conundrum is even more emphasised by the finding that roughly a third of this total number of genes is currently without known expression. It has been calculated that the glycome—the collective term for all the information stored in these sugars—carries 8x the amount of information than that which is stored in our genome. Even without a third of the genes expressing, that still leaves 12,540 functioning genes, which when multiplied by a 1,000 possible glycomic expressions gives a total number hypothetic genomic/glycomic combinations in the order of 12,540,000, comfortably more potential than required to build the tens of thousands of different proteins in the body. But with significantly less human genes than a banana, it suggests that the intelligence lies not in the genes but rather in the glycome that affectively operates the genes.

Cellular Communication

In cellular communication, tens of thousands of glycoforms are pushed up through the cell membrane, expressing specific needs. These are inserted through the cell wall, with their glycoforms protruding outside the surface of the cell, like the opening of thousands of tiny umbrellas. Their structures protrude into the super-conductive thin layer of structured water (H_3O_2) that surrounds each cell and line all the blood and lymph vessels. In essence, these glycoforms plug each cell into the information superhighway throughout the body.

Additionally, passing blood cells with their glycoforms read the messages like braille to initiate the response specific to their needs. Once the need is fulfilled, the corresponding glycoform is retracted back into the cytoplasm and its sugars recycled. Collectively, the web of glycoforms forms the cellular receptor sites for hormones, vitamins and drugs.

Through these mechanisms of cellular communication cells are able to maintain homeostasis, leading to optimal organ and immune system function. Thus, if a cell specifically needs sugars for energy or for making its glycoforms, amino acids for building peptides, lipids for making cellular membranes, vitamins and minerals for enzymic co-factors, not to mention maintaining the constant need for oxygen for cellular respiration, then it is able to instantaneously call out its needs. Similarly, it can deal with elimination requirements, with messages for carbon dioxide removal, nitrogenous waste disposal and countering toxins. There are glycoforms in relation to cellular regulation, such as temperature control and hydration.

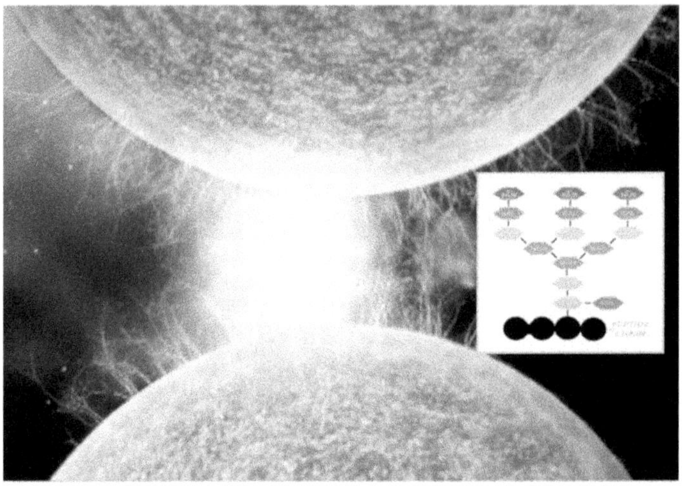

Figure 20.13: Cellular communication through touching glycoforms, after Mannatech

When nutritional formulations supplying all eight monosaccharides are introduced into the body the following beneficial changes have been identified: increased muscle mass, increased bone density, increased strength, increased aerobic capacity, decreased total cholesterol/HDL ratio, decreased percentage of body fat, decreased high blood pressure and increased blood glucose tolerance.

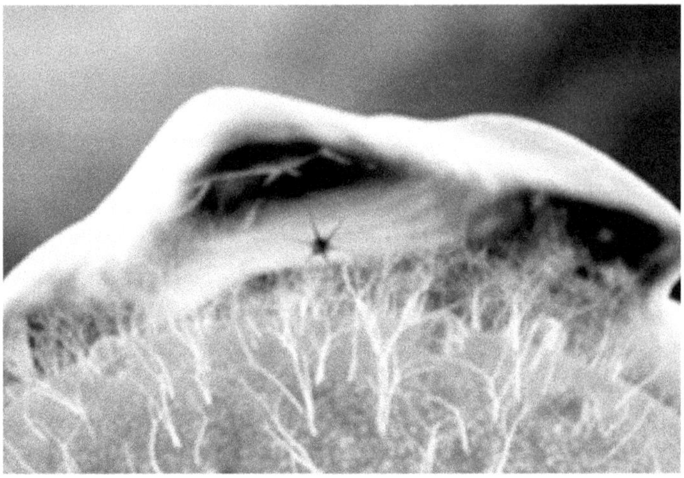

Figure 20.14: Macrophage phagocytosing a bacteria trapped in a glycoform mesh, after Mannatech

The integrity to the glycoform structures covering the cell membranes is very important. Their terminal sugars, with their negative electrical charge, repel each other, causing the glycoforms to fan out into a triangular shape and jostle for space between neighbouring structures. They collectively form a barricade against micro-biological attack. Any bacterium or virus that tries to penetrate the cell wall gets trapped, till phagocytic cells arrive to swallow it up.

Some viruses, however, such as influenza, have learnt how to deal with this obstacle. The nomenclature for classifying the different strains of influenza uses the letters H and N, referring to its protein coverings. The former is short for haemagglutinin (H), while the latter stands for neuraminidase (N), an enzyme capable of cutting off the terminal sugars of neuraminic acid. This collapses the glycoforms, giving much easier access to the virus penetrating through the cell membrane into its host cell.

In addition to the physical barricade, the glycoforms create specific messages calling for assistance from the immune system. Cells can even send out a rope of sugars to catch passing immune cells and then winch them to the specific cell that is under attack, where it can phagocytose the offending micro-organism.

Glycoforms play a significant role in cellular identification, for when covered with a full complement of glycoforms, a cell is able to express its full identity as a host cell. This enables passing immune cells, reading the glycoforms, to distinguish host cells from other invading micro-organisms. Similarly, the immune cells are able to recognise mutant cells and initiate apoptosis.

The biologist Bruce Lipton is correct when he says, *"The membrane is the brain of the cell."* The glycoforms confer to the cells a spatial awareness of both the internal and external environments and trigger epigenetic expression, enabling it to respond and adapt the cell to environmental changes. In a sense, every cell has its own pharmacy, which it utilises as soon as it senses it is out of balance.

Where deficiencies of these monosaccharides develop then it is easy to see how every metabolic pathway becomes compromised and functions less efficiently. Cells become more vulnerable to microbial attack and mutating cells are not adequately dealt with.

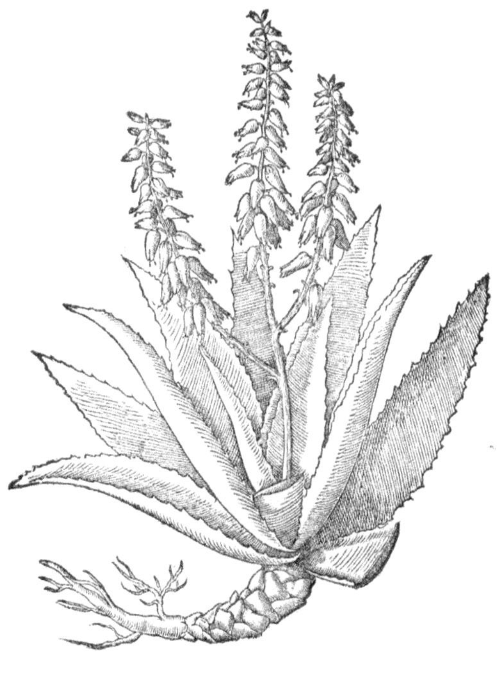

Figure 20.15: Woodcut of aloe from *Commentaries on the Six Books of Dioscorides* by Pietro Andrea Mattioli, 1665 Edition

Without mannose in particular, many of these glycoforms would not be able to be fully assembled, since it is often a key part of their mid-sections. The juice of aloes would supply a rich source of mannose, thereby triggering the completion of a whole range of glycoforms, restoring glycosylation of proteins, improving cellular communication and enhancing homoeostasis of the tissues. This is such a key part of the plant's unique healing properties. The monosaccharide function can thus be seen as a key mechanism for how certain herbs can work on the body.

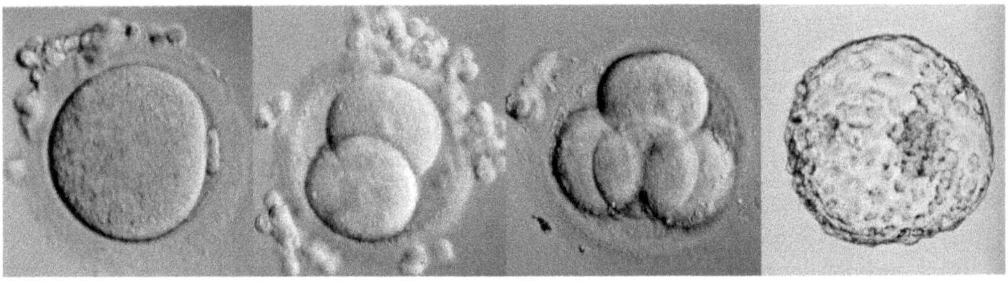

Figure 20.16: Stages of cellular division following fertilisation of an ovum

One of the key areas of cellular communications is apoptosis or cellular death, which plays a vital role in sculpting the tissues of the developing embryo into the shape of the future body.

The image shows the sequence of a fertilised ovum, on the left, undergoing binary cellular division, resulting in a ball of undifferentiated cells. What would happen if none of the cells died? Basically, we would just end up as a pulsating ball of cells that would be short-lived outside the womb from where it is implanted.

Paradoxically, it is the death of key cells within this cellular mass that enables the embryo to develop into the foetus. Where a cell dies, then no further cellular division can take place, leaving a gap or hollow space within the rest of the dividing mass of dividing cells, which carry on growing.

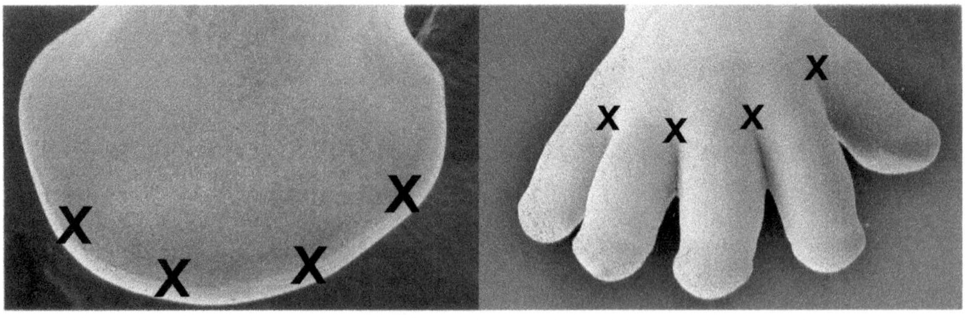

Figure 20.17: Role of apoptosis in the foetal development of the hand

A particularly good example of the role of apoptosis is shown in the embryological development of the hand. The hand starts to develop at 7 weeks, from just a pad, a sort of proto palm. It is the apoptosis of cells at key points (X) along the edge of the pad that leads to the development of the fingers and thumb, and the remaining cells on either of the points evolve into the digits. Amazingly, by 10 weeks the hand is fully formed with all its lines present, well before the muscles in the wrist develop sufficiently to begin the first primitive movements of the hand. It is about the size of a postage stamp.

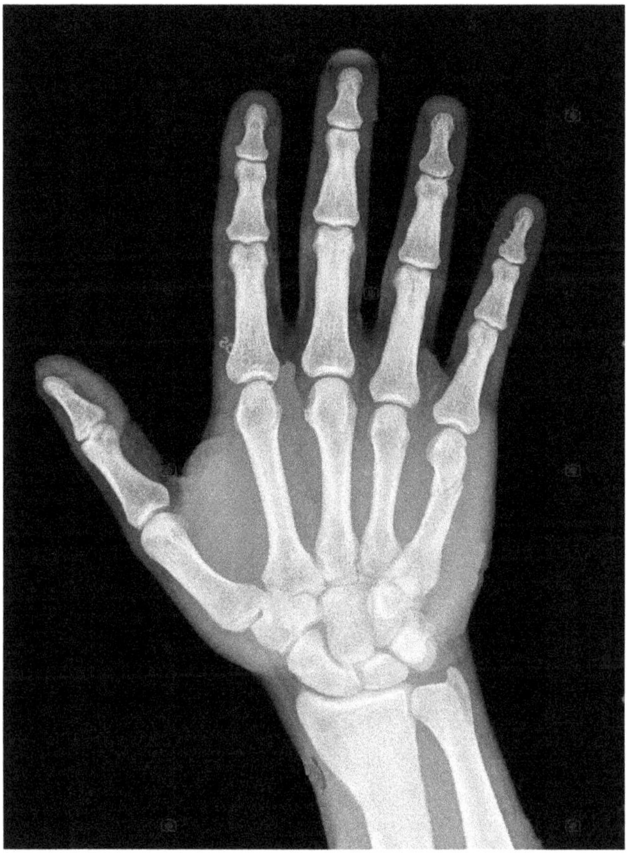

Figure 20.18: X-ray of a hand

So much of modern medical imaging gives us an unbalanced view of an individual. For example, X-rays have given medical science unprecedented insights into the structure of the bones in the skeletal system. But this is a view entirely devoid of any psychological or emotional insights. It creates a perspective of the body that is purely physical.

To gain an understanding of how consciousness influences the body, physicians need to cultivate a symbolic perspective. The premise of hand reading is that the form, structure and animation of the hand, and indeed the rest of the body, is an expression of the invisible inner psyche of the person. Both the outer form of the hand and the inner psyche can be visualised as having a parallel relationship to each other, just like an old-fashioned analogue slide projector.

When the projector is turned on, light shining through the slide carries the image to the screen. The image on the screen is essentially the same as the image on the slide.

By describing details observed in the image on the screen, you are simultaneously able to describe the image on the slide that is inaccessible within the projector. In this way a picture of a person's emotional, psychological and vitalistic perspective can be seen reflected in the hand.

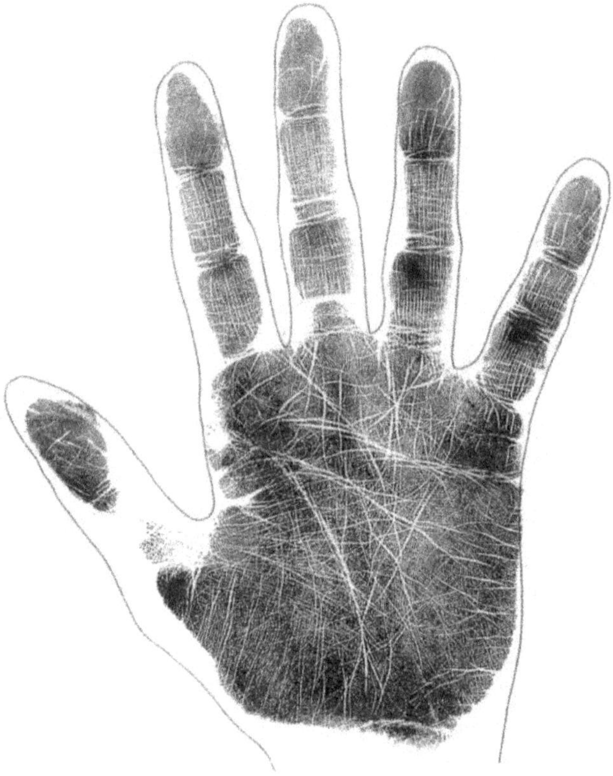

Figure 20.19: Hand print showing the palmar lines

Lines on the palm are not crease lines, as suggested in the labelling of the hand in many anatomy books, but formations that intricately reflect patterns of a person's consciousness. This is why in medieval times a physician was not considered properly trained unless he could read the lines of the palm. The alchemist and physician Paracelsus defined hand reading as *"the art of discovering what is within and hidden in man"*.

Their formations are highly dynamic, reflecting changes in a person's consciousness. New formations can be observed in as little as six weeks, which reflects the physiological time of the skin's growth, from its germinal layer to the outer horny layer. This link is most dramatically shown when a patient falls into a coma, and the lines on the palm have been observed to fade. Should the patient be fortunate enough to awaken from the coma again, then the lines reassert their presence on the palm over the next few weeks of their convalescence.

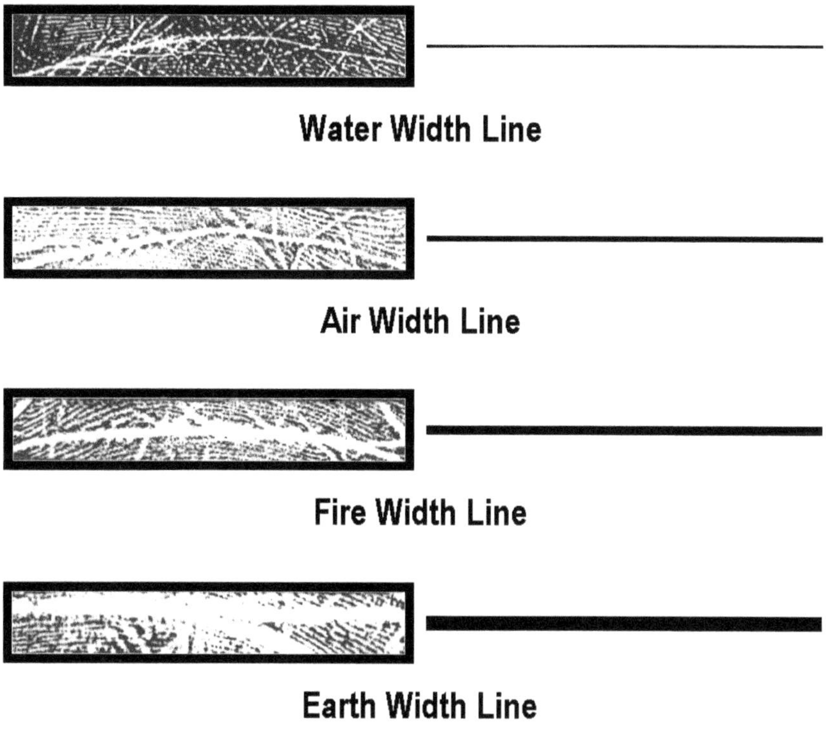

Figure 20.20: Elemental widths of the palmar lines

It should not be any surprise, in cheiromancy, that describing these patterns of consciousness involves the symbolism of the Planets and the Five Elements that are such a key part of medieval medicine. For example, using their quintessential relationship, the Four Elements are used to describe the spectrum of different widths of the palmar lines. Since Ether is synonymous with the flow of energy through the lines, this Elemental classification describes the quality of its flow.

The head line, which starts roughly halfway between the thumb and index finger, traverses the palm to the little finger side of the palm, and reflects the mental range, awareness and quality of thinking of a person. If there is a Fire width to the line, it shows someone who is quick-witted, direct, argumentative, pragmatic and critical in their thinking. By contrast, a Water width shows someone who is imaginative, artistic, sympathetic, tolerant and intuitive in their thinking.

The Air width shows someone who is much more philosophical, inventive, abstract, communicative and accommodating of different views. By contrast, the Earth width shows someone who is down-to-earth, literally, instinctive, simplistic, purposeful and reserved in thought.

We will not go into full details here, but the essential point is to appreciate how lines reflect patterns of consciousness and how symbolism is used to interpret what is happening in that person's consciousness. For more details. see my book *The Hand Reveals* and my "Introduction to Cheiromancy" webinar series.

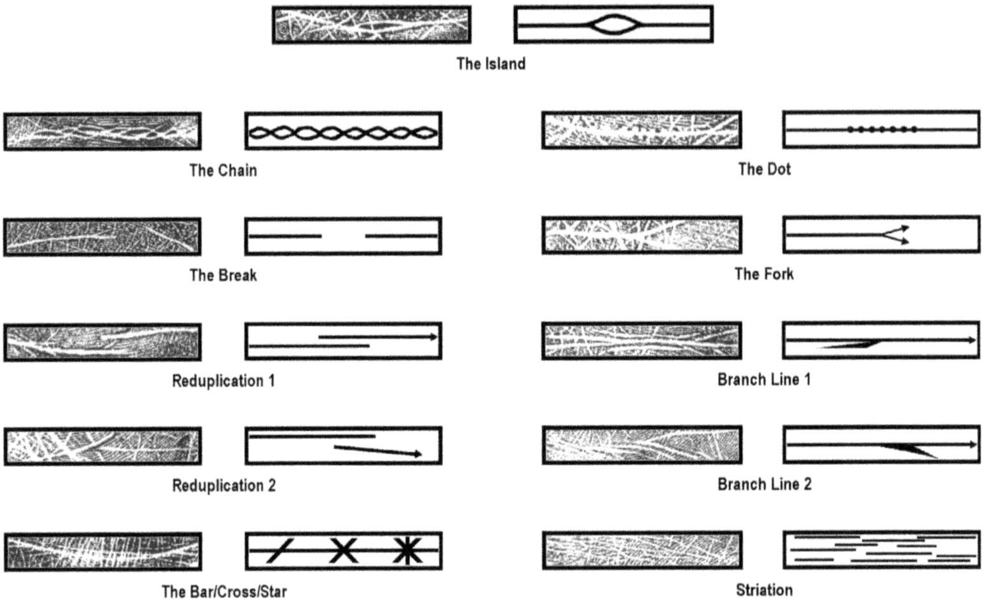

Figure 20.21: Principal markings found in the palmar lines

Markings punctuate the flow of energy through consciousness, describing events and experiences of that person. When a line is well defined, clear and free from markings, it shows that person's experience in life is flowing smoothly. All these markings indicate disruption to this harmonious flow and are characteristic of different types of experience.

An island reflects an obstruction to this flow, causing two different perspectives—thus on the head line it may describe a situation, say at college, where you want to study a particular topic, but the course does not include it, so you are torn between what you want to study and what you are able to.

A break or gap in the head line may describe a period of time when consciousness was not flowing at all, such as when a head injury leaves a person unconscious and possibly the further complication of concussion for a period of time.

The most important aspect to hand reading from a health point of view is the fact that lines change, so when remedial steps are followed that successfully heal a person, the dissonant features disappear and much clearer lines emerge.

The illustration shows the differences between two sets of handprints of the same person, taken six years apart. The first print reflects his former life as a homeless, insecure junkie who at the time of taking it had just become a monk. The second print was taken after he had applied himself to the rigorous daily discipline of meditation, hatha yoga, pranayama and hard physical labour on a farm.

Without going into detail about what all the features of the hand shows, it is easy to observe a marked improvement in the clarity of the palm in the second print. Clarity of mind is one of the important benefits of meditation, when, cleared of excessive thoughts, worries and conflict, the mind becomes still, calm and reflective. The clarity is perhaps most noticeable on the palm at the base of the thumb, in the area called the Venus mount.

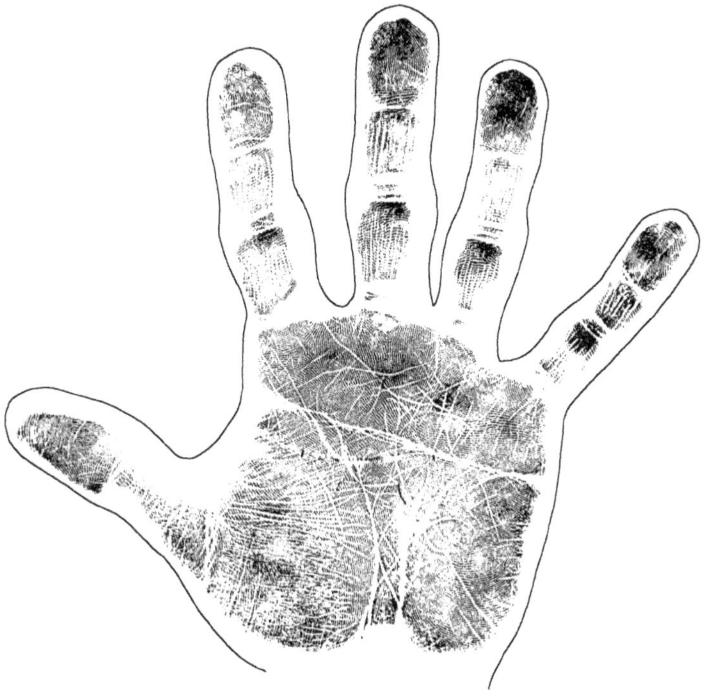

Figure 20.22a: Example of changes in the hand—1st print

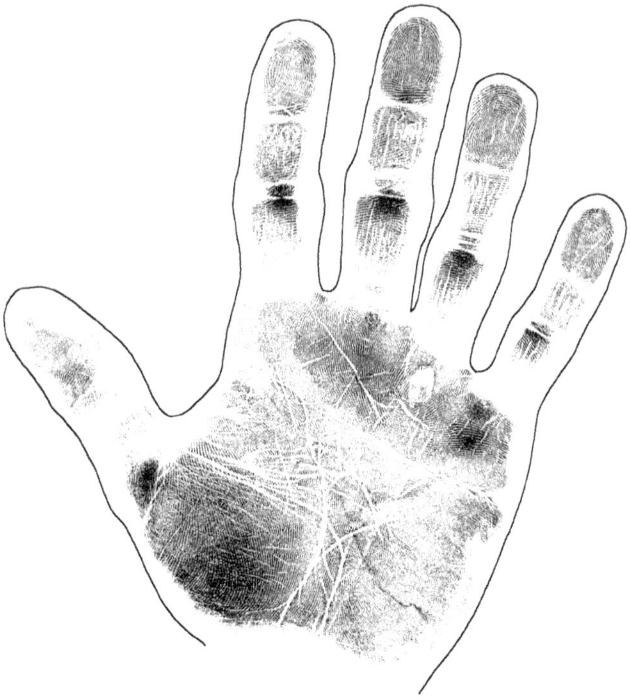

Figure 20.22b: Example of changes in the hand—2nd print

The thumb is associated with will power, so this region of the Venus mount is linked to where will is applied through the body, out into the world to achieve objectives. Without inner clarity, you can have no clear objectives of what you want to achieve and how you go about achieving them.

When the will power becomes thwarted, it creates an immense amount of stress and inner tension. This is shown by the many lines radiating down the Venus mount in the first print. By contrast, the clarity of the second print, where the number of the lines has decreased and faded, reflects just how much more relaxed the person had become.

In becoming a monk, he would have surrendered all his personal desires for achievement to the collective objectives of working for the monastery that had become his home.

This is just one of the many insights this case study provides, a fuller account of which can be found in *The Hand Reveals*. Though this is related to the changes brought about by the practice of yoga, it is typical of the changes that can also be seen in patients as a result of successful herbal treatment.

The study of the lines on the palm provides profound insights into the patterns of consciousness, affecting a person's life. You can appreciate why Paracelsus held the art in high regard. He additionally explains that not only is it important diagnostically, but when the principles of cheiromancy are transposed to the herbal world they enable the physician to understand how to use plants medicinally from the venation in their leaves:

> *... the physician should also study the lines of the herbs and the leaves, and by application of cheiromancy, he should discover their efficacy and virtues.*

Clearly, he saw the venation of the leaves reflecting the consciousness of the plant.

* * *

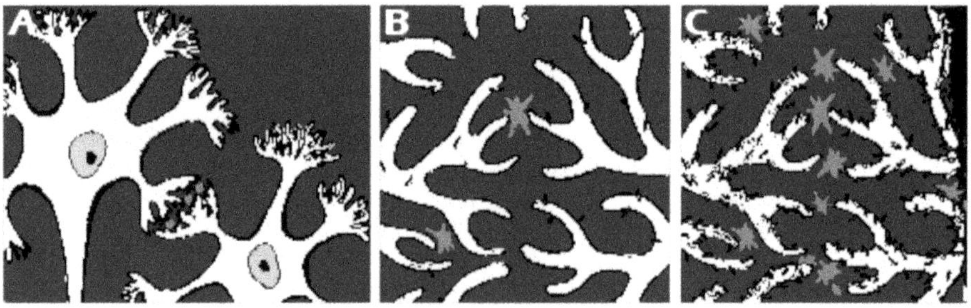

Figure 20.23: Neuroplasticity shown in formation of connections between brain cells

The plasticity of the brain provides fascinating insights into how consciousness is instrumental in neuronal development. In diagram (A), the dendrites of adjacent nerve cells are connected by synapses that transmit nervous impulses, shown by the gray flashes. During learning (B), the number of new terminals develop on the nerve cells along with new synapses, enabling an increase in nervous conduction and transmission.

As the will is focused towards learning a new task or information, so the brain responds by forging new synaptic connections between nerve cells, as in (C), increasing the possible nervous impulses. The glycoforms containing their monosaccharide sugars form the scaffolding that joins the dendrites together, so are key to the physiology of developing new connections between brain cells, resulting in a person being successful at learning new tasks, skills and gaining knowledge.

As well as mucilaginous herbs like aloe, fungi like lion's mane (*Hericium erinaceus*) contain complex polysaccharides, including glucans, xylans and diterpenes (hericenones, erinacenes). Hericenones promote nerve growth factor, which is a small peptide involved in the differentiation and development of mature neurons (nerve cells) through signalling tyrosine kinases.

Collectively, they help promote neuronal plasticity and survival, thereby protecting and enhancing memory. In addition to the protective effects on the central nervous system, the fungus is used as an immune modulator, for healing wounds, as an antimicrobial and antihypertensive. All these physiological functions are linked in part to the role of monosaccharide sugars.

Hopefully it is possible to see the value of Ether in uniting consciousness, its connection to nature and Vital Force, not forgetting its importance in connecting to our herbal heritage. When John D. Rockefeller sought to establish the market for pharmaceutical medicine around the world by influencing the training of doctors, he pushed to get Ether thrown out of their training, saying it was not a proper chemical element. He wanted medical students to be trained solely in a materialistic perspective of the body that suited the chemical basis of his petroleum-based medicines. Thus, when medical students are trained in this model, they obtain no metaphysical understanding of how the body works—instead they become merely medical technicians serving the needs of the pharmaceutical industry.

As we have seen in Chapter 8, medieval learning sought to create a spiritual awareness within the Soul. It was the integration of the Four Elements that encouraged a transcendent, intuitive understanding of life.

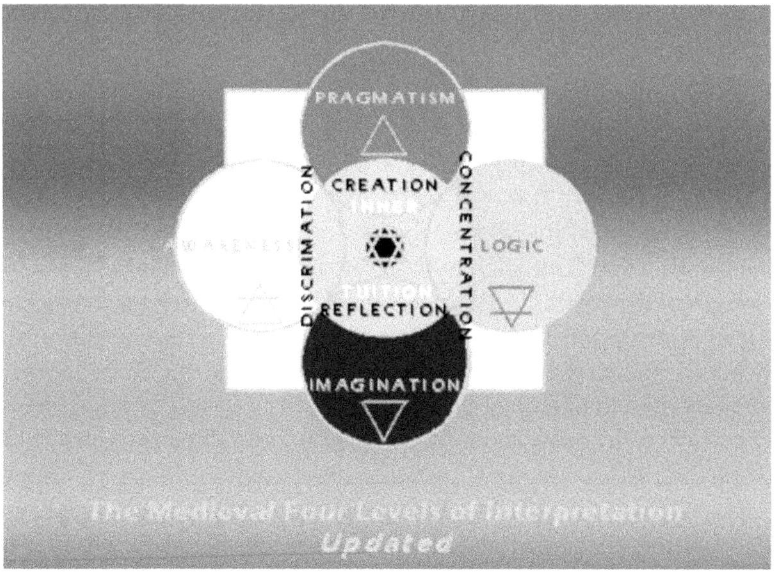

Figure 20.24: Medieval four levels of interpretation—updated

Since its infancy, science has symbolically emphasised the development of the Fire Element, at the expense of the other Elements. The Fire Element alone defines a very specific mode of consciousness. Fire burns at a substrate, taking the material apart and reducing it to ash. In so doing it gives off light, which derives more energy to perpetuate its burning. This image very much describes the nature of reductionist thinking, in taking a problem, ripping things apart, deriving insights and leaving whatever has been the focus of inquiry in pieces.

Water is the opposite to the Fire Element. If Fire takes things apart, Water is the Element that joins things together. If you watch how two drops coalesce to form a much larger drop, it demonstrates how Water is the Element of connection. Given their opposite natures, when the Fire Element is strong, the Water Element becomes weak. Similarly, when reductionist thinking is strong, then the understanding of connection and relationship becomes poor. The cultivation of reductionist, empirical thinking has created a lopsided and unbalanced view of life, dissociated from Nature, that as a consequence threatens our very existence upon the Planet.

Rational thinking, as the adjective implies, is limited. A symptom of its limitation is shown in the vast amounts of data it generates in its attempt to understand things. Just as a flame erupts, then dies, so rational thinking is defined by time. It is limited by the physical consciousness of the person.

Imagine driving a car: as you look through the windscreen, you see the future coming towards you. As you look through the side windows, you can see where you are at, in the present. As you look in the rear-view mirror, you see the past receding behind you. However, if instead you fly above the car in a helicopter, then everything from this higher perspective is now in the present, and the progression of time, past, present and future, is all in the now.

Such is the perspective of the intuitive mind. It shows the need to transcend the rational, logical part of our mind to develop our intuition and embrace our spiritual awareness. As Einstein so eloquently put it: *"The intuitive mind is a sacred gift, and the rational mind is a faithful servant. We have created a society that honours the servant and has forgotten the gift."*

* * *

The very word "petroleum" literally means the "oil from the rock". Petroleum is formed from dead vegetation that flourished millions of years ago, and had become compressed under the weight of the Earth's crust, in the absence of light, to form a toxic, thick, black liquid that does not support life in any way. In that sense oil is truly Saturnine. It is in stark contrast to herbal medicines derived from living herbs, for those drugs made from oil are completely devoid of any vitality.

When you see how readily just a few drops of petrol falling on grass kill it, how oil should become the basis of a medical system is utterly extraordinary. Its failure to heal is reflected in the fact that pharmaceutical medicine is now the third leading cause of death in the Western world, after heart attacks and strokes, closely followed by cancer as the fourth. In reality pharmaceutical medicine has its hands in all these other causes of death too. Saturn is the Lord of Death.

In humoral physiology the liver was considered to be the most important organ, in view of its role in maintaining the balance of the humours, thereby enhancing the flow of the Vital Force through the blood. In the avitalistic world of pharmaceutical drugs, it is notable that prolonged use of many synthetic drugs causes liver damage.

It is our dissociation of medicine from nature that has allowed this situation to flourish. Perhaps the biggest irony is found in the very name "pharmaceutical", for it is derived from the Greek *phamakia*, meaning "magic or sorcery". It is an idea that captures the excitement of the initial success of synthetic drugs—working as if by magic. Drugs have even been described as "magic bullets" targeting specific disease. But in Ancient Greece there were many forms of magic, and *phamakia* was more specifically the practice of making potions and poisons used for killing people!

This is all the more alarming given this quote by John D. Rockefeller in "The Secret Covenant":

> *The poisons will be hidden in everything that surrounds them, in what they drink, eat, breathe and wear. We must be ingenious in dispensing the poisons for they can see far. We will teach them poisons are good with fun images and musical tones. Those they look up to will help. We enlist them to push our poisons.*

There are those that dispute that Rockefeller said this, but all around us it is easy to see the destructive impact that this limited way of thinking, motivated by profit, has had on the natural world.

Pharmacology, the physiological explanation for how drugs work or are supposed to work, is the language of this exploitation. Defining herbs solely in terms of their constituents and associated pharmacology, while it might satisfy and appease minds that have been trained scientifically, in reality, has the result of further dissociating herbalists from understanding their true roots in nature.

The respective discoveries of the Outer Planets, Uranus, Neptune and Pluto, from the 18th century onwards disrupted the symmetry of their Zodiacal rulerships, as perceived within the Hermetic Three World view. Each new Planet too seemingly made the old Ptolemaic order of the Seven Planets increasingly obsolete.

When the Zodiac is considered with Aquarius and Capricorn at the top, you can see how the Planetary rulers are arranged in accordance with the sequence of the Planetary Spheres. Hence, accommodating these three extra Planets was very disruptive to the Hermetic Three World view, leading many to thinking it too was out of date.

However, astrologers have studied world events and discoveries since the time of their sightings from a symbolic perspective, revealing their significance within the developments of scientific thinking and its subsequent impact on the evolution of modern medicine.

Uranus was the first of the Outer Planets to be discovered, by Sir William Herschel in 1781. This was the era of Dalton's Atomic Theory and the conceptualisation of matter as tiny balls. In the glyph for Uranus, the letter H is added to the Cross of Matter, as a nod to the Planet's discoverer. It has the effect of emphasising this abstracted chemical classification of matter, which is removed from the Elemental or Material realm and elevated into the Intellectual World.

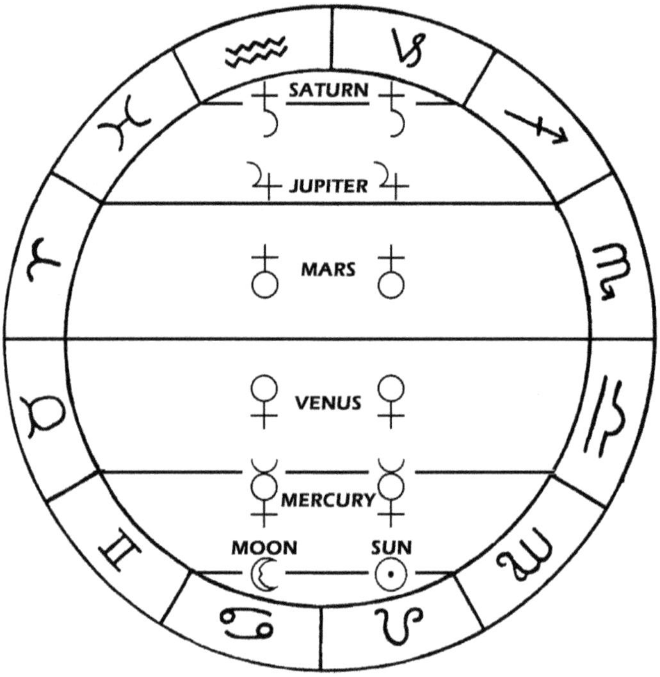

The Symmetry of the Traditional Planetary Rulers of the Zodiacal Signs

Figure 20.25: Planetary symmetry of Zodiacal rulerships

Through flying his kite through the Air in a thunderstorm in 1752, Benjamin Franklin became aware of the principles of electricity. Similarly, the upper part of the glyph too has been likened to an ariel, heralding the birth of electronics. This was the era when Luigi Galvani, through his experiments on frogs' legs, first proposed that the nervous system functioned by electricity.

The discovery of Neptune in 1846 coincided with development of anaesthesia. A cluster of different chemicals, including nitrous oxide in 1844, diethyl ether in 1846, chloroform in 1847 and ethyl chloride in 1848, were all explored. The phenomenon of anaesthesia in essence is the physical manifestation of the mind/body split, for in rendering a patient unconscious, the surgeon is able to penetrate the protective pain barrier to perform tasks inside the body.

The glyph for Neptune encapsulates this separation for it is composed of the Crescent of the Spirit largely detached from the Cross of Matter. The Circle of the Soul, which normally connects Spirit to Matter, is notably absent. This same era is also linked to the birth of microbiology, which came to replace the vitalistic, humoral causation of disease. It was also when organic chemistry—the chemistry of hydrocarbons—emerged as a specialist field of chemistry.

The discovery of Pluto in 1930 coincides with the era of the splitting of the structure of the atom. Rather than being a solid structure, as in the Daltonian conception of an atom, discoveries revealed that it is predominantly made up of space (99.99+%) and contained vast amounts of energy. The glyph for Pluto consists of a semicircle of the Soul linked to the Cross of Matter. It is like the "lid" has been taken off the structure of an atom, revealing the space, the nucleus and liberating the energy within it, whether it be light, X-rays or radiation.

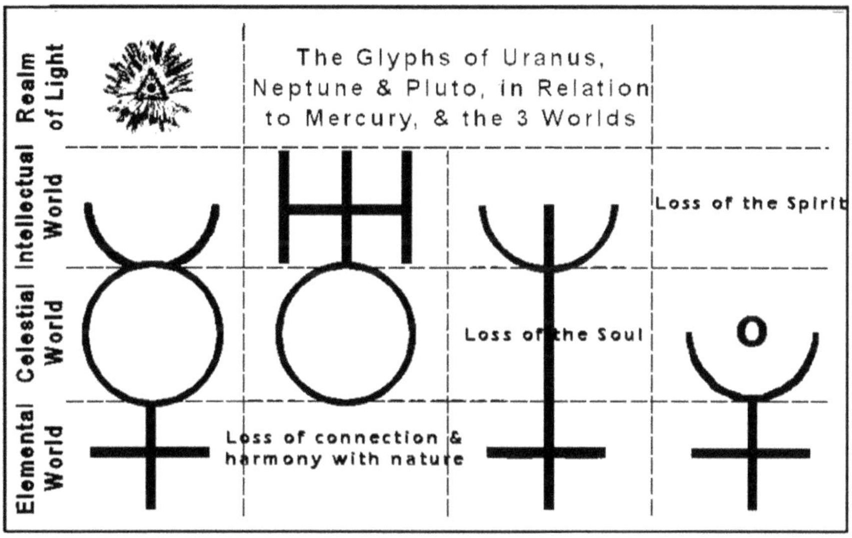

Figure 20.26: The Outer Planets and the evolution of medical science

The trans-saturnian Planets, in becoming descriptive of the evolution of medical science, also mirror the decline of herbal medicine.

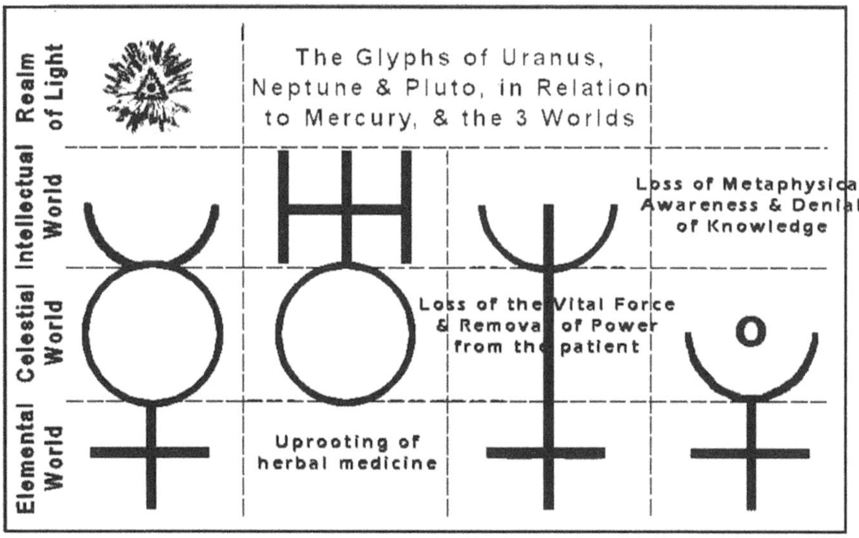

Figure 20.27: The Outer Planets and contemporary trends of herbal medicine

In this alien world of high-tech medicine, we need to get back to the root principles of physic—traditionally ruled by Mercury. Once again, physicians need to cultivate a symbolic awareness of life. We urgently need to respect and understand nature, in order to live in tune with it—as we and our herbs are intricately a part of it. We need to restore a vitalistic vision to both our understanding of herbs and to re-empower our patients in their journey back to health. We urgently need to cultivate this symbolic awareness to respect the wisdom of nature and enable herbal medicine to flourish.

Post-Covid, with the current lack of trust, and conspicuous profiteering from the vaccines, blind faith in the pharmaceutical industry has been completely shattered, creating a huge cultural vacuum and opportunity for natural medicines to flourish. From the immense harm that has been caused, people can starkly see the predatory and egregious profiteering of the industry, which far exceeds any supposed benefits of their medicines. Despite the glossy veneer, the industry has demonstrated little concern for the welfare of individual patients or taken any responsibility for the harm it has caused.

As people seek to reclaim responsibility for their own health, demand for herbal medicine is likely to become massive, but it will be difficult to sustain this demand on the herbal kingdom against the ecological and environmental degradation of the near future. However, if herbal medicine is not the medicine of the future, such is our dependence on the herbal kingdom that we as a species will not culturally survive.

CHAPTER TWENTY ONE

New horizons

In the previous chapter, herbal medicine today was shown to have two different perspectives: the metaphysical perspective and the reductionist, pharmacological perspective. Many herbs that we use today have been in use for millennia, so historically span these two perspectives. By putting both these perspectives together, we can derive an even richer appreciation of the value of physic.

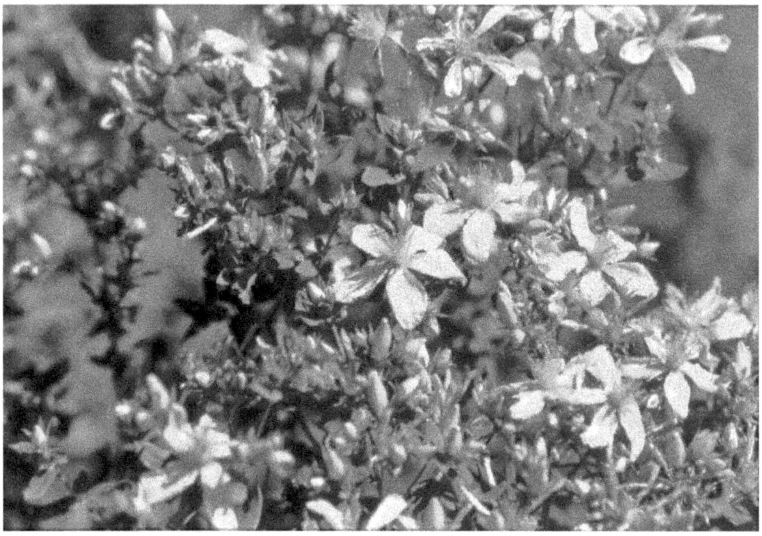

Figure 21.1: St John's wort in flower (*Hypericum perforatum*)

St John's wort (*Hypericum perforatum*) is an important example of a herb with a rich cultural heritage and one of our leading medicinal herbs. Prior to its adoption into

Christian teaching and mythology, it was a sacred herb to the Celts. With its golden flowers clearly linking the herb to the Sun, the Druids used it to celebrate the Summer Solstice, when the Sun reaches its zenith. This ritual is essentially giving thanks to the Sun for its generation of the Vital Force and the sustenance for all life—a memory that is preserved in Welsh as *Eurinllys*, meaning "leaf of the blessed".

In the Celtic tradition, at midsummer's eve, bunches of the freshly picked flowers were hung up above entrances and doorways to dwellings, to ward off evil spirits. The Solar virtue was essentially visualised as dispelling the darkness in which demons hide.

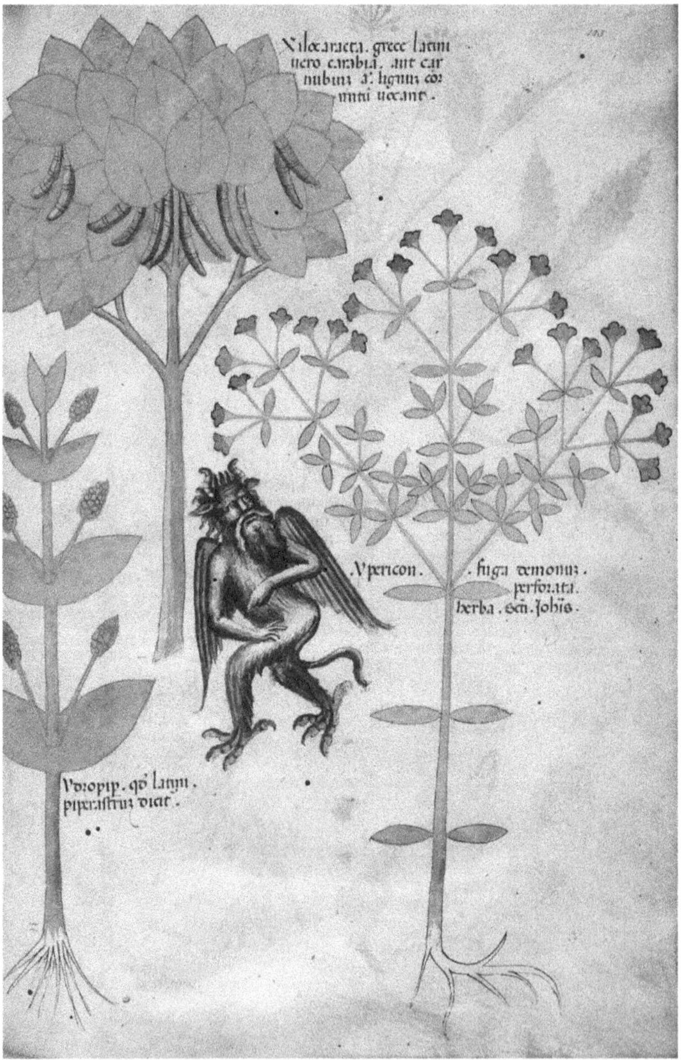

Figure 21.2: A page from Johannes Hartlieb's *Tractatus de Herbis*, Lombardy, 1440

The herb has a number of old names that give reference to this practice, such as *Demonem fugiens*, the devil chaser. This 15th-century illustration of St John's wort from the *Tractatus de Herbis* captures a demon clearly cowering away from the Solar herb. The Latin inscription says, "*Hypericum drives away poison. perforata herb of St John.*" The idea is still preserved in the Latin name for the herb, *Hypericum perforatum*.

The herb acquired its Christianised name in the Gothic era, for it possesses a unique signature reflecting the fate of St John the Baptist, who baptised Jesus in the water of the Jorden. At his daughter Salome's wedding, King Herod granted her a wish. Salome was said to have requested the head of John the Baptist as a wedding present. So, Herod ordered his men to capture John the Baptist and have his severed head brought to the wedding celebrations.

Truth is John the Baptist was a very successful spiritual teacher in his own right, who had already attracted a large following that potentially threatened Herod's authority. Clearly Herod was looking for an opportunity to get rid of him for political reasons. which his daughter's request provided.

By late summer, on 29 August, when the feast day of St John the Baptist was celebrated in the Christian calendar, the flowers have largely gone over—hence the herb too appears "beheaded". More than that, the lower leaves too start to acquire red blotches, as if blood from where his head had been removed had dripped down onto the body of the leaves below.

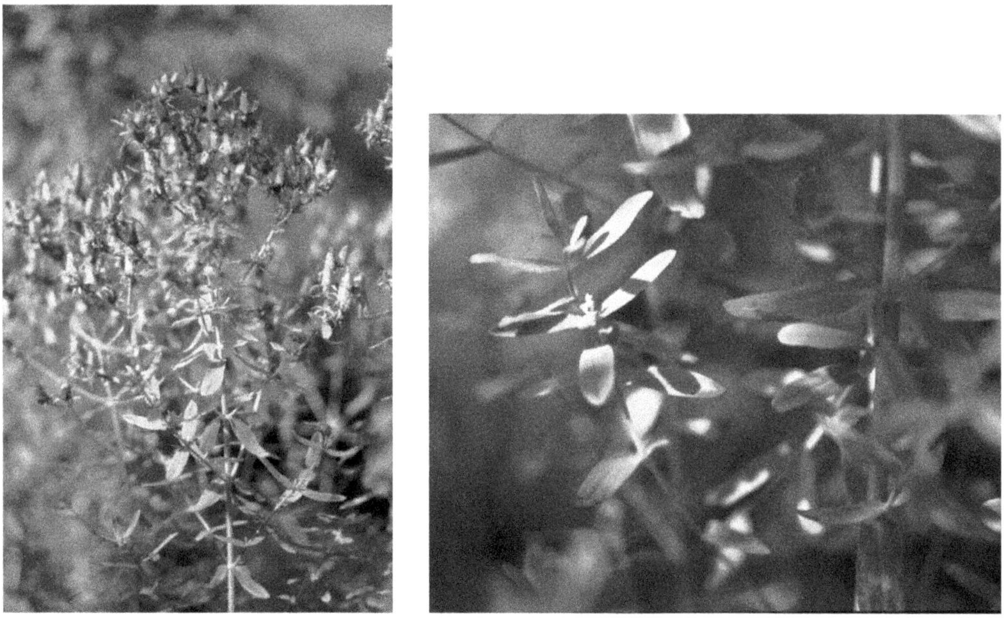

Figure 21.3: The Beheaded St John's wort, depicting the saint's blood on the leaves

In the early 12th century, the Knights Hospitallers arose. They were merchants from the Amalfi coast, of which Salerno is the principal city. They founded a hospital in Jerusalem, within the Muristan district, a hospital dedicated to St John the Baptist. It provided care for sick, poor or injured pilgrims visiting the Holy Land. In particular, it treated soldiers wounded in the Crusades.

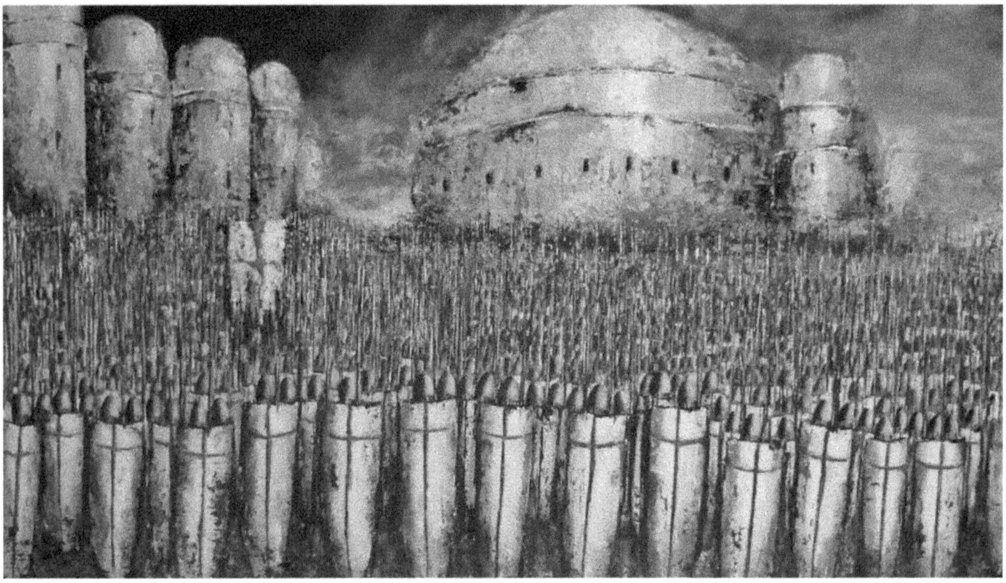

Figure 21.4: Kaye Miller-Dewing "Defence of Jerusalem". Reproduced with permission of the artist

When Jerusalem was conquered in 1099 in the First Crusade, a group of the crusading knights then formed a religious order in support of the hospital, hence the name "Knights Hospitallers".

With the order of the Knights Hospitallers dedicated to St John the Baptist, imagine the reverence they would have attached to this herb, which embodies the signature of the fate of St John.

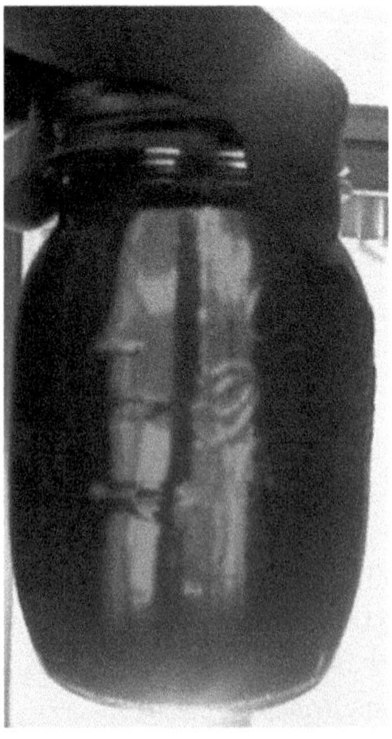

Figure 21.5: St John's wort oil (*Hypericum perforatum*). Photo credit Andrea Passini

Traditionally an infused oil from St John's wort, used as a vulnerary, is made by seeping the dried flowers in olive oil, leaving the glass jar in sunshine for 40 days and 40 nights.

The Sun was deliberately utilised to enhance the extraction of the Solar virtue of the herb. The resultant liquid takes on a wonderful red colour, from the red pigment hypericin.

With the herb symbolically connected to St John, the resultant oil would have been quite literally seen as the "Blood of St John", and further imbued with remarkable healing powers. What better remedy to heal the wounds sustained by the soldiers on the crusades? Many herbalists still use this oil today, for its remarkable healing properties.

The principal modern use of St John's wort has been for treating depression, or melancholia. Following the detailed description of melancholia in Chapter 14, it should be seen how the plant's powerful Solar virtue would dispel the darkness of Saturn's paralysing influence, thereby elevating a person's mood from the depression and despondency of their melancholia. Furthermore, the temperature of the herb is traditionally hot and dry to the 2nd degree. Hence the heat of the herb will help "thaw out" the coldness of the melancholia.

In Hartlieb's depiction of St John's wort, the illustrator shows, with a degree of artistic licence, that the symmetry of the herb was clearly important to understanding its virtue. You can see it in the three pairs of leaves that line up the main stem, whereupon the two lateral branching stems emerge from the central stem, creating three flowering stems in total.

This pattern is repeated, with three more pairs of leaves. From inside these leaves, axillary branching forms a pair of three leaves, at each level. At the top leaf pair, on each of the three stems the inflorescence forms, comprised of three florets. Thus, the number 3 is replicated through the symmetry of the plant's structure.

As Dürer showed in his Melancholia 1, so powerfully symbolised by his "Dürerhedron", an excess of the Melancholic humour crushes and distorts a person's experience of life. Once appreciating the importance of the symmetry in this illustration of St John's wort, you can see how the virtue of the herb similarly restores balance between the mind, emotions and the body. In essence, it will remind the person of their true inner wealth. The Devil chaser can now be seen as also dispelling the darkness of melancholia.

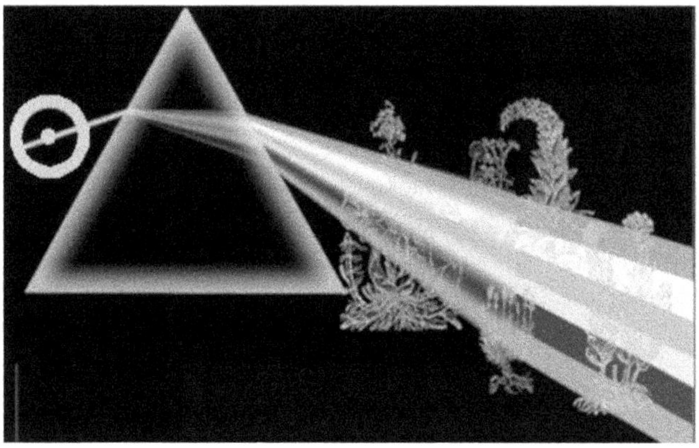

Figure 21.6: The tradition Idea of the Sun being the source of the healing virtues of herbs

An exciting new field of pharmacology, called photobiomodulation (PBM) is opening up, which reinforces the traditional astrological idea of the healing power of the Sun in the 10th house as the source of the healing virtue of herbs. This involves substances that are frequently described as antioxidants. In general, they include plant pigments, like curcumin, the yellow pigment found in turmeric rhizome, and ellagic acid, the red pigment found in pomegranates.

As these substances are absorbed and circulate in the blood, sunlight penetrating through the skin and eyes hits them. As pigments they absorb specific wavelengths of light. Thus, the yellow curcumin absorbs the blue component, becoming energised by it. Similarly, the red ellagic acid absorbs the green component.

Carotene, the yellow pigment found in carrots, when converted to rhodopsin, becomes the visual pigment inside the rods of the retina. Responding to light, it generates the electrical signals that travel from the eyes via the optic nerves to the visual cortex at the brain. This has been understood for many decades now, but the extent of photo-activation of other pigment molecules as they circulate in the blood is only just starting to be fully appreciated.

One of the functions of the photo-activated pigments is to enhance the role of glycolysis in the mitochondria of the cells, thereby increasing the production of adenosine triphosphate (ATP), the high energy-containing molecule that powers every cell in the body. Each colour pigment, once activated, has an effect on specific parts of the glycolytic pathway. Thus the modern trend of eating fruits and vegetables in accordance with the colours of the rainbow has profound physiological wisdom to it. Sunlight is essentially a form of nutrition for the body, of which its healing effects have been identified since the time of Hippocrates.

As we have seen, St John's wort has long been visualised as driving away the demon of melancholia or depression. Its Solar virtue is envisaged as dissolving the darkness of depression, restoring balance and harmony to the person. This releases the willpower needed to confront the obstacles in their life, so they can start moving forward again. Numerous clinical studies show that St John's wort is superior in action and safer than a number of conventional antidepressant drugs.

For several decades the red pigment hypericin has been identified as the active principle of St John's wort contributing to its antidepressive action, yet just how it has this action remained elusive.

Absorbing energy of the green part of the spectrum (496–570 nm) increases the production of ATP within the mitochondria. With more energy generated, this improves red blood cell function, enhances blood flow and increases oxygen delivery around the body, thereby delivering more blood, oxygen and energy to the brain cells, literally lifting their physiology out of the stagnation of depression.

While this new development of photobiomodulation is now confirming how this particular herb works, it also gives validity to the metaphysical knowledge that understood the nature of melancholia and identified this action of the herb in the first place.

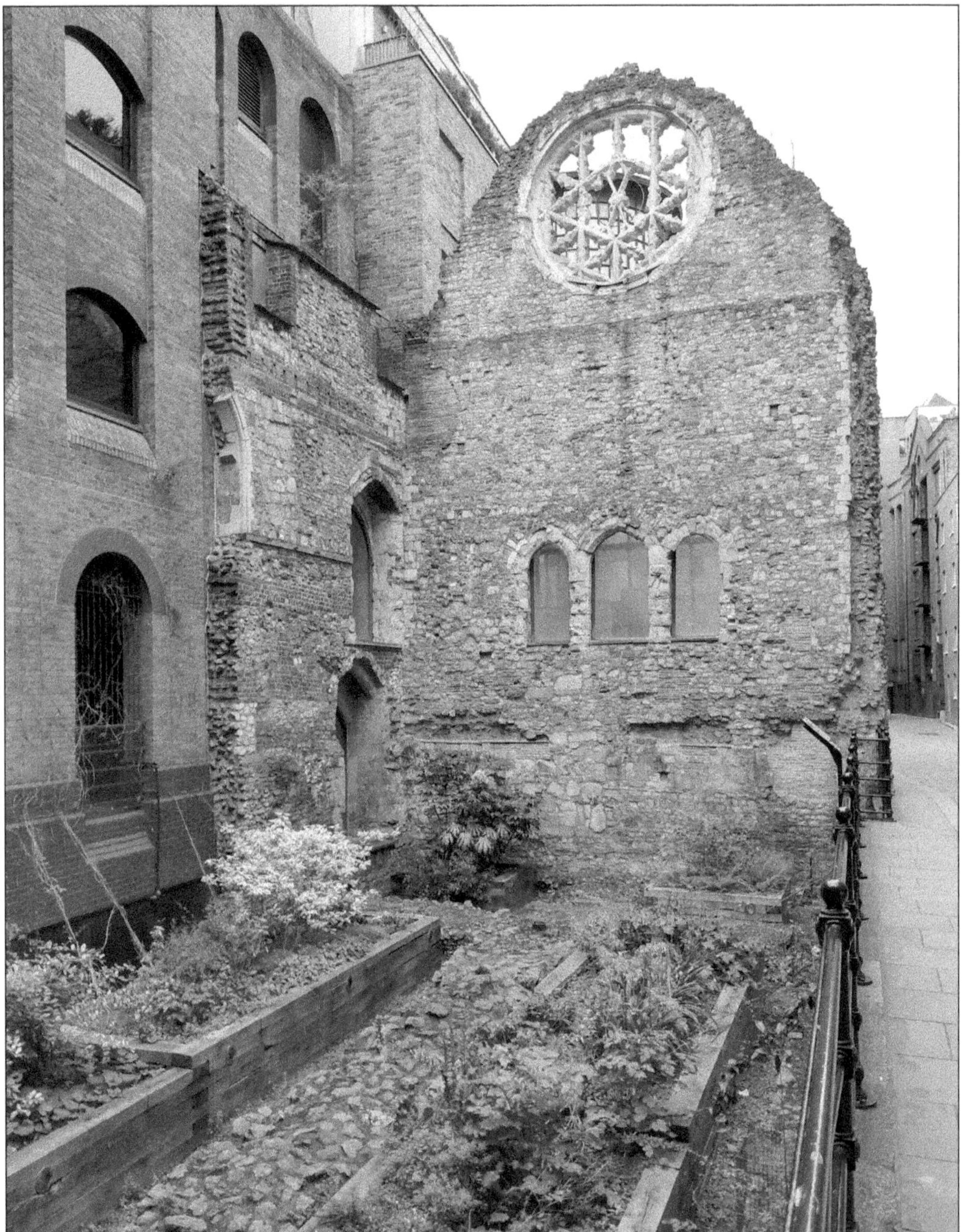

Winchester Palace Rose Window and Medieval Garden

EPILOGUE

Since writing this book, the site of Winchester Palace Rose Window, which was its inspiration when just a part of an ugly building site, fittingly has become transformed into a delightful little medieval garden! It is managed by Bankside Open Spaces Trust. Passers-by can take some time out from the hustle and bustle of London life and find a little sanctuary there. A great place, maybe, to read this book!

https://www.english-heritage.org.uk/visit/places/winchester-palace/

GLOSSARY OF ASTROLOGICAL TERMS

Aqua Vitae: The Four Elements have a quintessential relationship to the Fifth Element Ether, whereby the Four evolve out of the Fifth. Ether was known to the alchemists as the Aqua Vitae, meaning "the Water of Life".

Ascendant: Called the horoscope (Literally meaning, the "hour that comes into view") in traditional astrology. This is the eastern horizon and the first house cusp of the astrological chart, which commences there.

Aspect: The angular, geometric relationship between Planets located in the signs of the Zodiac. The principal aspects and their angles used in traditional astrology are conjunction = 0°, opposition = 180°, square or quartile = 90°, sextile = 60° and trine = 120°. Additionally, the quincunx = 135° is important in medical charts, since it is the angular relationship between the first house of health and vitality, and the sixth house of disease. [L. aspectus (adspicere = to look at)]

Benefic: A term used to describe Jupiter and Venus as Planets of good influence in an astrological chart.

Chart ruler: A term for a Planet which rules the Zodiac sign present at the Ascendant or horoscope of the chart, also traditionally known as "Lord of the Geniture".

Cheiromancy: The word comes from the Greek *chir*, meaning "hand", and *manteia*, meaning "divination"; literally meaning "divination through the hand".

Conjunction: A conjunction is when two or more Planets occupy the same degree of the Zodiac. They can be good or bad depending on the nature of the Planets involved. If their natures are similar, like the Moon and Venus, their combined energy powerfully works well together. If their natures are opposites, like Mars and Venus, then their energies are unstable and conflictive.

Descendant: The western horizon, and the seventh house cusp of an astrological chart.

Detriment: A Planet poorly placed in a particular sign is described as being in detriment.

Dexter: A Planet that has an aspect made to it by a faster-moving Planet further forwards in the sequence of the Zodiacal signs. [L. *dexter* = to the right]

Dispositor: A Planet which has essential dignity within a particular section of the Zodiac is capable of disposing any other Planet present within the section.

Essential dignity: A Planet strongly placed in a particular sign, usually a sign that it rules or in which it is in exaltation, is described as having essential dignity. A Planet may also have accidental dignity from its house position in the chart or through contacting the benefic Planets, Jupiter and Venus.

Exaltation: A particular placing of a Planet in a sign, different from the one it rules, in which it functions well. For example, Mars is exalted in Capricorn.

Fall: Where a Planet is placed in the opposite sign of the Zodiac to its exaltation, in which it functions poorly. For example, Mars has its fall in Cancer.

Glyphs: These are the graphic symbols used to represent the Elements, Planets and the signs of the Zodiac. [Gk. *glyphé* = carving]

Grand Trine: A particular astrological configuration whereby three Planets form a triangular pattern in the chart. Each Planet has a trine aspect (120°) with the other two Planets composing the triangle. A grand trine is usually formed between Planets occupying Zodiacal signs of the same Element or triplicity. Their collective energy is expressed powerfully through that Element.

Heiroglyph: Literally, "the sacred symbol". [Gk. heiros = sacred + *glyphé* = carving]

House: An astrological term for the division of the sky into 12 sections, as represented in an astrological chart.

House cusp: The division in an astrological chart between one house and its adjacent house.

House ruler: The Planet that rules the Zodiacal sign in which a house cusp falls, is called the house ruler. For example, if the third house cusp of a chart is at 15° Aries, then Mars is the ruler of the third house. In this case Mars may be referred to as the Lord of the third house.

Horoscope: See Ascendant.

IC: Short for *imum caelorum*, meaning "the depths of the heavens". It is located at the fourth house cusp at the bottom of an astrological chart.

Luminaries: The collective astrological term for both the Sun and Moon. [L. *lumen, luminis* = a light, an opening]

Macrocosm: The universe. [Gk. *makros* = large + *kosmos* = world]

Malefic: An astrological term used to describe Saturn and Mars as Planets of misfortune in an astrological chart.

MC: Short for *midi caelorum*, meaning "the middle of the heavens". It is placed at the tenth house cusp at the top of an astrological chart.

Microcosm: The view of Mankind as a reflection of the universe. [Gk. *mikros* = small + *kosmos* = world]

Mutual reception: A relationship between two Planets occupying positions of each other's dignity or exaltation, whereby they can symbolically swap places.

Opposition: An opposition is when two Planets oppose each other across the Zodiac occupy, the same degree. In general, this is a contentious aspect, irrespective of the nature of the Planets involved.

Orb: A halo of influence surrounding each Planet in which it is effective. This influence extends a number of degrees either side of the position of the Planet. Each half of the orb is called the Planet's moiety. In modern astrology it is the aspects that have the orbs.

Peregrine: A Planet that has no essential dignity. [L. *peregrinator* = a wanderer]

Prima Materia: An alchemical term for the Fifth Element of Ether meaning "the First Matter" since it is the matrix from which the Elemental World was born.

Retrograde: The perceived backwards movement of a Planet through the Zodiacal signs. Symbolically, the retrograde motion detracts from the essential dignity of the Planet. The retrograde motion of a Planet is denoted by the symbol (℞).

Sextile: A sextile 60° aspect is usually formed between Planets occupying Zodiacal signs of compatible Elements. Their combined energy is expressed harmoniously together.

Sinister: Aspects between Planets made forwards in sequence of the Zodiacal signs. [L. *sinister* = to the left]

Square: A square 90° aspect is usually formed between Planets occupying Zodiacal signs of incompatible Elements. Their combined energy is expressed conflictive and disruptive ways.

BIBLIOGRAPHY AND RESOURCES

Culpeper, Nicholas, *A Physical Directory, or A Translation of the London Dispensatory Made by the Colledge of Physicians in London* (1649)
—— *The English Physitian* (1652), known as *Culpeper's Herbal*
—— *Astrologicall Judgement of Diseases, from the Decumbiture of the Sick* (1655)
Lilly, William, *Christian Astrology* (1647); reissued by Regulus Books (1985)
Taylor, Stephen, *The Humoral Herbal*, Aeon Books (2021)
Warren-Davis, Dylan, *The Hand Reveals*, Aeon Books, 4th edn (2021)
Yates, Frances, *Giordano Bruno and the Hermetic Tradition*, RKP (1964)

Contact

For teaching, lecturing, mentoring, in person or via Zoom, a full pdf list of current topics is available from Dylan on d.warren-davis@outlook.com

Webinars

https://www.aeoneducation.co.uk/course/livinghistory
https://www.aeoneducation.co.uk/course/st-johns-wort-1
https://www.aeoneducation.co.uk/course/alchemyofherbs
https://www.aeoneducation.co.uk/course/culpeper
https://www.aeoneducation.co.uk/course/cheiromancy

INDEX

www.ingramcontent.com/pod-product-compliance
Ingram Content Group UK Ltd.
Pitfield, Milton Keynes, MK11 3LW, UK
UKHW052326221026
9535IPUK00004B/8

9 781912 807970